Oxford Dictionary of Medical Quotations

Preface

The *Oxford Dictionary of Medical Quotations* is intended to be a rich source of quotations covering a variety of medically related topics. Those selected have been deliberately kept short in an effort to highlight the pithiest phrase or the sharpest insight. Some are witty, some are maudlin, some merely factual. They have been selected on the basis of their usefulness to modern medical authors, journalists, politicians, nurses, physios, lecturers, and even health managers, who will always have need to season their works with the clever or witty phrases of former colleagues whose intuitions still say as much today as when they were first published. Many reflect the compiler's tastes and prejudices but there will be something for everyone within these pages.

Browsing through many texts to find the most appropriate quotations to include in the *Oxford Dictionary of Medical Quotations* has afforded an insight into both medical history as well as the nature of the doctors and others who have chiselled these phrases. A glance for the casual reader not looking for a specific quote will be rewarding in itself.

Quotations are listed under author, with an index of keywords that permits the reader to access a number of quotes with the same keyword. Wherever possible, biographical information about the author and whence the quote originated are included, although it is acknowledged that there are several omissions in this regard. When the original source is not clear, the secondary source has been substituted if it was thought useful for further study for the reader. If the quotation was deemed to merit a place in the *Dictionary* even without full reference being available, it was included. Indeed, it is not necessary for an author to be particularly well known to be in the dictionary if he or she had given birth to a *bon mot* or a succinct phrase.

The majority of the quotations come from the English-speaking medical worlds of Great Britain, Ireland, and North America but several quotes from other rich medical cultures have been included in translation.

Whether readers are looking for a suitable quotation on surgery, science, kidneys, or kindness, they should find much here to satisfy. Medicine is both the narrowest and broadest of subjects, and I have included examples of both the specific and the general. If I have failed to find that favourite concise quote, please send it fully referenced and it will be included in the next edition. Any corrections of birth dates and deaths will be most welcome and acknowledged in subsequent editions.

July 2002

Peter McDonald MBBS MS FRCS
Northwick Park and St. Mark's Hospital, Harrow, Middlesex, UK
pmcdo69277@aol.com

Acknowledgements

Sister Annie Driscoll of St. Mark's Hospital, Harrow, Middlesex, UK; Dr Neville P. Robinson, Northwick Park and St. Mark's Hospital, Harrow, Middlesex, UK; and Dr John Ballantyne, Kensington, London, UK; Martin Baum and Kate Smith of the Oxford University Press.

Contents

How to Use the Dictionary

The sequence of entries is by alphabetical order of author, usually by surname but with occasional exceptions such as imperial or royal titles, authors known by a pseudonym ('Zeta') or a nickname (Caligula). In general authors' names are given in the form by which they are best known, so we have Mark Twain (not Samuel L. Clemens), and T. S. Eliot (not Thomas Stearns Eliot). Collections such as Anonymous, the Bible, the Book of Common Prayer, and so forth, are included in the alphabetical sequence.

Within each author entry, quotations are arranged by alphabetical order of the titles of the works from which they are taken: books, plays, poems. These titles are given in italic type; titles of pieces which comprise part of a published volume or collection (e.g. essays, short stories, poems not published as volumes in their own right) are given in roman type inside inverted commas. For example, *Sweeney Agonistes*, but 'Fragmert of an Agon'; often the two forms will be found together.

All numbers in source references are given in arabic numerals, with the exception of lower-case roman numerals denoting quotations from prefatory matter, whose page numbering is separate from that of the main text. The numbering itself relates to the beginning of the quotation, whether or not it runs on to another stanza or page in the original. Where possible, chapter numbers have been offered for prose works, since pagination varies from one edition to another. In very long prose works with minimal subdivisions, attempts have been made to provide page references to specified editions.

A date in brackets indicates first publication in volume form of the work cited. Unless otherwise stated, the dates thus offered are intended as chronological guides only and do not necessarily indicate the date of the text cited; where the latter is of significance, this has been stated. Where neither date of publication nor of composition is known, an approximate date (e.g. '*c*.1625') indicates the likely date of composition. Where there is a large discrepancy between date of composition (or performance) and of publication, in most cases the former only has been given (e.g. 'written 1725', 'performed 1622').

Spellings have been Anglicized and modernized except in those cases, such as ballads, where this would have been inappropriate; capitalization has been retained only for personifications; with rare exceptions, verse has been aligned with the left hand margin. Italic type has been used for all foreign-language originals.

The Index

Both the keywords and the entries following each keyword, including those in foreign languages, are in strict alphabetical order. Singular and plural nouns (with their possessive forms) are grouped separately: for 'you choose your disease' see 'disease'; for 'coughs and sneezes spread diseases' see 'diseases'. Variant forms of common words (doctor, Dr) are grouped under a single heading: 'doctor'.

The references show the author's name, usually in abbreviated form (SHAK/Shakespeare), followed by the page number.

Dedication

To my late father George McDonald (1918–1983) whose love of words both ancient and modern was as fine a legacy as any son could ask for.

OXFORD

UNIVERSITY PRESS

Great Clarendon Street, Oxford OX2 6DP

Oxford University Press is a department of the University of Oxford.
It furthers the University's objective of excellence in research, scholarship,
and education by publishing worldwide in

Oxford New York

Auckland Bangkok Buenos Aires Cape Town Chennai
Dar es Salaam Delhi Hong Kong Istanbul Karachi Kolkata
Kuala Lumpur Madrid Melbourne Mexico City Mumbai Nairobi
São Paulo Shanghai Taipei Tokyo Toronto

Oxford is a registered trade mark of Oxford University Press
in the UK and in certain other countries

Published in the United States
by Oxford University Press Inc., New York

A catalogue record for this title is available from the British Library

ISBN 0 19 263047 4 (Hbk)

10 9 8 7 6 5 4 3 2 1

Typeset by Newgen Imaging Systems (P) Ltd., Chennai, India
Printed in Great Britain
on acid-free paper by
T.J. International, Padstow

Oxford Medical Publications

Oxford Dictionary of Medical Quotations

Peter McDonald

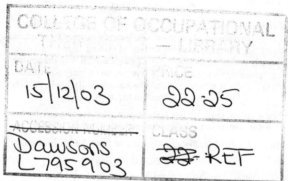
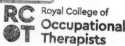
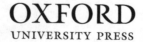
OXFORD
UNIVERSITY PRESS

Quotations

William O. Abbot 1902–43
US physician and inventor of intestinal tube

As an adult she had her organs removed one by one. Now she is a mere shell with symptoms where her organs used to be.

Quoting the dangers of overzealous treatment of non-organic disease in: *Dictionary of Medical Eponyms*, (2nd edn), p. 267, Firkin and Whitworth. The Parthenon, Lancashire, UK (1996)

John Abernethy 1764–1831
English Surgeon, St. Bartholomew's Hospital, London

Private patients, if they do not like me, can go elsewhere; but the poor devils in the hospital I am bound to take care of.

Memoirs of John Abernethy Ch. 5, George Macilwain

The hospital is the only proper College in which to rear a true disciple of Aesculapius.

Memoirs of John Abernethy Ch. 5, George Macilwain

There is no short cut, nor 'royal road' to the attainment of medical knowledge.

Hunterian Oration (1819)

Sir Adolf Abrams
British physician, Westminster Hospital, London

In my experience of anorexia nervosa it is exclusively a disease of private patients.

Attributed

Goodman Ace 1899–1982

You know, my father died of cancer when I was a teenager. He had it before it became popular.

The New Yorker (1977)

Samuel Hopkins Adams 1871–1958
US journalist and author

Ignorance and credulous hope make the market for most proprietary remedies.

Collier's Weekly 7 October (1905)

With a few honorable exceptions the press of the United States is at the beck and call of the patent medicines. Not only do the newspapers modify news possibly affecting these interests, but they sometimes become their agents.

Collier's Weekly 7 October (1905)

With the exception of lawyers, there is no profession which considers itself above the law so widely as the medical profession.

The Health Master Ch. 1

Medicine would be the ideal profession if it did not involve giving pain.

The Health Master Ch. 3

Any physician who advertises a positive cure for any disease, who issues nostrum testimonials, who sells his services to a secret remedy, or who diagnoses and treats by mail patients he has never seen, is a quack.

The Great American Fraud p. 39. Collier and Sons (1905)

Thomas Addis 1881–1949
US physician, San Francisco

When the patient dies the kidneys may go to the pathologist, but while he lives the urine is ours. It can provide us day by day, month by month, and year by year, with a serial story of the major events going on within the kidney.

Glomerular Nephritis, Diagnosis and Treatment Ch. 1

A clinician is complex. He is part craftsman, part practical scientist, and part historian.

Glomerular Nephritis, Diagnosis and Treatment Ch. 5

Joseph Addison 1672–1719
English literary figure

Physick, for the most part, is nothing else but the Substitute of Exercise or Temperance.

The Spectator Vol. III, No. 195, 13 October (1711)

Health and cheerfulness naturally beget each other.

The Spectator Vol. V, No. 387 (1712)

Our sight is the most perfect and most delightful of all our senses.

The Spectator Vol. V No. 411 (1712)

Francis Heed Adler 1895–1975
US ophthalmologist and researcher, Philadelphia

The faculties developed by doing research are those most needed in diagnosis.

Transactions of the American Academy of Ophthalmology and Otolaryngology **70**: 17 (1966)

African proverbs

Filthy water cannot be washed.

If you are too smart to pay the doctor, you had better be too smart to get ill.
Transvaal

If you intend to give a sick man medicine, let him get very ill first, so that he may see the benefit of your medicine.
Nupe

In the midst of your illness you will promise a goat, but when you have recovered, a chicken will seem sufficient.
Jukun

Loss of teeth and marriage spoil a woman's beauty.

Poison should be tried out on a frog.
Bantu

Visitor's footfalls are like medicine; they heal the sick.
Bantu

Fuller Albright 1900–69
US professor of medicine, Harvard

As with eggs, there is no such thing as a poor doctor, doctors are either good or bad.
Textbook of Medicine

Any theory is better than no theory.
Textbook of Medicine

Alexander (III) the Great of Macedon 356–323 BC

I am dying with the help of too many physicians.
Comment on his deathbed

Alexander of Tralles AD 525–605
Greek physician

The physician should look upon the patient as a besieged city and try to rescue him with every means that art and science place at his command.

Sir Thomas Clifford Allbutt 1836–1925
English physician, historian, Professor of Medicine, Cambridge, and inventor of the short thermometer

Lister saw the vast importance of the discoveries of Pasteur. He saw it because he was watching on the heights, and he was watching there alone.
Attributed

Another source of fallacy is the vicious circle of illusions which consists on the one hand of believing what we see, and on the other in seeing what we believe.
Attributed

In science, law is not a rule imposed from without, but an expression of an intrinsic process. The laws of the lawgiver are impotent beside the laws of human nature, as to his disillusion many a lawgiver has discovered.
Attributed

We are led to think of diseases as isolated disturbances in a healthy body, not as the phases of certain periods of bodily development.
Attributed

Thus we work not in the light of public opinion but in the secrecy of the bedchamber; and perhaps the best of us are apt at times to forget the delicacies and sincerities which under these conditions are essential to harmony and honour.
On Professional Education with Special Reference to Medicine

Woody Allen 1935–
US comedian and film director

I am not afraid to die. I just don't want to be there when it happens.
Death p. 63 (1975)

American proverbs

Everybody loves a fat man.

It will never get well if you pick it.

Nobody loves a fat man.

The California climate makes the sick well and the well sick, the old young and the young old.

Henri Amiel 1821–81
Swiss writer and philosopher

Health is the first of all liberties, and happiness gives us the energy which is the basis of health.
Journal Intime 3 April (1865)

Dreams are excursions into the limbo of things, a semi-deliverance from the human prison.
Journal Intime 3 December (1872)

To me the ideal doctor would be a man endowed with profound knowledge of life and of the soul, intuitively divining any suffering or disorder of whatever kind, and restoring peace by his mere presence.
Journal Intime 22 August (1873)

There is no curing a sick man who believes himself to be in health.
Journal Intime 6 February (1877)

To know how to grow old is the master-work of wisdom, and one of the most difficult chapters in the great art of living.
Journal Intime 21 September (1874)

John Allan Dalrymple Anderson
1926–
British pharmacologist

The view that a peptic ulcer may be the hole in a man's stomach through which he crawls to escape from his wife has fairly wide acceptance.
A New Look at Social Medicine. London (1965)

Sir Christopher Andrews 1903–86
Director, World Influenza Centre, London

Influenza is something unique. It behaves epidemiologically in a way different from that of any other known infection.

Foreword to Influenza: The Last Great Plague, W.I.B. Beveridge. Heinemann, London (1977)

Professor 'Tommy' Annandale
1838–1907
Professor of Surgery, Edinburgh

They say it doesn't matter how long one washes one's hands, because there will still be organisms in the sweat glands and hair follicles, so I rub my hands with Vaseline.

Harley Street p. 31, Reginald Pound. Michael Joseph, London (1967)

Anonymous

An adult is one who has ceased to grow vertically but not horizontally.

A consultant is a man sent in after the battle to bayonet the wounded.

Penguin Dictionary of Modern Humorous Quotations p. 60, Fred Metcalf. Penguin Books, London (2001)

A doctor who cannot take a good history and a patient who cannot give one are in danger of giving and receiving bad treatment.

Clues in the Diagnosis and Treatment of Heart Diseases Introduction, Paul Dudley White

An epidemiologist is a doctor broken down by age and sex.

A faithful friend is the medicine of life.

A fool lives as long as his destiny allows him.

The Sunday Times 15 July 2001, as a phrase of the suicide Svetozar Milošović, father of Slobodan Milošović, President of Serbia on trial for war crimes

A man's liver is his carburettor.

An observant parent's evidence may be disproved but should never be ignored.

Lancet I: 688 (1951)

A minor operation: one performed on somebody else.

Penguin Dictionary of Modern Humorous Quotations p. 191, Fred Metcalf. Penguin Books, London (2001)

A physician is someone who knows everything and does nothing.
A surgeon is someone who does everything and knows nothing.
A psychiatrist is someone who knows nothing and does nothing.
A pathologist is someone who knows everything and does everything too late.

A surgeon should give as little pain as possible while he is treating the patient, and no pain at all when he charges his fee.

'FRCS' in *The Times*, quoted by Reginald Pound in *Harley Street*. Michael Joseph, London (1967)

Abstinence is a good thing, but it should always be practised in moderation.

A rash of dermatologists, a hive of allergists, a scrub of interns, a giggle of nurses, a flood of urologists, a pile of proctologists, an eyeful of ophthalmologists, a whiff of anesthesiologists, a cast of orthopaedic rheumatologists, a gargle of laryngologists.

Asthma is a disease that has practically the same symptoms as passion except that with asthma it lasts longer.

Journal of the American Medical Association **190**: 392 (1964)

By the year 2000 the commonest killers such as coronary heart disease, stroke, respiratory, diseases and many cancers will be wiped out.

Irish Times 24 April (1987)

Children are one third of our population and all our future.

US Select Panel for Promotion of Child Health (1981)

Choose your specialist and you choose your disease.

The Westminster Review 18 May (1908)

Coughs and sneezes spread diseases.

British wartime slogan (1942)

Dermatology is the best specialty. The patient never—dies and never gets well.

Medical Quotes, J. Dantith and A. Isaacs. Market House Books, Oxford (1989)

Dr Bell fell down the well
And broke his collar bone
Doctors should attend the sick
And leave the well alone

Doctor says he would be a very sick man if were still alive today.

Even a good operation done poorly is still a poor operation.

Everyone faces at all times two fateful possibilities: one is to grow older, the other not.

Exploratory operation: a remunerative reconnaissance.

Fifty years ago the successful doctor was said to need three things; a top hat to give him Authority, a paunch to give him Dignity, and piles to give him an Anxious Expression.

Lancet I: 169 (1951)

Get up at five, have lunch at nine,
Supper at five, retire at nine,
And you will live to ninety-nine.

Continued

Anonymous *continued*

Have faith in the Lord but use sulphur for the itch.

Here lies one who for medicines would not give
A little gold, and so his life he lost;
I fancy now he'd wish again to live,
Could he but guess how much his funeral cost.

Homeopathy waged a war of radicalism against
the profession. Very different would have been the
profession's attitude toward homeopathy if it had
aimed, like other doctrines advanced by
physicians, to gain a foothold among medical men
alone or chiefly, instead of making its appeal to the
popular favour and against the profession.
> Report to the Connecticut Medical Society (1852), quoted by
> Coulter in *Divided Legacy*

If I were summing up the qualities of a good
teacher of medicine, I would enumerate human
sympathy, moral and intellectual integrity,
enthusiasm, and ability to talk, in addition, of
course, to knowledge of his subject.

If three simple questions and one well chosen
laboratory test lead to an unambiguous diagnosis,
why harry the patient with more?
> Editorial, Clinical decision by numbers. *Lancet* 1: 1077 (1975)

If you resolve to give up smoking, drinking and
loving, you don't actually live longer; it just seems
that way.

In diagnosis, the young are positive and the
middle-aged tentative; only the old have flair.
> *Lancet* 1: 795 (1951)

In the nineteenth century men lost their fear of
God and acquired a fear of microbes.

It is better to employ a doubtful remedy than to
condemn the patient to a certain death.

It is not what disease the patient has but which
patient has the disease.

Late children, early orphans.

Let out the blood, let out the disease.
> Popular aphorism for hundreds of years until the end of
> the nineteenth century

Man has an inalienable right to die of something.
> Quack cures for cancer, *Cardiff Mail* 20 October (1923)

Many physicians would prefer passing a small
kidney stone to presenting a paper.
> *Journal of the American Medical Association* **174**: 292 (1960)

Marriage—a stage between infancy and adultery.
> *Commentary on adolescence*

Medical statistics are like a bikini. What they
reveal is interesting but what they conceal is vital.

Medicine, like every useful science, should be
thrown open to the observation and study of all.
> *New York Evening Star* 27 December (1833), reflecting the
> Thomsonian populist philosophy of the time

Mind over matter.

My friend was sick: I attended him. He died; I
dissected him.

My God all that reality!
> Thespian to doctor on discovering his trade.

Never let the sun set or rise on a small bowel
obstruction.
> P. Mucha Jr, Small intestinal obstruction. *Surgical Clinics of
> North America* **67**: 597–620 (1987)

Not so much attention is paid to our children's
minds as is paid to their feet.
> Quoted by A.V. Neale in *The Advancement of Child Health*

No woman wants an abortion. Either she wants a
child or she wishes to avoid pregnancy.
> Letter to the *Lancet*

Palliative care should not be associated exclusively
with terminal care. Many patients need it early in
the course of their disease.
> Report of the Expert Advisory Group on Cancer to the Chief
> Medical Officers of England and Wales, Calman-Hine (1995)

Parenthood is the only profession that has been
left exclusively to amateurs.

Patients and their families will forgive you for
wrong diagnoses, but will rarely forgive you for
wrong prognoses; the older you grow in medicine,
the more chary you get about offering iron clad
prognoses, good or bad.
> David Seegal *Journal of Chronic Diseases* **16**: 443 (1963)

Physicians and politicians resemble one another
in this respect, that some defend the constitution
and others destroy it.
> *Acton or the Circle of Life*

Physicians are rather like undescended testicles,
they are difficult to locate and when they are
found, they are pretty ineffective.
> *Book of Humorous Medical Anecdotes* p. 47. Springwood
> Books, Ascot, Berkshire, UK (1989)

Poverty is a virtue greatly exaggerated by
physicians no longer forced to practise it.

Removing the teeth will cure something,
including the foolish belief that removing the
teeth will cure everything.

Rheumatic fever licks at the joints, but bites at the
heart.

Science without conscience is the death of the soul.

Sepsis is an insult to a surgeon.

Surgeons get long lives and short memories.
> Comment at The Association of Coloproctology Meeting,
> Harrogate, June (2001)

The best patient is a millionaire with a positive
Wassermann.
> Commentary before the era of antibiotics

The best physicians are Dr. Diet, Dr. Quiet and
Dr. Merryman.

The British Medical Association is a club of London
physicians and surgeons who once a year visit and
patronize their professional friends in the country.
> *Medical Times and Gazette* p. 37, 18 January (1870)

The comforting, if spurious, precision of laboratory results has the same appeal as the lifebelt to the weak swimmer.

Lancet I: 539–40 (1981)

The fact is that in creating towns, men create the materials for an immense hotbed of disease, and this effect can only be neutralised by extraordinary artificial precautions.

The Times 8 October (1868)

The inhabitants of Harley Street and Wimpole Street have been so taken up with their private practices that they have neglected to add to knowledge. The pursuit of learning has been handicapped by the pursuit of gain.

Royal Commission on University Education (1915)

The National Health Service is rotting before our eyes, with a lack of political will to make the tough choices for a first-class service for an ever more demanding population.

Leader, *The Times* July (2000)

The new definition of psychiatry is the care of the id by the odd.

The principal objection to old age is that there is no future in it.

The psychiatrist is the obstetrician of the mind.

The publication of a long list of authors' names after the title is a little like having all a vessel's ballast hanging from the masthead, as if to counterbalance the barnacles.

New England Journal of Medicine **271**: 1068 (1964)

The reason that academic disputes are so bitter is that the stakes are so small.

There are two kinds of sleep. The sleep of the just and the sleep of the just after.

There is no bed shortage – most people have their own.

Capital Doctor Issue 5, December (2000)

There is no short cut from chemical laboratory to clinic, except one that passes too close to the morgue.

American Medical Association (1929) as quoted in *Cured to Death*, Arabella Melville and Colin Johnson. Secker and Warburg Ltd, London (1982)

The sick are still in General Mixed Workhouses—the maternity cases, the cancerous, the venereal, the chronically infirm, and even the infectious, all together in one building, often in the same ward where they cannot be treated.

The Failure of the Poor Law, UK National Committee to Promote the Break-up of the Poor Laws (1909)

The spine is a series of bones running down your back. You sit on one end of it and your head sits on the other.

The wound is granulating well, the matter formed is diminishing in quantity and is laudable. But the wound is still deep and must be dressed from the bottom to ensure sound healing.

British Medical Journal (1901) of the postoperative recovery after appendicectomy of Edward VII

They shall lay their hands on the sick, and they shall recover.

Book of Common prayer (1708), describing Queen Anne's 'healings'

Thou to whom the sick and dying
Ever came, nor came in vain,
With thy healing hands replying
To their wearied cry of pain.

The New English Hymnal p. 331. Canterbury Press, Norwich (1986)

'Tis better than riches
To scratch when it itches

Today's facts are tomorrow's fallacies.

We forever have to walk the tightrope between what is seen to be the need and what is thought to be the demand . . . that's all part of setting priorities and having a rational debate.

A NHS Chief Executive Officer in *Primary Care and Public Involvement*, Timothy Milewa and Michael Calnan *Journal of the Royal Society of Medicine* **93**: 3–5 (2000)

You shall not eat or drink in the company of other people but with lepers alone, and you shall know that when you shall have died you will not be buried in the church.

Advice to lepers in the Middle Ages in Treves. Quoted in O. Schell, *Zur Geschichte des Aussatzes am Niederrhein, Ardir für Geschichte der Medezin* **iii**: 335–46 (1910)

You Surgeons of London, who puzzle your Pates,
To ride in your Coaches, and purchase Estates,
Give over, for Shame, for your Pride has a Fall,
And ye Doctress of Epsom has outdone you all.

Gentleman's Magazine October (1732), sardonically commenting on the rise of quackery in the eighteenth century with this line from 'The Husband's Relief', quoted in *Sidelights of Medical History* by Zachary Cope, The Royal Society of Medicine (1957)

Antiphanes 408–334? BC
Greek philosopher and playwright, Athens

All pain is one malady with many names.
The Doctor

John Apley 1909–80
Consultant paediatrician, Bristol, UK

The further away the chronic abdominal pain in a child is from the umbilicus the more likely an organic cause.

Attributed

Apocrypha

Perfect health is above gold; a sound body before riches.

Ecclesiasticus

Arabic proverbs

He who has health has hope; and he who has hope has everything.

No man is a good physician who has never been sick.

Love and pregnancy and riding on a camel cannot be hid.   *Continued*

Arabic proverbs *continued*

For most diagnoses all that is needed is an ounce of knowledge, an ounce of intelligence, and a pound of thoroughness.

Exercise is good for your health, but like everything else it can be overdone.
Shape Magazine, USA

When fate arrives the physician becomes a fool.

John Arbuthnot 1667–1735
Scottish physician and satirist

The first Care in building of Cities, is to make them airy and well perflated; Infectious Distempers must necessarily be propagated amongst Mankind living close together.
An Essay Concerning the Effects of Air on Human Bodies
Ch. 9, No. 20

Aretaeus of Cappadocia AD 120–180
Greek physician

This is a mighty wonder: in the discharge from the lungs alone, which is not particularly dangerous, the patients do not despair of themselves, even although near the last.
On the Causes and Symptoms of Acute Diseases II.ii.18 (on Tuberculosis)

When he can render no further aid, the physician alone can mourn as a man with his incurable patient. This is the physician's sad lot.
Attributed

In diabetes the thirst is greater for the fluid dries the body . . . For the thirst there is need of a powerful remedy, for in kind it is the greatest of all sufferings, and when a fluid is drunk, it stimulates the discharge of urine.
Therapeutics of chronic diseases II, Ch. II, 485–6

Aristophanes 448–380 BC
Greek philosopher and playwright

Old age is but a second childhood.
Clouds (1417) (transl. Thomas Mitchell)

Aristotle 384–322 BC
Greek phliosopher

The physician himself, if sick, actually calls in another physician, knowing that he cannot reason correctly if required to judge his own condition while suffering.
De Republica iii.16

Nature does nothing without a purpose.

In children may be observed the traces and seeds of what will one day be settled psychological habits, though psychologically a child hardly differs for the time being from an animal.
Historia Animalium VIII.1 (transl. D. W. Thompson)

Nature proceeds little by little from things lifeless to animal life in such a way that it is impossible to determine the exact line of demarcation, nor on which side thereof an intermediate form should lie.
Historia Animalium VIII.I

While it is true that the suicide braves death, he does it not for some noble object but to escape some ill.
Nicomachean Ethics 3

It is no part of a physician's business to use either persuasion or compulsion upon the patients.
Politics VII.ii

The body is most fully developed from thirty to thirty-five years of age, the mind at about forty-nine.
Rhetoric II.xiv

Rising before daylight is also to be commended; it is a healthy habit, and gives more time for the management of the household as well as for liberal studies.
Economics I

Conscientious and careful physicians allocate causes of disease to natural laws, while the ablest scientists go back to medicine for their first principles.
Attributed

Speeches are like babies—easy to conceive but hard to deliver.
Attributed

It is well to be up before daybreak, for such habits contribute to health, wealth and wisdom.
Attributed

John Armstrong 1710–79
English physician and poet

For want of timely care
Millions have died of medicable wounds.
Art of Preserving Health

Many more Englishmen die by the lancet at home, than by the sword abroad.
Attributed

Matthew Arnold 1822–88
British poet and critic

Nor bring to see me cease to live,
Some doctor full of phrase and fame,
To shake his sapient head, and give
The ill he cannot cure a name.
New Poems 'A Wish'

Ar-Rumi 836–896

The blunders of a doctor are felt not by himself but by others.
Attributed

Antonin Artaud 1896–1948
French actor and producer

I know each conversation with a psychiatrist in the morning made me want to hang myself because I knew I could not strangle him.
Attributed

Asclepiades 1st century BC
Greek-born Roman physician

To cure safely, swiftly and pleasantly.
Attributed

A man is a poor physician who has not two or three remedies ready for use in every case of illness.
Attributed

Richard Asher 1912–69
British physician and writer

Too often a sister puts all her patients back to bed as a housewife puts all her plates back in the plate-rack – to make a generally tidy appearance.
British Medical Journal **2**: 967 (1947)

Despair is better treated with hope, not dope.
Lancet 1: 954 (1958)

For many doctors the achievement of a published article is a tedious duty to be surmounted as a necessary hurdle in a medical career.
British Medical Journal **2**: 502 (1958)

The modern haematologist, instead of describing in English what he can see, prefers to describe in Greek what he can't.
British Medical Journal **2**: 359 (1959)

Gynaecologists are very smooth indeed. Because they have to listen to woeful and sordid symptoms they develop an expression of refinement and sympathy.
A Sense of Asher p. 86. Pitman Medical, UK (1972)

It is not always worth the discomforts of major surgery to get minor recovery.
A Sense of Asher p. 86. Pitman Medical, UK (1972)

The only similarity between the car and the human body is that if something is seriously wrong with the design of the former you can send it back to its maker.
A Sense of Asher p. 86. Pitman Medical, UK (1972)

Isaac Asimov 1920–92
US science fiction writer

If my doctor told me I had only six minutes to live, I wouldn't brood. I'd type a little faster.
Life (1984)

Dana W. Atchley 1892–?
US physician

The principles of medical management are essentially the same for individuals of all ages, albeit the same problem is handled differently in different patients.
Attributed

W. H. Auden 1907–73
English poet

A professor is one who talks in someone else's sleep.
Attributed

Leopold Auenbrugger 1722–1809
Austrian physician and discoverer of the percussion of the thorax

I here present the reader with a new sign which I have discovered for detecting diseases of the chest. This consists in percussion of the human thorax, whereby, according to the character of the particular sounds then elicited, an opinion is formed of the internal state of that cavity.
New Invention by Means of Percussing the Human Thorax for Detecting Signs of Obscure Disease of the Interior of the Chest (Inventum novum ex percussione), 31 December (1761)

St. Augustine AD 354–430
Bishop of Hippo, early Christian Theologian

The greatest evil is physical pain.
Soliloquies I.21

Marcus Aurelius AD 121–180
Roman emperor and Stoic philosopher

Nowhere can man find a quieter or more untroubled retreat than in his own soul.
Meditations

Tranquility is nothing else than the good ordering of the mind.
Meditations IV.3

Death is a release from the impressions of sense, and from impulses that make us their puppets, from the vagaries of the mind, and the hard service of the flesh.
Meditations VI.28

Jane Austen 1775–1817
English novelist

My sore throats, you know, are always worse than anybody's.
Persuasion Ch. 18 (1815)

Avicenna 980–1037
Persian physician, Baghdad school

The physical signs of measles are nearly the same as those of smallpox, but nausea and inflammation is more severe, though the pains in the back are less.
The Canon Bk IV

The different sorts of madness are innumerable.
The Canon Bk IV

Leeches should be kept a day before applying them. They should be squeezed to make them eject the contents of their stomachs.
The Canon Bk IV

Washington Ayer
19th century US Surgeon

Here the most sublime scene ever witnessed in the operating room was presented when the patient placed himself voluntarily upon the table, which was to become the altar of future fame.
Description of the first public demonstration of ether at the Massachussetts General Hospital, 16 October 1846

The heroic bravery of the man who voluntarily placed himself upon the table, a subject for the surgeon's knife, should be recorded and his name enrolled upon parchment, which should be hung upon the walls of the surgical amphitheatre in which the operation was performed. His name was Gilbert Abbott.
Description of the first public demonstration of ether at the Massachussetts General Hospital, 16 October 1846

Pam Ayres 1947–
English poet and humorist
Medicinal discovery,
It moves in mighty leaps,
It leapt straight past the common cold
And gave it us for keeps.
Oh no! I got a cold (1976)

Sir Francis Bacon 1551–1626
English philosopher and politician

Medical men do not know the drugs they use, nor their prices.
De Erroribus Medicorum

It is as natural to die as to be born; and to a little infant, perhaps, the one is as painful as the other.
Essays 'Of Death'

Men fear Death, as children fear to go in the dark; and as that natural fear in children is increased with tales, so is the other.
Essays

Cure the disease and kill the patient.
Essays 'Of Friendship'

Surely every medicine is an innovation, and he that will not apply new remedies, must expect new evils.
Essays 'Of Innovations'

The remedy is worse than the disease.
Essays 'Of Seditions and Troubles'

A man that is young in years may be old in hours, if he has lost no time.
Essays 'Of Youth and Age'

The men of experiment are like the ant; they only collect and use: the reasoners resemble spiders, who make cobwebs out of their own substance. But the bee takes a middle course; it gathers its material from the flowers of the garden and of the field, but transforms and digests it by a power of its own.
Novum Organum 'Aphorisms'

Brutes by their natural instinct have produced many discoveries, whereas men by discussion and the conclusions of reason have given birth to few or none.
Novum Organum LXXIII

They are the best physicians, who being great in learning most incline to the traditions of experience, or being distinguished in practice do not reflect the methods and generalities of art.
The Advancement of Learning Bk IV, Ch. II

Deformed persons commonly take revenge on nature.
The Advancement of Learning Bk VI, Ch. 3

Walter Bagehot 1826–77
English economist and journalist

Writers, like teeth, are divided into, incisors and grinders.
Literary Studies 'The First Edinburgh Reviewers'

Giorgio Baglivi 1669–1707
Professor of Anatomy at Sapienza, Papal University, Rome

Let the young know they will never find a more interesting, more instructive book than the patient himself.
Attributed

The doctor is the servant and the interpreter of nature. Whatever he thinks or does, if he follows not in nature's footsteps he will never be able to control her.
Introduction to De Praxi Medica (1696)

The origin and the causes of disease are far too recondite for the human mind to unravel them.
Introduction to De Praxi Medica

The two fulcra of medicine are reason and observation. Observation is the clue to guide the physician in his thinking.
Introduction to De Praxi Medica

Mary Baines 1934–
Palliative care physician, London, UK

One cannot help a man to come to accept his impending death if he remains in severe pain, one cannot give spiritual counsel to a woman who is vomiting, or help a wife and children say their goodbyes to a father who is so drugged that he cannot respond.
Quoted in *Clinical Pharmacology* by D. R. Lawrence, P. N. Bennett, and M. J. Brown. Churchhill Livingstone, Edinburgh (1997)

Jacob Balde c. 1658
German preacher

What difference is there between a smoker and a suicide, except that the one takes longer to kill himself than the other.
Attributed

Honoré de Balzac 1799–1850
French novelist

The glory of surgeons is like that of actors, who exist only in their lifetime and whose talent is no longer appreciable once they have disappeared.
The Atheist's Mass

Physically, a man is a man for a much longer time than a woman is a woman.
The Physiology of Marriage

No man should marry until he has studied anatomy and dissected at least one woman.
The Physiology of Marriage Meditation V, Aphorism 28

Six weeks with a fever is an eternity.
Attributed

Alvan L. Barach 1895–?
US physician, New York

An alcoholic has been lightly defined as a man who drinks more than his own doctor.
Journal of the American Medical Association **181**: 393 (1962)

Middle age has been said to be the time of a man's life when, if he has two choices for an evening, he takes the one that gets him home earlier.
Journal of the American Medical Association **181**: 393 (1962)

Asaph ben Barachiah 6th century

The humour and illnesses are already on the sperm and are transmitted to the embryo.
Attributed

Sam Bardell 1915–

Psychiatrist: A man who asks you a lot of expensive questions your wife asks you for nothing.
Attributed

Christian Barnard 1922–2001

Pioneer South African heart surgeon

The prime goal is to alleviate suffering, and not to prolong life. And if your treatment does not alleviate suffering, but only prolongs life, that treatment should be stopped.
Attributed

Norman Barrett 1904–?

UK surgeon, St. Thomas's Hospital, London

It is the doctors who desert the dying and there is so much to be learned about pain.
Quoted in *Journal of the Royal Society of Medicine* **94**: 430 (2001)

Sir James Matthew Barrie 1860–1937

British playwright

When the first baby laughed for the first time, the laugh broke into a thousand pieces and they all went skipping about, and that was the beginning of fairies.
Peter Pan Act 1 (1904)

The scientific man is the only person who has anything new to say and who does not know how to say it.
Attributed

John Barrymore 1882–1942

US actor

He neither drank, smoked, nor rode a bicycle. Living frugally, saving his money, he died early, surrounded by greedy relatives. It was a great lesson to me.
The Stage January (1941) (J. P. McEvoy)

Elisha Bartlett 1804–1855

US professor of medicine, editor and educator

Certainly it is by their signs and symptoms, that internal diseases are revealed to the physician.
Philosophy of Medical Science Pt II, Ch. 10

Bernard Baruch 1870–1965

US financier

There are no such things as incurable, there are only things for which man has not found a cure.
Quoted by his son, Simon Baruch, the surgeon, in a speech, 30 April (1954)

Sir Henry Howarth Bashford ('Peter Harding') 1880–1961

After all we are merely the servants of the public, in spite of our M.D.'s and our hospital appointments.
The Corner of Harley Street Ch. 8

General practice is at least as difficult, if it is to be carried on well and successfully, as any special practice can be, and probably more so; for the G.P. has to live continually, as it were, with the results of his handiwork.
The Corner of Harley Street Ch. 26

If your news must be bad, tell it soberly and promptly.
The Corner of Harley Street Ch. 26

St. Basil the Great c. 330–379

Bishop of Caesarea in Cappadocia

Drunkenness, the ruin of reason, the destruction of strength, premature old age, momentary death.
Homilies No. XIV, Ch. 7

Charles Baudelaire 1821–67

French poet

Sexuality is the lyricism of the masses.
Journaux intimes (1887) 93

Richard Baxter 1615–91

English non-conformist divine

An aching tooth is better out than in,
To lose a rotting member is a gain.
Poetical Fragments 'Man'

Sir William Maddock Bayliss 1860–1937

British physiologist

The greatness of a scientific investigator does not rest on the fact of his having never made a mistake, but rather on his readiness to admit that he has done so, whenever the contrary evidence is cogent enough.
Principles of General Physiology, Preface

William B. Bean 1909–89

US physician

The so-called medical literature is stuffed to bursting with junk, written in a hopscotch style characterised by a Brownian movement of uncontrolled parts of speech which seethe in restless unintelligibility.
Journal of Laboratory and Clinical Medicine **39**: 3 (1952)

G. H. Beaton

Contemporary US professor of nutrition

The interactions of man with his environment are so complex that only an ecological approach to nutrition permits an understanding of the whole spectrum of factors determining the nutritional problems that exist in human societies.
Nutrition in Preventive Medicine p. 15. WHO (1976)

Lindsey E. Beaton 1911–
US psychiatrist

We are physicians. It is a proud title. It carries prerogatives; it carries privileges. Most of all it carries accountability, not only for the future of a great profession but for the very lives of our fellow sufferers from the human condition.
Journal of Medical Education **40**: 35 (1965)

Pierre de Beaumarchais 1732–99
French dramatist

That which distinguishes man from the beast is drinking without being thirsty and making love at all seasons.
Le Marriage de Figaro II. xxi

William Beaumont 1785–1853
US physician

Of all the lessons which a young man entering upon the profession of medicine needs to learn, this is perhaps the first – that he should resist the fascination of doctrines and hypotheses till he has won the privilege of such studies by honest labour and faithful pursuit of real and useful knowledge.
Notebook

Simone de Beauvoir 1908–86
French feminist writer

One is not born a woman, one becomes one.
The Second Sex Ch. 2 (1949)

There is no such thing as a natural death: nothing that happens to a man is ever natural, since his presence calls the world into question.
A Very Easy Death

Samuel Becket 1906–89
Irish novelist and playwright

We are all born mad. Some remain so.
Waiting for Godot II (1955)

George Howard Bell 1905
Scottish physician (Dundee)

In the practice of medicine more mistakes are made from lack of accurate observation and deduction than from lack of knowledge.
Experimental Physiology

John Bell 1796–1872
Edinburgh surgeon

Of the two forms of arthritis or articular inflammation, rheumatism is the tax most frequently paid by the vulgar dram and grog drinker; gout, that incurred by the genteel and sometimes the literary wine-bibber.
Lectures on Theory and Practice of Physic Lect. CLXVII

Peter Bell 1938–
Professor of Surgery and Chairman of Research at Royal College of Surgeons of England

There are few people who have not benefited in some way, either directly or indirectly, from advances made in surgical research.
Research Report 2001. Royal College of Surgeons of England

Nicholas de Belleville 1753–1831

When you are called to a sick man, be sure you know what the matter is—if you do not know, nature can do a great deal better than you can guess.
Help-Bringers 'Belleville' by Fr B. Rogers

Hilaire Belloc 1870–1953
French-born British poet, essayist and historian

Physicians of the Utmost Fame
Were called at once; but when they came
They answered, as they took their Fees,
'There is no cure for this disease.'
Cautionary Tales for Children 'Henry King' (1907)

The Microbe is so very small
You cannot make him out at all,
But many sanguine people hope
To see him through a microscope
More Beasts for Worse Children 'The Microbe' (1897)

Stephen Vincent Benét 1898–1943
US writer

So it was all modern and scientific and well arranged. You could die very nearly as privately in a modern hospital as you could in the Grand Central Station, and with much better care.
Tales of our Time 'No Visitors'

Alan Bennet 1934–
British dramatist and actor

There are more microbes per person than the entire population of the world.
The Old Country II

Billy Bennett 1887–?
British comedian

You can't part the skin of a sausage,
Or a dad from his fond son and heir.
And you can't part the hair on
a bald-headed man,
For there'll be no parting there.
Quoted from Bennett's monologue Daddy (1929)

Jeremy Bentham 1748–1832
English philosopher and reformer

Nature has placed mankind under the governances of two sovereign masters, pain and pleasure.
Introduction to the Principles of Morals and Legislation Ch. 1

A man may be said to be in a state of health when he is not conscious of any uneasy sensations, the primary seat of which can be perceived to be anywhere in his body.

Introduction to the Principles of Morals and Legislation Ch. 6

Pain is in itself an evil; and, indeed, without exception, the only evil.

Introduction to the Principles of Morals and Legislation Ch. X

Bernard Berenson 1865–1959

US art critic

Psychoanalysts are not occupied with the minds of their patients; they do not believe in the mind but in a cerebral intestine.

Quoted by Umberto Morra in Conversations with Berenson
8 February (1931)

Frank M. Berger 1913–

US pharmacologist

Tranquilizers at times do much more than eliminate agitation; they may facilitate social adjustment, eliminate delusions and hallucinations, or make mute patients communicative.

Drugs and Behavior Ch. 3, Leonard Uhr and James
G. Miller (ed.)

Claude Bernard 1813–78

French physiologist and founder of experimental medicine

Put off your imagination as you take off your overcoat, when you enter the laboratory.

Introduction to the Study of Experimental Medicine (1865)

True science teaches us to doubt and, in ignorance, refrain.

Introduction to the Study of Experimental Medicine (1865)
Pt I, Ch. I, Sect. ii

A scientific hypothesis is merely a scientific idea, preconceived or previsioned. A theory is merely a scientific idea controlled by experiment.

Introduction to the Study of Experimental Medicine (1865)
Pt I, Ch. I, Sect. vi

In biological sciences, the role of method is even more important than in other sciences, because of the immense complexity of the phenomena and the countless sources of error which complexity brings into experimentation.

Introduction to the Study of Experimental Medicine (1865)
Pt I, Ch. 2, Sect. ii

If an idea presents itself to us, we must not reject it simply because it does not agree with the logical deductions of a reigning theory.

Introduction to the Study of Experimental Medicine (1865)
Pt I, Ch. 2, Sect. iii

A discovery is generally an unforeseen relation not included in theory, for otherwise it would be foreseen.

Introduction to the Study of Experimental Medicine (1865)

Men who have excessive faith in their theories or ideas are not only ill prepared for making discoveries; they also make very poor observations.

Introduction to the Study of Experimental Medicine (1865)
Pt I, Ch. 2, Sect. iii

It is in the darker regions of science that great men are recognised; they are marked by ideas which light up phenomena hitherto obscure and carry science forward.

Introduction to the Study of Experimental Medicine (1865)
Pt I, Ch. 2, Sect. iv

Experiment is fundamentally only induced observation.

Introduction to the Study of Experimental Medicine (1865)
Pt I, Sect. v

The doubter is a true man of science; he doubts only himself and his interpretations, but he believes in science.

Introduction to the Study of Experimental Medicine (1865)
Pt I, Ch. 2, Sect. vi

True science teaches us to doubt and, in ignorance, to refrain.

Introduction to the Study of Experimental Medicine (1865)
Pt I, Ch. 2, Sect. vii

Systems do not exist in Nature but only in men's minds.

Introduction to the Study of Experimental Medicine (1865)

In experimentation it is always necessary to start from a particular fact and proceed to the generalization ... But above all one must observe.

Manuscript Collège de France

Medicine is destined to get away from empiricism little by little; like all other sciences, it will get away by scientific method.

Attributed

I consider the hospital to be a vestibule for scientific medicine; it is the first field of observation to which a physician is exposed. However, the laboratory is the temple of science.

Written in 1844 when splitting from his collaborator
François Magendie

In pathology, as in physiology, the true worth of an investigator consists in pursuing not only what he seeks in an experiment, but also what he did not seek.

Attributed

Jeffrey Bernard 1932–97

British journalist and wit

I read that a member of the General Medical Council has called on his colleagues for quicker identification and treatment for alcoholic doctors. They apparently consider heavy drinking to be more than four pints of beer a day, or four doubles or a bottle of wine a day. I should have thought that to be the national average lunchtime consumption.

Low Life

Aneurin Bevan 1897–1960

British Statesman

Our hospital organization has grown up with no plan, with no system. I would rather be kept alive in the efficient if cold altruism of a large hospital than expire in a gush of warm sympathy in a small one.

Speech in the House of Commons, 30 April (1946)

The doctors are too narrowly educated.

Attributed to Bevan in Harley Street p. 178, Reginald
Pound. Michael Joseph, London (1967)

W. I. B. Beveridge 1908–

Professor of veterinary science

People whose minds are not disciplined by training often tend to notice and remember events that support their views and forget others.
The Art of Scientific Investigations Preface

Probably the majority of discoveries in biology and medicine have been come upon unexpectedly, or at least had an element of chance in them, especially the most important and revolutionary ones.
The Art of Scientific Investigation Ch. III

There is an interesting saying that no one believes an hypothesis except its originator but everyone believes an experiment except the experimenter.
The Art of Scientific Investigation Ch. V

He is a bold man who submits his paper for publication without it having first been put under the microscope of friendly criticism by colleagues.
The Art of Scientific Investigation Ch. IX

Gareth Beynon 1940–

British physician

Early to bed, early to rise, work like hell and advertise.
Quoted in *Consultant Care* (1998), BUPA communications about private practice

The Bible

The eye is not satisfied with seeing.
Ecclesiasticus 1: 8

Be not slow to visit the sick: for that shall make thee to be beloved.
Ecclesiasticus 7: 35

The Lord hath created medicines out of the earth; and he that is wise will not abhor them.
Ecclesiasticus 38: 4

Honour a physician with the honour due unto him for the uses which ye may have of him: for the Lord hath created him. For of the most High cometh healing, and he shall receive honour of the king.
Ecclesiasticus 38: 1–2

And God said, Let us make man in our image, after our likeness: and let them have dominion over the fish of the seas, and over the fowl of the air, and over the cattle, and over all the earth, and over every creeping thing that creepeth upon the earth.
Genesis 1: 26

Unto the woman he said, I will greatly multiply thy sorrow and thy conception; in sorrow thou shalt bring forth children.
Genesis 3: 16

Man's days shall be to one hundred and twenty years.
Genesis 6: 3

But the men of Sodom were wicked and sinners before the Lord exceedingly.
Genesis 13: 13

Ye shall circumcise the flesh of your foreskin; and it shall be a token of the covenant betwixt me and you.
Genesis 17: 11

Isaac was old, and his eyes were dim, so that he could not see.
Genesis 27: 1

Give me children or else I die. (Rachel)
Genesis 30: 1

Let us eat and drink; for tomorrow we die.
Isaiah 22: 13

We have made a covenant with death.
Isaiah 28: 15

The prayer of faith shall save the sick.
James 5: 15

A woman when she is in travail hath sorrow, because her hour is come: but as soon as she is delivered of the child, she remembereth no more the anguish, for joy that a man is born into the world.
John 16: 21

But Ahijah could not see; for his eyes were set by reason of his age.
1 Kings 14: 4

The leper in whom the plague is, his clothes shall be rent, and his head bare, and he shall put a covering upon his upper lip, and shall cry, Unclean, unclean.
Leviticus 13: 45

Physician, heal thyself.
Luke 4: 23

Man shall not live by bread alone.
Matthew 4: 4 and *Luke* 4: 4

The light of the body is the eye.
Matthew 6: 22

They that be whole need not a physician, but they that are sick.
Matthew 9: 12

And if the blind lead the blind, both shall fall into the ditch.
Matthew 15: 14

The glory of young men is their strength.
Proverbs 20: 29

The wringing of the nose shall bring forth blood.
Proverbs 30: 33

Bodily exercise profiteth little.
1 Timothy 4: 8

Drink no longer water, but use a little wine for thy stomach's sake and thine often infirmities.
1 Timothy 5: 23

Xavier Bichat 1771–1802

French surgeon, Paris

Life is the sum of the functions that resist death.
Attributed

We cannot therefore deny that a change in just one of an organ's tissues is frequently enough to disturb the functions in all the others; yet likewise, it is in only one of them that the evil originates.
Attributed

August Bier 1861–1949
German professor of surgery

A smart mother makes often a better diagnosis than a poor doctor.
Attributed

Medical scientists are nice people, but you should not let them treat you.
Attributed

Medicine is like a woman who changes with the fashions.
Attributed

In America there exist professional anaesthetists. This specialty is being praised in Germany. I cannot think of anything more dull.
Attributed

Ambrose Bierce 1842–1914
US writer and journalist

ABSTAINER, n. A weak person who yields to the temptation of denying himself a pleasure.
The Devil's Dictionary

DENTIST, n. A prestidigitator who, putting metal into your mouth, pulls coins out of your pocket.
The Devil's Dictionary

GOUT, n. A physician's name for the rheumatism of a rich patient.
The Devil's Dictionary

GRAVE, n. A place in which the dead are laid to await the coming of the medical student.
The Devil's Dictionary

All are lunatics, but he who can analyze his delusion is called a philosopher.
Epigrams

Jacob Bigelow 1786–1879
US physician, Harvard

A far more just definition would be that medicine is the art of understanding diseases, and of curing or relieving them when possible.
Nature in Disease Ch. 2

When we know that a case is self-limited or incurable, we are to consider how far it is in our power to palliate or diminish sufferings which we are not competent to remove.
Nature in Disease Ch. 2

He is a great physician who, above other men, understands diagnosis.
Nature in Disease Ch. 2

Hermann M. Biggs 1859–1923
Professor of Medicine, New York

The human body is the only machine for which there are no spare parts.
Radio Talk (quoted in *Doctor's Legacy*)

John Shaw Billings 1838–1913
British reformer

You cannot legislate a new layer of cortical gray matter into, or a cirrhosed liver out of, a man.
Boston Medical and Surgical Journal **131**: 125 (1894)

The education of the doctor which goes on after he has his degree, is, after all, the most important part of his education.
Boston Medical and Surgical Journal **131**: 140 (1894)

It has been considered from the point of view of the hygienist, the physician, the architect, the taxpayer, the superintendents, and the nurse . . . but I do not remember to have seen one from the point of view of the patient.
Public Health Reports **2**: 384 (1874–75)

The public is not always sagacious, but in the long run, it does somehow contrive to find out who are the skilled lawyers and doctors.
Public Health Reports **2**: 384 (1874–75)

Theodor Billroth 1829–94
Prussian-born Professor of Surgery, Vienna

It is quite correct to distinguish between medical science and the physician's art.
The Medical Sciences in the German Universities Pt I, 'The Early Universities'

Can there be a better preparatory school for the physician than the study of the natural sciences? I think not!
The Medical Sciences in the German Universities Pt II, Ch. 2

It is a most gratifying sign of the rapid progress of our time that our best text-books become antiquated so quickly.
The Medical Sciences in the German Universities Pt II

The physician can do all he has to do with speed and precision, but he must never appear to be in a hurry, and never absent-minded.
The Medical Sciences in the German Universities Pt III

The principal method and goal of investigations is recognition of truth, even though the truth may be in conflict with our social, ethical and political circumstances.
The Medical Sciences in the German Universities

Solitary, meditative observation is the first step in the poetry of research, in the formation of scientific fantasies, the reality of which we then test with the tools of logic, mathematics, physics and chemistry.
The Medical Sciences in the German Universities

We are entitled to operate when there are reasonable chances of success. To use the knife when these chances are lacking is to prostitute the splendid art of surgery, and to render it suspect among the laity and among one's colleagues.
Quoted in *The Great Doctors—A Biographical History of Medicine* p. 383, Henry E. Sigerist. Dover Publications, New York (1971) (original W.W. Norton & Co. Ltd, 1933)

Statistics are like women; mirrors of purest virtue and truth, or like whores to use as one pleases.
Attributed

Kenneth T. Bird 1917–
US physician

A medical chest specialist is long-winded about the short-winded.
> *Familiar Medical Quotations* Maurice B. Strauss (ed.). Little, Brown and Company, Boston (1968)

Prince Otto von Bismarck 1815–98
German statesman

You can do anything with children if you only play with them.
> Attributed

Give the worker the right to work as he is healthy, look after him when he is ill, take care of him when he is old.
> Attributed

Sir William Blackstone 1723–80
English jurist

Mala praxis is a great misdemeanor and offence at common law, whether it be for curiosity and experiment, or by neglect; because it breaks the trust which the party had placed in his physician, and tends to the patient's destruction.
> *Commentaries on the Laws of England* Bk III, Ch. 8 (1765)

William Blake 1757–1827
Painter and poet

The eye altering alters all.
> *The Mental Traveller*

Sir John Bland-Sutton 1855–1936
President of the Royal College of Surgeons of England

I divided my life into three parts: in the first I learned my profession, in the second I taught it, in the third I enjoy it.
> *The Story of a Surgeon*

The most dangerous items in a surgical operation were the instruments and the surgeon's fingers.
> Quoted in *Harley Street* p.6, Reginald Pound: Michael Joseph, London (1967)

Arthur L. Bloomfield 1888–1962
US physician

There are some patients whom we cannot help; there are none whom we cannot harm.
> *Familiar Medical Quotations* Maurice B. Strauss (ed.). Little, Brown and Company, Boston (1968)

Giovanni Boccaccio 1313–75
Italian writer

To the cure of this disease, neither the knowledge of medicine nor the power of drugs was of any effect, whether because the disease was itself fatal or because the physicians, whose number was increased by quacks and woman pretenders, could discover neither cause nor cure, and so few escaped.
> *Decameron* describing the plague

Hermann Boerhaave 1668–1738
Dutch physician and chemist

He that desires to learn truth should teach himself by facts and experiments; by which means he will learn more in a year than by abstract reasoning in an age.
> *Academical Lectures on the Theory of Physic* Vol. I (1751)

A disease which new and obscure to you, Doctor, will be known only after death; and even then not without an autopsy will you examine it with exacting pains. But rare are those among the extremely busy clinicians who are willing or capable of doing this correctly.
> *Atrocis, nec Descipti Prius, Morbi Historia* transl. in *Bulletin of the Medical Library Association* **43**: 217 (1944)

A good Doctor can foresee the fatal outcome of an incurable illness, when he cannot help, the experienced Doctor will take care not to aggravate the sick person's malady by tiring and injurious efforts; and in an impossible case he will not frustrate himself further with ineffective solicitude.
> *Atrocis, nec Descipti Prius, Morbi Historia* transl. in *Bulletin of the Medical Library Association* **43**: 217 (1944)

Keep the head cool, the feet warm and the bowels open.
> Attributed

Curtis Bok 1897–1962
US physician

We are convinced that the only genuine medical insurance for this country lies in making the benefits of science available to all practitioners and to all patients.
> Foreword to *Medial Research, A Mid-century Survey*

Book of Common Prayer

Man that is born of woman, hath but a short time to live.
> *Burial of the Dead*

From lightning and tempest; from plague, pestilence and famine; from battle and murder, and from sudden death, Good Lord, deliver us.
> *The Litany*

Andrew Boorde 1490–1549
English physician and Carthusian monk

It is extremely difficult for a physician who puts too much trust in what he reads to form a proper decision from what he sees.

George Borrow 1803–81
English author

If you must commit suicide, always contrive to do it as decorously as possible; the decencies, whether of life or of death, should never be lost sight of.
> *Lavengro* Ch. XXIII

Keith Botsford
Contemporary

Americans are indeed in a constant state of alarm about the immortality to which they seem to think they are constitutionally entitled.
Independent 27 October (1990)

William Boyd 1885–1979
British-born Canadian pathologist, Toronto

Of all the ailments which may blow out life's little candle, heart disease is the chief.
Pathology for the Surgeon (1925)

Edward Hickling Bradford 1848–1926
US physician

Neither the precision of science nor the efficiency of business methods will suffice, for above all else the practitioner must preserve and exercise the kindly indulgence of a considerate friend.
Harvard Graduate Magazine **35**: 70 (1926)

A. C. Bradley 1851–1935
Professor of Poetry, Oxford, England

Research, though toilsome, is easy; imaginative vision, though delightful, is difficult.
Oxford Lectures on Poetry, 'Shakespeare's Theatre and Audience'

Brahmanic saying

In illness the physician is a father; in convalescence, a friend; when health is restored, he is a guardian.

W. Russell, Lord Brain 1895–1966
British neurologist

In the post-mortem room we witness the final result of disease, the failure of the body to solve its problems, and there is an obvious limit to what one can learn about normal business transactions from even a daily visit to the bankruptcy court.
Canadian Medical Association Journal **83**: 349 (1960)

Freud's discovery of unconscious motivation, and the importance of the experiences of early infancy for the subsequent development of the personality, has profoundly influenced our conception of human nature, and had lasting effects on ethics.
Doctors Past and Present 'The Doctor's Place in Society' (1964)

The doctor occupies a seat in the front row of the stalls of the human drama, and is constantly watching, and even intervening in, the tragedies, comedies and tragi-comedies which form the raw material of the literary art.
The Quiet Art: A Doctor's Anthology Foreword, R. Coope

William Cooper Brann 1855–98

No man can be a patriot on an empty stomach.
Brann, The Iconoclast, 'Old Glory', 4 July (1893)

Nicholas Breton 1545–1626
English poet

There is no pain like the Gout.
Crossing of Proverbs

Richard Bright 1789–1858
English physician, Guy's Hospital, London

To connect accurate and faithful observations after death with symptoms displayed during life must be in some degree to forward the objects of our noble art.
Reports of Medical Cases

Acute disease must be seen at least once a day by those who wish to learn; in many cases twice a day will not be too often.
Lecture on the Practice of Medicine

One of the most ready means of detecting albumin is the application of heat by taking a small quantity of urine in a spoon and holding over a flame of a candle.
Describing a test for nephritis in 1830

Anthelme Brillat-Savarin 1755–1826
French gastronome

Tell me what you eat, and I will tell you what you are.
La Physiologie du Goût (1825)

Edouard Brissaud 1852–1909
French neurologist

A symptom that cannot be simulated cannot be a symptom of hysteria.
Attributed

Paul Broca 1824–80
French surgeon and anthropologist

Private practice and marriage—those twin extinguishers of science.
Letter, 10 April (1851)

A. Gerard Brom 1915–

It is with coarctation surgery as with love: rather easy to do but difficult to understand.
Journal of Thoracic and Cardiovascular Surgery **50**: 166 (1965)

Jacob Bronowski 1908–74
Polish-born British biologist and broadcaster

At bottom, the society of scientists is more important than their discoveries. What science has to teach us here is not its techniques but its spirit: the irresistible need to explore.
Science and Human Values Ch. 3

Science has nothing to be ashamed of, even in the ruins of Nagasaki.
Science and Human Values

Charles Brook
UK surgeon

The good physician is a disciple of Paracelsus, who was a sceptic, while the good surgeon is a disciple of Galen, who was a good dogmatist.
Battling Surgeon Ch. 1 (1945)

Michael Brook
Contemporary British physician, London

When medicine is practised in the tropics, with little or no aid from laboratory tests, clinical acumen is the most important tool used in arriving at the correct diagnosis.
Symptoms and Signs in Tropical Medicine In: *Manson's Tropical Diseases* (20th edn), G. C. Cook (ed.). W. B. Saunders (1996)

François Joseph Victor Broussais
1772–1838
Paris physician and protagonist of the erroneous 'physiological medicine'

There is no essential distinction between one malady and another. What determines the difference between particular diseases is nothing but the degree of excitation, stimulation or irritation.
The Great Doctors—A Biographical History of Medicine p. 288, Henry E. Sigerist. W. W. Norton & Co. Ltd (1933)

There are no such diseases. They are but the products of a disordered imagination.
The Great Doctors—A Biographical History of Medicine p. 288, Henry E. Sigerist. W. W. Norton & Co. Ltd (1933) (in response to the Ontologists, e.g. Pinel who were busy classifying diseases)

J. Howard Brown 1884–?
US haematologist

A man may do research for the fun of doing it but he can not expect to be supported for the fun of doing it.
Journal of Bacteriology **23**: 1 (1932)

John Brown 1810–82
Edinburgh physician and author

It is not a case we are treating; it is a living, palpitating, alas, too often suffering fellow creature.
Lancet **1**: 464 (1904)

Symptoms are the body's mother tongue; signs are in a foreign language.
Horae Subsecivae Series I, Introduction

Science and Art are the offspring of light and truth, of intelligence and will; they are the parents of philosophy—that its father, this its mother.
Attributed

Sir Dennis Browne 1892–1967
Paediatric surgeon, Great Ormond Street Hospital, London

The one eternal jibe at our profession is that it ignores any advance originating outside its own members.
Quoted with reference to osteopathy by Reginald Pound in *Harley Street*, Michael Joseph, London (1967)

Sir Thomas Browne 1605–82
English physician, writer and rhetorician

For the world, I count it not an inn, but an hospital, and a place, not to live, but to die in.
Religio Medici ii, Sect. 11 (1643)

We all labour against our own cure, for death is the cure of all diseases.
Religio Medici ii, Sect. 11 (1643)

With what shift and pains we come into the World we remember not; but 'tis commonly found no easy matter to get out of it.
Christian Morals Pt II, Sect. 13

I do not believe that any man fears to be dead, but only the stroke of death.
An Essay on Death

The ancient Inhabitants of this Island were less troubled with Coughs when they went naked, and slept in Caves and Woods, than Men now in Chambers and Feather beds.
Letter to a friend

The common fallacy of consumptive Persons, who feel not themselves dying, and therefore still hope to live.
Letter to a friend

No one should approach the temple of science with the soul of a money changer.
Attributed

Philip A. Bruce 1856–1933
US physician

Drinking was much more general than card playing, since it required no previous scientific training for its indulgence.
History of the University of Virginia Vol. II, Ch. 28

Ernst Wilhelm von Brücke 1819–92
Austrian physiologist

Teleology is a lady without whom no biologist can live. Yet he is ashamed to show himself with her in public.
Bulletin of the Johns Hopkins Hospital **95**: 45 (1954)

Jean de La Bruyère 1645–96
French author

There are but three events which concern man: birth, life and death. They are unconscious of their birth, they suffer when they die, and they neglect to live.
Characters 'Of Mankind' (transl. Henri van Laun) (1688)

A long illness seems to be placed between life and death, in order to make death a comfort both to those who die and to those who remain.
Characters 'Of Mankind' (transl. Henri van Laun) (1688) Ch. XI

Those who are well get sick; they need people whose business it is to assure them they will not die: as long as men go on dying, and love living, the doctor will be made game of and well paid.
Characters 'Of Mankind' (transl. Henri van Laun) (1688) Ch. XIV

Sir James Bryce 1838–1922
British liberal politician

Medicine is the only profession that labours incessantly to destroy the reason for its own existence.
  Address, 23 March (1914)

William Buchan 1729–1805
Scottish physician and medical reformer

No discovery can be of general utility while the practice of it is kept in the hands of a few.
  Domestic Medicine (2nd edn), p. 171. Philadephia (1771)

It appears from the annual register of the dead that almost one half of the children born in Great Britain die under twelve years of age.
  Domestic Medicine (8th edn) (1784)

Physicians should be consulted when needed, but they should be needed very rarely.
  Domestic Medicine (8th edn), X, vii (1784)

Pearl Buck 1892–1973
US novelist

Euthanasia is a long, smooth-sounding word, and it conceals its danger as long, smooth words do, but the danger is there, nevertheless.
  The Child Who Never Grew Ch. 2

Henry Thomas Buckle 1821–62
English historian

Among the arts, medicine, on account of its eminent utility, must always hold the highest place.
  Miscellaneous and Posthumous Works Vol. II, Fragment 7

Henry Lytton Bulwer 1801–72
Diplomatist and author

A man's ancestry is a positive property to him. How much, not only of acres, but of his constitution, his temper, his conduct, character and nature he may inherit from some progenitor ten times removed!
  The Caxtons Pt XI, Ch. VII

There are two things in life that a sage must preserve at every sacrifice, the coats of his stomach and the enamel of his teeth. Some evils admit of consolations, but there are no comforters for dyspepsia and the toothache.
  The Caxtons Pt XI, Ch. VII

Edward Bulwer-Lytton 1831–91 ('Owen Meredith')
English poet, diplomatist and statesman

In science, address the few, in literature, the many. In science, the few must dictate opinion to the many; in literature, the many, sooner or later, force their judgment on the few.
  Caxtoniana 'Readers and Writers'

There's nothing certain in man's life but this: That he must lose it.
  Clytemnestra Pt XX

John Bunyan 1628–88
English writer, non-conformist preacher, and philosopher

The captain of all these men of death that came against him to take him away was the consumption; for it was that brought him down to the grave.
  The Life and Death of Mr. Badman

Anthony Burgess 1917–93
British novelist

Keep away from physicians. It is all probing and guessing and pretending with them. They leave it to Nature to cure in her own time, but they take the credit. As well as very fat fees.
  Nothing Like the Sun (1964)

Edmund Burke 1729–97
British politician

People will not look forward to posterity, who never look backward to their ancestors.
  Reflections on the Revolution in France

Dennis Burkitt 1911–93
Northern Irish surgeon and African missionary doctor and nutritionist

Big stools, small hospitals,
Small stools, big hospitals.
  Attributed

Robert Burton 1577–1640
English divine and author

Diseases crucify the soul of man, attenuate our bodies, dry them, wither them, rivel them up like old apples, make them as so many Anatomies.
  The Anatomy of Melancholy I

Tobacco, divine, rare, superexcellent

Tobacco, which goes far beyond all their

Panaceas, potable gold, and Philosphers stones, a sovereign remedy to all disease.
  The Anatomy of Melancholy II, Sect. 2, Memb. 2, Subsect. 2

Health indeed is a precious thing, to recover and preserve which, we undergo any misery, drink bitter potions, freely give our goods: restore a man to his health, his purse lies open to thee.
  The Anatomy of Melancholy III, Sect. 1

If there be a hell upon earth, it is to be found in a melancholy man's heart.
  The Anatomy of Melancholy III, Sect. 1

In letting of blood, three main circumstances are to be considered, who, how much, when?
  The Anatomy of Melancholy III, Sect. 1

George W. Bush 1946–
President of the USA

Drug therapies are replacing a lot of medicines as we used to know them.
Quoted October 2000

Nicholas Murray Butler 1862–1947
US professor of philosophy

An expert is one who knows more and more about less and less.
Commencement Address, Columbia University

Samuel Butler 1835–1902
British writer

Parents are the last people on earth who ought to have children.
Notebooks (1912)

Life is one long process of getting tired.
Notebooks (1912) Ch. I, 'Life'

Death in anything like luxury is one of the most expensive things a man can indulge himself in. It costs a lot of money to die comfortably, unless one goes off pretty quickly.
Notebooks (1912) Ch. II, 'A Luxurious Death'

A physician's physiology has much the same relation to his power of healing as a cleric's divinity has to his power of influencing conduct.
Notebooks (1912) Ch. XIV

The body is but a pair of pincers set over a bellows and a stew pan and the whole fixed upon stilts.
Notebooks (1912) Ch. XIV

The more a thing knows its own mind, the more living it becomes.
Notebooks (1912) Ch. XIV

I reckon being ill as one of the greatest pleasures of life, provided one is not too ill and is not obliged to work until one is better.
The Way All Fresh (1903) Ch. 80

George Gordon Lord Byron 1788–1824
English poet

What deep wounds ever closed without a scar?
Child Harold's Pilgrimage Canto III, Stanza 84

What men call gallantry, and gods adultery,
Is much more common where the climate's sultry.
Don Juan Canto I, Stanza 63

Pierre Cabanis 1757–1808
French physician and philosopher

Impressions arriving at the brain make it enter into activity, just as food falling into the stomach excites it to more abundant secretion of gastric juice.
Traité du physique et du moral de l'homme, Second Mémoir (1802)

Richard Clarke Cabot 1868–1939
US physician and sociologist

Ethics and Science need to shake hands.
The Meaning of Right and Wrong, Introduction

There are two kinds of appendicitis – acute appendicitis and appendicitis for revenue only.
Clinical pathological conference discussion (c. 1925)

As I look over twenty five years of medical work, I can remember but two patients whose lives I saved.
Rewards and Training of a Physician

William Cadogan 1711–97
English physician

The gout is so common a disease, that there is scarcely a man in the world, whether he has had it or not, but thinks he knows perfectly what it is.
A Dissertation on the Gout, and All Chronic Diseases, Jointly Considered

Children, in general, are overclothed and overfed. To these causes, I impute most of their diseases.
Essays upon Nursing and Management of Children

John Caffey 1895–1966
Professor of Radiology, New York

Shadows are but dark holes in radiant streams twisted rifts beyond the substance, meaningless in themselves. He who would comprehend Röntgen's pallid shades, needs always to know well the solid matrix whence they spring.
Introduction to Paediatric Radiology

Sir Hugh Cairns 1896–1952
Australian-born British neurosurgeon and Professor of Surgery, Oxford, UK

. . . a good doctor is one who is shrewd in diagnosis and wise treatment; but, more than that, he is a person who never spares himself in the interest of his patients . . .
Lancet **2**: 665 (1949)

Joseph A. Califano Jr
US Secretary of Health, Education and Welfare 1976–80

The physician is the central decision maker for more than 70% of health care services.
Governing America Simon and Schuster, New York (1981)

James S. Calnan 1919–
British plastic surgeon, London

Since nearly every surgical operation begins with an incision in the skin and ends with closure of the wound, knowledge of the healing of skin wounds is of fundamental importance.
British Journal of Plastic Surgery **16**: 118 (1963)

Rohan Candappa 1962–
London-born writer

Eat less fresh food.
Eat more things containing preservatives.
Preservatives are called preservatives because they
   help you live longer.
   The Little Book of Stress 'Diet Hard' (1998)

A. Benson Cannon 1889–1950

It is a good thing for a physician to have
prematurely grey hair and itching piles. The first
makes him appear to know more than he does,
and the second gives him an expression of
concern which the patient interprets as being on
his behalf.
   Attributed

Walter Bradford Cannon 1871–1945
US physiologist

What the experimenter is really trying to do is to
learn whether facts can be established which will
be recognised as facts by others and which will
support some theory that in imagination he has
projected.
   The Way of an Investigator 'Fitness for the Enterprise'

Al Capp (Alfred Gerald Caplin)
1909–79
US strip cartoonist

Psychiatrists are often amusing company,
especially when they are drunk.
   Tufts folia Medica **9**: 97 (1963)

Thomas Carlyle 1795–1881
Scottish historian and philosopher

Self-contemplation is infallibly the symptom of
disease.
   Characteristics

Quackery gives birth to nothing; gives death to all
things.
   Heroes and Hero-Worship Lect. I

A man is not strong who takes convulsion-fits;
though six men cannot hold him then.
   Lecture in London, 19 May, (1840)

A stammering man is never a worthless one.
Physiology can tell you why. It is an excess of
sensibility to the presence of his fellow creature,
that makes him stammer.
   Letter to Ralph Waldo Emerson, 17 November (1843)

Lewis Carroll (Charles L. Dodgson)
1832–98
English author

Speak roughly to your little boy,
And beat him when he sneezes:
He only does it to annoy,
Because he knows it teases.
   Alice in Wonderland Ch. 6

William H. Carruth 1859–1924
US physician

Some call it Evolution
And others call it God.
   Each in His Own Tongue

Malcolm Carruthers 1938–
UK chemical pathologist

It is an ironic fact that while half the world's
population is dying as a result of diseases
of poverty (largely starvation and infection)
the other half is succumbing to diseases of
affluence.
   Introduction to *The Western Way of Death*. Davis Poynter,
   London (1974)

Alice Cary 1820–71
US poet and storyteller

My soul is full of whispered song;
My blindness is my sight;
The shadows that I feared so long
Are all alive with light.
   Dying Hymn

William B. Castle 1897–?
US physician and teacher

An expert is a man who tells you a simple thing in
a confused way in such a fashion as to make you
think the confusion is your own fault.
   Harvard Medical Alumni Bulletin **29**: 18 (1955)

Catalan proverb

From the bitterness of disease man learns the
sweetness of health.

David W. Cathell 1839–1925
US physician

If, at your office and elsewhere, you make use of
instruments of precision they will not only assist
you in diagnosis but will also aid you greatly in
curing people by heightening their confidence in
you and enlisting their cooperation.
   *The Physician Himself and What He Should Add to the Strictly
   Scientific* Baltimore (1882)

Conviviality has a levelling effect, and divests the
physician of his proper prestige.
   *The Physician Himself and What He Should Add to the Strictly
   Scientific* Baltimore (1882)

A badly set limb or an unnecessary or bungled
amputation injures our whole profession.
And the limb or stump may be held up in court
in a suit for damages. Unless you are a fool,
Xray them all.
   Book on the Physician Himself Philadelphia (1924)

Catherine II 1729–96
Empress of Russia

Reduce the mortality rate, consult doctors, do something about the care of young children. They run about naked in their shifts in the snow and ice. Those who survive are healthy, but nineteen out of twenty die, and what a loss to the state.
  Catherine the Great Ch. 35 (Zoe Oldenbourg)

Dionysius Cato 14th century
Unknown author

Become old early if you wish to stay old long.
  Moral Precepts

Benvenuto Cellini 1500–71
Florentine sculptor

Oh the powers of nature. She knows what we need, and the doctors know nothing.
  Autobiography

Aulus Cornelius Celsus 53 BC–AD 7
Roman encyclopaedist and physician

Now a surgeon should be youthful with a strong and steady hand which never trembles, with vision sharp and clear, and spirit undaunted; filled with pity, so that he wishes to cure his patient, yet is not moved by his cries, to go too fast, or cut less than is necessary; but he does everything just as if the cries of pain cause him no emotion.
  De Medicina VIII Proaemium (transl. W.G. Spencer)

The blood vessels that are pouring out blood are to be grasped, and about the wounded spot they are to be tied in two places, and cut across in between, so that each may retract and yet have its opening closed.
  De Medicina VIII Proaemium (transl. W. G. Spencer)— perhaps the first description of dividing and ligating blood vessels

Rubor, et tumor cum calor et dolor. (Redness and swelling with heat and pain)
  De Medicina—the four signs of inflammation

It is impossible to remedy a severe malady unless by a remedy likewise severe.
  De Medicina II.xi.6

The art of medicine has almost no constant rule.
  De Medicina Proaemium

For major ills, major remedies.
  De Medicina Proaemium i.3

Always aid the organ that suffers most.
  De Medicina Proaemium ii.11

Miguel de Cervantes 1547–1616
Spanish novelist

Every tooth in a man's head is more valuable than a diamond.
  Don Quixote I, Ch. 4 (1605)

Well, now, there's a remedy for everything except death.
  Don Quixote II, Ch. 10 (1605)

Sleep covers a Man all over, Thoughts and all, like a Cloak; 'tis Meat for the Hungry, Drink for the Thirsty, Heat for the Cold, and Cold for the Hot.
  Dan Quixote II, Ch. 68 (1605)

The guts carry the feet not the feet the guts.
  Don Quixote (1605)

Nicolas Chamfort 1741–94
French writer and wit

Man arrives as a novice at each age of his life.
  Caracteres et anecdotes p. 176 (1825)

Philosophy, like medicine, has plenty of drugs, few good remedies, and hardly any specific cures.
  Maximes et penseés (1825)

Living is a sickness from which sleep provides relief every sixteen hours. It's a palliative. The remedy is death.
  Attributed

Chang Ch'ao c. 1676
Chinese sage

It is easy to stand a pain, but difficult to stand an itch.
  Sweet Dream Shadows, quoted in *Familiar Medical Quotations* Maurice B. Strauss (ed.). Little, Brown and Company, Boston (1968)

Charles V. Chapin 1856–1941
US epidemiologist

As it takes two to make a quarrel, so it takes two to make a disease, the microbe and its host.
  Papers 'The Principles of Epidemiology'

Jean Martin Charcot 1825–93
Paris neurologist

Disease is very old, and nothing about it has changed. It is we who change, as we learn to recognise what was formerly imperceptible.
  De l'expectation en médecine

Symptoms, then are in reality nothing but the cry from suffering organs.
  Leçons cliniques sur les maladies des vieillards et les maldies chroniques, Introduction, Sect. I

It is the mind which is really alive and sees things, yet it hardly sees anything without preliminary instruction.
  Attributed

In the last analysis, we see only what we are ready to see, what we have been taught to see. We eliminate and ignore everything that is not a part of our prejudices.
  Attributed

Charles II 1630–85
King of England

He had been, he said, a most unconscionable time dying; but he hoped that they would excuse it.
  Quoted on his deathbed in *History of England* (Macaulay), Vol. I, Ch. 4

Charles, Prince of Wales 1948–
First in line to British throne

I believe it is most certainly possible to design features in such buildings that are positively healing … The spirit needs healing as well as the body.
BBC Television Documentary (1988)

The whole imposing edifice of modern medicine is like the celebrated tower of Pisa—slightly off balance.
Attributed

Is the whole of the health care system—and the confidence of the public in it—not undermined by the publicity given to what goes wrong rather than the tiny miracles wrought day in day out by an expert, kind and dedicated staff?
Speech to newspaper editors and proprietors in Fleet Street, 11 March (2002)

Guy de Chauliac 1300–70
French surgeon

The conditions necessary for the surgeon are four: first, he should be learned: second, he should be expert: third, he must be ingenious, and fourth, he should be able to adapt himself.
Ars Chururgic Introduction

A blind man works on wood the same way as a surgeon on the body, when he is ignorant of anatomy.
Chirurgia Magna, Treatise I, Doctrine I, Ch. I

Anton Chekhov 1860–1904
Russian dramatist and doctor

When a lot of remedies are suggested for a disease, that means it cannot be cured.
The Cherry Orchard II

Doctors are just the same as lawyers; the only difference is that lawyers merely rob you, whereas doctors rob you and kill you, too.
Ivanov I

I realise I have two professions, not one. Medicine is my lawful wife and literature my mistress. When I grow weary of one, I pass the night with the other. Neither of them suffers because of my infidelity.
Letter, 11 October (1889)

Chen Jen
Chinese sage

When you treat a disease, first treat the mind.

Earl of Chesterfield 1694–1773
English statesman

Advice is seldom welcome; and those that want it the most always like it the least.
Letter to his son, 29 January (1748)

The pleasure is momentary, the position ridiculous and the expense damnable.
Nature **227**: 772 (1970)

G. K. Chesterton 1874–1936
British writer

Psychoanalysis is confession without absolution.
Attributed

It seems a pity that psychology should have destroyed all our knowledge of human nature.
Observer 9 December (1934)

Drink because you are happy, but never because you are miserable.
Attributed

Sir Watson Cheyne 1852–1932
Surgeon, Professor of Surgery, King's College, London, scientist and assistant to Joseph Lister

The human form is a very delicate organization. It is not a thing which should be meddled with by people who do not know it as intimately as it is possible to know it.
Quoted with reference to a quack bone setter in *Harley Street* p. 76 Reginald Pound. Michael Joseph, London (1967)

Chinese proverbs

Before thirty, men seek disease; after thirty, diseases seek men.

Before you tell the 'truth' to the patient, be sure you know the 'truth' and that the patient wants to hear it.

For colic, get the bowels open.

He that takes medicine and neglects to diet himself wastes the skill of the physician.

However strong a mother may be, she becomes afraid when she is pregnant for the third time.

If a child is constantly sick, it is due to overfeeding.

In typhoid treat the beginning; in consumption do not treat the end.

It is easy to get a thousand prescriptions, but hard to get one single remedy.

Medicine cures the man who is fated not to die.

Nine out of every ten men have piles.

No man is a good doctor who has never been sick himself.

Only the healing art enables one to make a name for himself and at the same time give benefit to others.

The appearance of a disease is swift as an arrow; its disappearance slow, like a thread.

The body may be healed but not the mind.

The patient has two sleeves, one containing a diagnostic and the other a therapeutic armamentarium; these sleeves should rarely be emptied in one move; keep some techniques in reserve; time your manoeuvres to best serve the status and special needs of your patient. *Continued*

Chinese proverbs *continued*

The unlucky doctor treats the head of a disease; the lucky doctor its tail.

To be uncertain is to be uncomfortable, but to be certain is to be ridiculous.

When a disease relapses there is no cure.

Ch'in Yueh-jen *c.* 225 BC

The skillful doctor treats those who are well but the inferior doctor treats those who are ill.
   Attributed

W. W. Chipman 1866–1950
US physician

Parturition is a physiological process—the same in the countess and in the cow.
   Quoted in *Familiar Medical Quotations* Maurice B. Strauss (ed.). Little, Brown and Company, Boston (1968)

A. B. Christie 1908–
British infectious disease physician

Man is a creature composed of countless millions of cells: a microbe is composed of only one, yet throughout the ages the two have been in ceaseless conflict.
   Infectious Disease, Epidemiology and Clinical Practice p. 1. The Epidemiologist and the Clinician (4th edn) (1987)

The history of epidemics is the history of wars and wanderings, of famine and drought and of man's exposure to inhospitable surroundings. When man has travelled rough, microorganisms have always been ready to take advantage of his discomfitures.
   Infectious Disease, Epidemiology and Clinical Practice p. 1. The Epidemiologist and the Clinician (4th edn) (1987)

Christina of Sweden 1626–89
Queen of Sweden

We grow old more through indolence than through age.
   Maxims (1660–80)

St. John Chrysostom *c.*345–407
Bishop of Constantinople

Fasting is a medicine.
   Homilies on the Statutes III

The heart is the most noble of all the members in our body.
   Homilies on the Statutes IX

Chu Hui Weng
Chinese sage

To avoid sickness eat less; to prolong life worry less.

Charles Churchill 1731–64
English satirical poet

Most of those evils we poor mortals know

From doctors and imagination flow.
   The Prophecy of Famine (1763)

Dreams, Children of night, of indigestion bred,

Which, Reason clouded, seize and turn the head.
   The Candidate

Sir Winston Churchill 1874–1965
British statesman

I must point out that my rule of life prescribes as an absolutely sacred rite smoking cigars and also the drinking of alcohol before, after, and if need be during all meals and in the intervals between.
   Uttered during a lunch with the Arab leader, Ibn Saud

There is no finer investment for any community than putting milk into babies.
   Radio broadcast, 21 March (1943)

I can think of no better step to signalize the inauguration of the National Health Service than that a person who so obviously needs psychiatric attention should be among the first of its patients.
   Speech, July (1948) about Labour's Health Secretary Aneurin Bevan

Science bestowed immense new powers on man, and, at the same time, created conditions which were largely beyond his comprehension and still more beyond his control.
   Speech at the Massachusetts Institute of Technology, 31 March (1949)

Scientists should be on tap, but not on top.
   Twenty-one Years by Randolph Churchill

Cicero 106–43 BC
Roman orator and statesman

It is not by muscle, speed, or physical dexterity that great things are achieved, but by reflection, force of character, and judgement; in these qualities old age is usually not only not poorer, but is even richer.
   On Old Age VI (transl. W. A. Falconer)

No one is so old as to think he cannot live one more year.
   On Old Age VII.24

Exercise and temperance can preserve something of our early strength even in old age.
   On Old Age X.34

It is our duty, my young friends, to resist old age.
   On Old Age XI.35

The keenest of all our senses is the sense of sight.
   On the Orator II.lxxxvii.357

The appetites of the belly and the palate, far from diminishing as men grow older, go on increasing.
   Pro Caelio 191

One should eat to live, not live to eat.
   Rhetoricorum LV

In a disordered mind, as in a disordered body, soundness of health is impossible.
Tusculanarum Disputationum Bk III

Diseases of the soul are more dangerous and more numerous than those of the body.
Tusculanarum Disputationum Bk III, Ch. 3

Physicians, when the cause of disease is discovered, consider that the cure is discovered.
Tusculanarum Disputationum Bk III, Ch. 3

Alonzo Clark 1807–87
US physician and Professor of Medicine, New York

Every man's disease is his personal property.
Bulletin of the New York Academy of Medicine **5**: 154 (1929)

The medical errors of one century constitute the popular faith of the next.
Attributed

You may know the intractability of a disease by its long list of remedies.
Attributed

There is no courtesy in science.
Attributed

Symptoms which cannot be readily marshalled must be credited to the nerves.
Attributed

Michael Clark 1935–
Gastroenterologist, St. Bartholomew's Hospital, London

The young gastroenterologist of today is only happy if he can learn another endoscopic technique, the excitement of the 1960's has been replaced by the decade of the Peeping Tom.
Lancet **1**: 629 (1985)

Sir Stanley Clayton 1900?–?
British obstetrician

Until the end of the last century, and indeed, until the early years of the present one, the vast bulk of midwifery was done in the home and nearly all babies were born under the care of an untrained or self-trained woman or midwife.
Obstetrics by Ten Teachers (12th edn, p. 2 Edward Arnold, London (1972)

Logan Clendening 1884–1945
Medical historian

Surgery does the ideal thing—it separates the patient from his disease. It puts the patient back to bed and the disease in a bottle.
Modern Methods of Treatment Ch. 1

Rest in bed will do more for more diseases than any other single procedure.
Attributed

Men are not going to embrace eugenics. They are going to embrace the first likely, trim-figured girl with limpid eyes and flashing teeth who comes along, in spite of the fact that her germ plasm is probably reeking with hypertension, cancer, haemophilia, colour blindness, hay fever, epilepsy, and amyotrophic lateral sclerosis.
Attributed

Arthur Hugh Clough 1819–61
British poet

Thou shalt not kill; but need'st not strive Officiously to keep alive.
The Latest Decalogue 11

John of Clyn 14th century
Irish friar

In scarcely any house did only one die, but all together, man and wife with their children and household, traversed the same road, the road of death.
Annals of Ireland (relating the effects of the Black Death in Kilkenny)

Irvin S. Cobb 1876–1944
US physician

I would rather that any white rabbit on earth should have Asiatic cholera twice than that I should have it just once.
Quoted in *Familiar Medical Quotations* Maurice B. Strauss (ed.). by Little, Brown and Company, Boston (1968)

Forrester Cockburn 1936–
Professor Child Health, Glasgow, Scotland

The origins of physical and mental health and disease lie predominantly in the early development of the child.
Preface to *Children's Medicine and Surgery* (1996)

Jean Baptiste Coffinhal-Dubail 1760?–1820?
French revolutionary tribune

The Republic has no need for scientists.
Comment at trial of Antoine Lavoisier, Paris (1794)

Thomas Cogan c.1545–1607
English physician

Drink wine and have the gout drink none and have the gout.
Haven of Health, Dedication

Henry, Lord Cohen of Birkenhead 1900–77
British physician

All diagnoses are provisional formulae for action.
Lancet **1**: 23–5 (1943)

The feasibility of an operation is not the best indication for its performance.
Annals of the Royal College of Surgeons of England **6**: 3 (1950)

Warren H. Cole 1898–?

US surgeon

Too often surgical therapy for elective conditions is postponed in elderly patients in the hope, I presume, that the patient will die of some other disease before the present one threatens his life.

Annals of Surgery **138**: 145 (1953)

Samuel Taylor Coleridge 1772–1834

British poet

The history of man for the nine months preceding his birth would, probably, be far more interesting and contain events of greater moment than all the three score and ten years that follow it.

Miscellanies, Aesthetic and Literary

Oh sleep! it is a gentle thing,

Beloved from pole to pole.

The Rime of the Ancient Mariner V

The man's desire is for the woman; but the woman's desire is rarely other than for the desire of the man.

Table Talk 23 July (1827)

Abraham Colles 1773–1843

Irish surgeon

Be assured, that no man can know his own profession perfectly, who knows nothing else; and that he who aspires to eminence in any particular science must first acquire the habit of philosophising on matters of science in general.

A Treatise on Surgical Anatomy Pt I, Sect. I

Richard Collier 1924–

British journalist

The disease took at least half a million American lives—ten times as many as the Germans took during the war—yet only in the hardest-hit cities did it ever win through to the newspapers' front pages.

Epilogue to *The Plague of the Spanish Lady* (influenza epidemic October 1918–January 1919)

John Churton Collins 1848–1908

Professor of Literature, Birmingham, UK

Suicide is the worst form of murder, because it leaves no opportunity for repentance.

Life and Memoirs of John Churton Collins Appendix VII (quoted by L. C. Collins)

Mortimer Collins 1827–76

British writer

A man is as old as he's feeling,
A woman as old as she looks.

The Unknown Quantity

The true way to render age vigorous is to prolong the youth of the mind.

The Village Comedy Vol. I

Death a friend that alone can bring the peace his treasures cannot purchase, and remove the pain his physicians cannot cure.

The Village Comedy Vol. II, Ch. 110

Hypochondriacs squander large sums of time in search of nostrums by which they vainly hope they may get more time to squander.

The Village Comedy Vol. II

Professors in every branch of the sciences prefer their own theories to truth: the reason is that their theories are private property but the truth is common stock.

The Village Comedy Vol. II

Charles Caleb Colton 1780–1832

English clergyman, sportsman, author, and suicide

Examinations are formidable even to the best prepared for the greatest fool may ask more than the wisest man can answer.

Lacon Vol. I, p. 170 (1820–22)

The poorest man would not part with health for money, but the richest would gladly part with all their money for health.

Lacon Vol. I, Ch. 225

Body and mind, like man and wife, do not always agree to die together.

Lacon Vol. I, Ch. 324

It is better to have recourse to a quack, if he can cure our disorder, although he cannot explain it, than to a physician, if he can explain our disease but cannot cure it.

Lacon Vol. I, Ch. 323

Andrew Combe 1797–1847

Physician to Queen Victoria

What we desire our children to become,
we must endeavour to be before them.

Physiological and Moral Management of Infancy (1834)

Alex Comfort 1920–

English physician and sexologist

The idea of the human responsibility of the doctor has been present since medicine was indistinguishable from magic.

The Listener 29 November (1951)

Auguste Comte 1798–1857

French philosopher and sociologist, and founder of Positivism

To understand a science it is necessary to know its history.

Positive Philosophy (1832–42)

Arthur Conan Doyle 1856–1930

British crime novelist

Education never ends, Watson. It is a series of lessons with the greatest for the last.

His Last Bow 'The Adventure of the Red Circle'

When a doctor does go wrong he is the first of criminals. He has nerve and he has knowledge.
The Speckled Band

Confucius 551–478 BC
Chinese sage and philosopher

Learning without thinking is useless. Thinking without learning is dangerous.
Analects Bk II, Ch. XV

Cyril Connolly 1903–74
British journalist and writer

The one way to get thin is to re-establish a purpose in life.
The Unquiet Grave Pt I

Obesity is a mental state, a disease brought on by boredom and disappointment.
The Unquiet Grave Pt I

A mistake which is commonly made about neurotics is to suppose that they are interesting. It is not interesting to be always unhappy, engrossed with oneself, malignant and ungrateful, and never quite in touch with reality.
The Unquiet Grave Pt II

There are many who dare not kill themselves for fear of what the neighbours will say.
The Unquiet Grave Pt II

Mike Connolly?

Psychoanalysis is spending forty dollars an hour to squeal on your mother.
Bartlett's Unfamiliar Quotations

Sir Edward Cook 1857–1919
Editor of the Westminster Gazette

The doctors all say we eat too much. My experience is that they do too.
Quoted after dining with Sir Thomas Barlow MD, by Reginald Pound in *Harley Street* p. 108. Michael Joseph, London (1967)

Robin Coombs 1921–
Professor of Immunology, Cambridge, UK

Erythrocytes were primarily designed by God as tools for the immunologist and only secondarily as carriers of haemoglobin.
Attributed

Sir Astley Paston Cooper 1768–1841
English surgeon, Guy's Hospital, London and President of the Royal College Surgeons (Eng) (1827 and 1836)

The best surgeon, like the best general, is the one who makes the fewest mistakes.
Attributed

Nothing is known in our profession by guess; and I do not believe, that from the first dawn of medical science to the present moment, a single correct idea has ever emanated from conjecture.
A Treatise on Dislocations and Fractures of the Joints

If you are too fond of new remedies, first you will not cure your patients; secondly, you will have no patients to cure.

By means of my finger nail, I scratched through the peritoneum on the left side of the aorta, and then gradually passed my finger between the aorta and the spine, and again penetrated the peritoneum, on the right side of the aorta.
The Lectures on the Principles and Practice of Surgery with Additional Notes and Cases by Frederick Tyrell, Vol. 2. Thomas and George Underwood, London (1824) (Description of the first ligation of the aorta in 1817 for left femoral aneurysm)

Sir (Vincent) Zachary Cope
1884–1974
See Zeta

Charles T. Copeland 1860–1952

To eat is human, to digest divine.
Attributed

Robert Copeland
Contemporary US commentator

To get something done a committee should consist of no more than three men, two of whom are absent.
Penguin Dictionary of Modern Humorous Quotations p. 55, Fred Metcalf. Penguin Books, London (2001)

Alan Coren 1938–
British humorist and writer

The Act of God designation on all insurance policies; which means, roughly, that you cannot be insured for the accidents that are most likely to happen to you.
The Lady from Stalingrad Mansions 'A Short History of Insurance'

Pierre Corneille 1606–84
French playwright

What destroys one man preserves another.
Cinna II.1

Jean Nicolas Corvisart 1755–1821
Professor of Medicine, College de France, Paris

The physician who fails to combine pathological physiology with his anatomy will never be anything more than a more or less adroit, diligent and patient prosector.
The Great Doctors—A Biographical History of Medicine p. 125, Henry E. Sigerist. Dover Publications, New York (1971) (original W. W. Norton & Co. Ltd 1933)

Bill Cosby
Contemporary US comedian

Did you ever see the customers in health-food stores? They are pale, skinny people who look half dead. In a steak house, you see robust, ruddy people. They're dying, of course, but they look terrific.
Penguin Dictionary of Modern Humorous Quotations p. 139, Fred Metcalf. Penguin Books, London (2001)

Nathaniel Cotton 1705–88
British physician and poet

Would you extend your narrow span,
And make the most of life you can;
Would you, when medicines cannot save,
Descend with ease into the grave;
Calmly retire, like the evening light,

And cheerful bid the world goodnight?
Visions in Verse III 'Health'

Émile Coué 1857–1926
French psychologist

Every day, in every way, I am getting better and
better.
My Method Ch. 3

Abraham Cowley 1618–67
English poet

Life is an incurable Disease.
Pindarique Odes 'To Dr. Scarborough' VI

William Cowper 1666–1709
English surgeon and anatomist

Grief is itself a medicine.
Charity

John Redman Coxe
1773–1864

The longer I live the less confidence I have in
drugs and the greater is my confidence in the
regulation and administration of diet and
regimen.
*A Short View of the Importance and Respectability of the
Science of Medicine.* An address to the Philadelphia Medical
Society, 7 February (1800)

Creole proverb

Sickness comes riding upon a hare, but goes away
riding upon a tortoise.

Sir James Crichton-Brown
1840–1938
British physician and psychiatrist

There is no short-cut to longevity. To win it is the
work of a lifetime, and the promotion of it is a
branch of preventive medicine.
The Prevention of Senility

Francis H. C. Crick 1916–
UK molecular biologist, discoverer of DNA structure

We think we have found the basic mechanism by
which life comes from life.
Letter to his son, Michael Crick, 19 March (1953)

Quentin Crisp 1910–98
English-born writer

Life was a funny thing that occurred on the way
to the grave.
The Naked Civil Servant

Colin Cromar 1910–?
Scottish-born US surgeon, Pasadena, Texas

Deliberate colostomy, first performed a bare
century and a half ago, was conceived as a
desperate means to relieve total obstruction of the
colon or rectum when all lesser remedies had
failed.
A History of Colostomy (1968)

A. J. Cronin 1896–?

As a doctor you would be well advised to acquaint
yourself with your patients' interests if not their
prejudices.
Advice to Dr Finlay from Dr Cameron in *Dr Finlay's
Casebook*

William Cullen 1710–90
*Scottish professor of medicine and pioneer in
psychological medicine*

Persons living very entirely on vegetables are
seldom of a plump and succulent habit.
First lines of the *Practice of Physic* Pt III, Bk 1 (1776)

It is said to be the manner of hypochondriacs to
change often their physician.
Practice of Physic Pt II, Bk II, Ch. 3

I propose to comprehend, under the title of
neuroses, all those preternatural affections of
sense or motion, which are without pyrexia as a
part of the primary disease.
Quoted on 'neurosis' in *The Oxford English Dictionary*

Bishop Richard Cumberland
1631–1718
Bishop of Peterborough, England

It is better to wear out than to rust out.
The Duty of Contending for the Faith, by Bishop
George Horne

Marie Curie 1867–1934
Polish-born doctor and scientist

In science we must be interested in things, not in
persons.
Quoted by Eve Curie in *Madame Curie* Ch. XVI (transl.
Vincent Sheean)

Thomas Curling 1811–88
President of the Royal College of Surgeons of England

An artificial anus in the loin, well established is
attended with little inconvenience or trouble in a
healthy state of the alimentary canal.
Lancet **I**: 3–5 (1865) (first description of a colostomy in
English)

Edwina Currie 1946–

English Conservative politician

My message to businessmen of this country when they go abroad on business is that there is one thing above all they can take with them to stop them catching AIDS, and that is the wife.

British Minister of State for Health as quoted in *The Observer* 15 February (1987)

The strongest possible piece of advice I would give to any young woman is: Don't screw around, and don't smoke.

The Observer 'Sayings of the Week', 3 April (1988)

George William Curtis 1824–92

US novelist and journalist

Happiness lies, first of all, in health.

Lotus-Eating Ch. 4

Harvey Cushing 1869–1939

US surgeon and founder of neurosurgery, Professor of Surgery, Harvard

A physician is obligated to consider more than a diseased organ, more even than the whole man – he must view the man in his world.

Man Adapting Ch. 12 (René J. Dubois)

There is only one ultimate and effectual preventive for the maladies to which flesh is heir, and that is death.

The Medical Career and Other Papers 'Medicine at the Crossroads'

Three fifths of the practice of medicine depends on common sense, a knowledge of people and of human reactions.

The Medical Career and Other Papers 'Medicine at the Crossroads'

I would like to see the day when somebody would be appointed surgeon somewhere who had no hands, for the operative part is the least part of the work.

Letter to Dr Henry Christian, 20 November (1911)

Nature saw fit to enclose the central nervous system in a bony case lined by a tough, protecting membrane, and within this case she concealed a tiny organ which lies enveloped by an additional bony capsule and membrane like the nugget in the innermost of a series of Chinese boxes.

Neurohypophysial Membrane From a Clinical Standpoint Yale University Press (1969)

Baron Georges Cuvier 1769–1832

French anatomist

The observer listens to Nature; the experimenter questions and forces her to unveil herself.

Attributed

Czech proverb

Small children stamp on your lap, big ones on your heart.

A. S. Daar

Contemporary medical anthropologist

Medicine cannot be practised without reference to social and cultural values, even in this post-modern era.

Brain death and transplantation: a reply. *Current Anthropology* **35**: 245–6 (1994)

J. Chalmers Da Costa 1863–1933

Surgeon and writer

Objectionable people are numerous. They have one trait in common, that is, a most unfortunate tendency to longevity.

Selected Papers and Speeches 'Behind the Office Doors'

A fashionable surgeon like a pelican can be recognized by the size of his bill.

The Trials and Triumphs of the Surgeon Ch. 1

Diagnosis by intuition is a rapid method of reaching a wrong conclusion.

The Trials and Triumphs of the Surgeon Ch. 1

What we call experience is often a dreadful list of ghastly mistakes.

The Trials and Triumphs of the Surgeon Ch. 1

They know nothing of the haunting anxieties, the keen disappointments, the baffling perplexities, the dread responsibilities, and the numerous self-reproaches of one who spends his life as an operating surgeon.

The Trials and Triumphs of the Surgeon Ch. 1

Sometimes when a doctor gets too lazy to work he becomes a politician.

The Trials and Triumphs of the Surgeon Ch. 1

A man who has a theory which he tries to fit to facts is like a drunkard who tries his key haphazard in door after door, hoping to find one it fits.

The trials and Triumphs of the Surgeon Ch. 1

Kennedy Dalziel 1875?–?

Scottish surgeon and discoverer of ulcerative colitis

The affected bowel gives the consistence and smoothness of an eel in a state of rigor mortis and the glands, though enlarged, are evidently not caseous.

British Medical Journal **2**: 1068–70 (1913) (Describing Crohn's disease for the first time)

Danish proverb

Fresh air impoverishes the doctor.

C. D. Darlington 1903–81

British geneticist

A large proportion of mankind, like pigeons and partridges, on reaching maturity, having passed through a period of playfulness or promiscuity, establish what they hope and expect will be a permanent and fertile mating relationship. This we call marriage.

Genetics and Man Ch. 16

Clarence Darrow 1857–1938
US lawyer

The first half of our lives is ruined by our parents, and the second half by our children.
Attributed

Charles Darwin 1809–82
British naturalist and author

Science consists in grouping facts so that general laws or conclusions may be drawn from them.
Charles Darwin Ch. 2 by Francis Darwin

We must, however, acknowledge, as it seems to me, that man with all his noble qualities, still bears in his bodily frame the indelible stamp of his lowly origin.
Descent of Man Ch. 21, Appleton, New York (1871)

False facts are highly injurious to the progress of science, for they often endure long; but false views, if supported by some evidence, do little harm, for every one takes salutary pleasure proving their falseness.
Descent of Man Ch. 21, Appleton, New York (1871)

I have called this principle, by which each slight variation, if useful, is preserved, by the term of Natural Selection.
Origin of Species Ch. 3, Appleton, New York (1881)

Life was originally from so simple a beginning (that) endless forms most beautiful and most wonderful have been and are being evolved.
Origin of Species Ch. 3, Appleton, New York (1881)

Vivisection is justifiable for real investigations on physiology; but not for mere damnable and detestable curiosity.
Letter, 22 March (1871)

I must begin with a good body of facts and not from a principle (in which I always suspect some fallacy) and then as much deduction as you please.
Letter to J. Fiske, 8 December (1874)

Sir Francis Darwin 1848–1925
British scientist

But in science the credit goes to the man who convinces the world, not to the man to whom the idea first occurs.
Eugenics Review **6**: 1 (1914)

W. H. Davies 1871–1940
British poet

Teetotallers lack the sympathy and generosity of men that drink.
Shorter Lyrics of the 20th Century, Introduction

Elmer Davis 1890–1958
US journalist

When a middle-aged man says in a moment of weariness that he is half dead, he is telling the truth.
On not being Dead, as Reported

Professor John Davis
Contemporary British anaesthetist

You are more likely to die on the first day of your life than on any other than your last.
The Anaesthetic Aide-Mémoire
John Urquhart. Oxford University Press, Oxford (1996)

Kingsley Davis
Contemporary US sociologist

When one contemplates procreation as a future act, it is always someone else who is going to be created; but when one contemplates death, it is one's own extinction that is involved.
Human Society The Macmillan Company (1948)

Sir Humphry Davy 1778–1829
English chemist and discoverer of anaesthesia

I have this day made a discovery, which, if you please, you may announce in your Physical Journal, namely that the nitrous phosoxyd or gaseous oxyd of azote, is respirable when perfectly freed from nitric phosoxyd (nitrous gas).
Letter to *Nicholson's Journal*, 17 April (1799)

John Blair Deaver 1855–1931
US Professor of Surgery, University of Pennsylvania

Cut well, get well, stay well.
Quoted by Marvin Corman in Classic articles in colonic and rectal surgery. *Diseases of the Colon and Rectum* **30**: 66–71 (1987)

Daniel Defoe 1660–1731
English writer

Self-destruction is the effect of cowardice in the highest extreme.
An Essay Upon projects 'Of Projectors'

Middle age is youth without its levity, and age without decay.
Attributed

Mervyn Deitel 1930?–
Professor of Surgery and of Nutritional Sciences at the University of Toronto

The commonest form of malnutrition in the western world is obesity.
Surgery of the Morbidly Obese Patient Preface. Lee and Febiger, Philadelphia (1989)

Thomas Dekker 1572–1641
English dramatist

Gold that buys health can never be ill spent.
Westward Hoe! Act V (1604)

Jean Baptiste de la Salle 1651–1719

The ears should be kept perfectly clean; but it must never be done in company. It should never be done with a pin, and still less with the fingers, but always with an ear-picker.
The Rules of Christian Manners and Civility I

Campbell Greig De Morgan 1811–76
Professor of Anatomy, Middlesex Hospital, London

Today the glands may be free; tomorrow they may be affected. Today all disease may be distributed far beyond.
Retrospect of Medicine **69**: 34–9 (1874) (Referring to the spread of cancer)

Jerry Dennis
Contemporary US comedian

A consultant is a man who knows 129 ways to make love, but doesn't know any women.
Penguin Dictionary of Modern Humorous Quotations p. 61, Fred Metcalf. Penguin Books, London (2001)

Joyce Dennys
20th century US physician

The only person to whom a Doctor can say exactly what he thinks about another Doctor is his Wife. That is why practically all Doctors are married.
The Over-Dose

Chauncey Depew 1834–1928
US politician

I get my exercise acting as a pallbearer to my friends who exercise.
Attributed

Lord Devlin 1905–
Appeal court judge, House of Lords

In strict legal terminology I doubt if doctors ever assault; they batter.
Samples 84

John Dewey 1859–1952
US philosopher

Popular psychology is a mass of cant, of slush and of superstition worthy of the most flourishing days of the medicine man
The Public and Its Problems Ch. 5

Every great advance in science has issued from a new audacity of imagination.
The Quest for Certainty Ch. 11

John Diamond 1950–2001
British journalist

In some aspects of alternative medicine we are fighting an almost medieval belief in magic but debunking such beliefs is like telling people that the tooth fairy is sniffing glue.
Attributed

In the face of such overwhelming statistical possibilities hypochondria has always seemed to me to be the only rational position to take on life.
C by John Diamond p. 17. Vermilion, London (1998)

Cancer is a word, not a sentence.
C by John Diamond p. 75. Vermilion, London (1998)

Charles Dickens 1812–70
British novelist

Minds like bodies, will often fall into a pimpled, ill-conditioned state from mere excess of comfort.
Barnaby Rudge Ch. 7

Every baby born into the world is a finer one than the last.
Nicholas Nickleby Ch. 36

A tall thin, large bowed, old gentleman, with an appearance at first sight of being hard-featured; but at second glance, the mild expression of his face and some particular touches of sweetness and patience about his mouth, corrected this impression and assigned his long professional rides, by day and night, in the bleak hill-weather, as the true cause of that appearance.
The Long Tour of the Two Idle Apprentices Ch.2 (1857) (written with Wilkie Collins) describing the features of a country doctor

There is something in sickness that breaks down the pride of manhood.
Attributed

Niall Dickson 1953–
BBC television health correspondent

You would have to be on another planet not to see that something is changing in the state of medicine. I suggest that the most important change is the collapse of deference.
Lecture at the Royal College of Physicians, London, May (2002)

As time goes by a new set of relationships between the medical profession and the public will emerge.
Lecture at the Royal College of Physicians, London, May (2002)

Denis Diderot 1713–84
French writer

Doctors are always working to preserve our health and cooks to destroy it, but the latter are the more often successful.
Attributed

Johann Friedrich Dieffenbach 1794–1847
Professor of Surgery, Berlin

That beautiful dream has become a reality: operations can now be performed painlessly.
On using ether anaesthesia.

Joseph Dietl 1804–78
Polish-born Austrian physician

A physician should not be judged by the success of his treatment but by the extent of his knowledge.
Attributed (1851)

As long as medicine is an art, it will not become a science. As long as there are successful physicians there will be no scientific physicians.
Attributed

Diphilus 4th century BC
Athenian writer

Time is a physician that heals every grief.
Attributed

Benjamin Disraeli, Lord Beaconsfield 1804–81
British Prime minister and novelist

Youth is a blunder; manhood a struggle; old age a regret.
Coningsby Bk III, Ch. 1

What Art was to the ancient world,
Science is to the modern.
Coningsby Bk IV, Ch. 1

Time is the great physician.
Henrietta Temple Bk VI, Ch. 9

The question is this: Is man an ape or an angel? I, my lord, am on the side of the angels.
Speech, 25 November (1864)

The health of a people is really the foundation upon which all their happiness and all their power as a State depend.
Speech, 23 June (1877)

There is no index of character so sure as the voice.
Tancred Bk II, Ch. 1

There are three kinds of lies: lies, damned lies and statistics.
Attributed

I had rather live, but I am not afraid to die.
Disraeli's last words, quoted by Moneypenny in his *Life of Disraeli* Bk IV, Ch. XVI

J. Frank Dobie 1888–1964
US educator, writer, and folklorist

Putting on the spectacles of science in expectation of finding the answer to everything looked at signifies inner blindness.
The Voice of the Coyote Introduction

Alphonse Raymond Dochez 1882–1964
US microbiologist, Columbia University

It is difficult, often impossible, to estimate the ultimate value of a new scientific fact.
P & S Quarterly **11**: 18, June (1996)

You do one experiment in medicine to convince yourself, then ninety nine more to convince others.
P & S Quarterly **11**: 18, June (1966)

William Dock 1898–?
US physician

The physician must look beyond the picture, now widely cherished, of the lonely, great-hearted doctor, bowed impotent beside the dying child.
The Next Half Century in Medicine

Ian Dodds-Smith

The provision of information is a corollary of the patient's right to self-determination which is a right recognised by law.
Clinical Pharmacology, D.R. Lawrence, P.N. Bennett, and M.J. Brown. Churchill Livingstone, Edinburgh (1997)

John Donne 1572–1631
English poet

That learning, thine ambassador
From thine allegiance we never tempt,
That beauty, paradise's flower
For physic made, from poison be exempt.
A Litany: The Doctors

Solitude is a torment which is not threatened in hell itselfe.
Awakenings

Colin Douglas 1948?–
Scottish doctor and writer

Heal the sick and comfort the dying, but do not get them mixed up!
British Medical Journal (2001), quoting an old consultant boss

John Langdon Down 1828–96
British psychiatrist and physician

The face is flat and broad, and destitute of prominence. The cheeks are rounded and extended laterally. The eyes are obliquely placed, and the internal canthi more than normally distant from one another.
Observations on an ethnic classification of idiots. *London Hospital Reports* **3**: 259–62 (1862)

The Mongolian type of idiocy occurs in more than 10% of the cases which are presented to me. They are always congenitally based and never result from accidents in uterine life.
Observations on an ethnic classification of idiots. *London Hospital Reports* **3**: 259–62 (1862)

Len Doyal
Contemporary British professor of medical ethics

It is time we stopped avoiding real debate on the possible legalisation of active euthanasia by pretending that the double effect argument will somehow resolve it for us. It will not.
British Medical Journal **318**: 1433 (1999)

Daniel Drake 1785–1852
US physician, Kentucky

The first acts of a graduate are apt to be his precedents through coming years, for there is no era in his life in which his self-complacency is so exalted as the time which passes between receiving his diploma with its blue ribbon, and receiving crape and gloves, to wear at the funeral of his first patient.
Western Journal of Medicine and Surgery **2**: 354 (1844)

Michael Drayton 1563–1631
English poet

Past cure, past care.
    England's Heroical Epistles 'Richard the Second to Queene Isabel' (1597)

John Dryden 1631–1700
English poet and playwright

There is pleasure, sure,
In being mad, which none but madmen know.
    The Spanish Friar II. ii

Louis I. Dublin *c.* 1890–1970
US epidemiologist

Each advancing age period of life shows a steady and consistent rise in suicide frequency.
    Attributed

Rene J. Dubos 1901–82
French-born US bacteriologist

Physicians and public health officials, like soldiers, are always equipped to fight the last war.
    The Dreams of Reason Ch. IV

In medicine even more than in other fields of science, theories and practice have always been under the sway of *a priori* philosophical attitudes and rationalized beliefs.
    The Dreams of Reason Ch. IV

The mind can be a piercing search-light which reveals many of the hidden mysteries of the world, but unfortunately, it often causes such a glare that it prevents the eyes from seeing the natural objects which should serve as guideposts in following the ways of nature.
    Louis Pasteur, Free Lance of Science Ch. V

The epidemic of syphilis which spread through all of Europe in the late fifteenth and early sixteenth century gave many physicians frequent occasions to observe, often in the form of a personal experience, that a given disease can pass from one individual to another.
    Louis Pasteur, Free Lance of Science Ch. IX

It can be said that each civilization has a pattern of disease peculiar to it.
    Industrial Medicine and Surgery **30**: 369 (1961)

Throughout nature, infection without disease is the rule rather than the exception.
    Man Adapting Ch. VII

If men allow themselves to continue breeding like rabbits, their fate will inevitably be to live like rabbits, a precarious and limited existence.
    Man Adapting Ch. IX

DDT went further toward the eradication of malariologists than of mosquitoes.
    Man Adapting Ch. XIV

Epidemics have often been more influential than statesmen and soldiers in shaping the course of political history, and diseases may also colour the moods of civilizations.
    The White Plague Ch. V

There is no evidence that tuberculosis breeds genius. The probability is rather, that eagerness for achievement often leads to a way of life that renders the body less resistant to infection.
    The White Plague Ch. V

Louis Adolphus Duhring 1845–1913
US dermatologist

The power of making a correct diagnosis is the key to all success in the treatment of skin diseases; without this faculty, the physician can never be a thorough dermatologist, and therapeutics at once cease to hold their proper position, and become empirical.
    American Journal of Syphilography and Dermatology **2**: 104 (1871)

Alexandre Dumas 1802–70
French novelist

A good surgeon operates with his hand, not with his heart.
    Attributed

Dr Dunlop

You notice that the tabetic has the power of holding water for an indefinite period. He also is impotent—in fact two excellent properties to possess for a quiet day on the river.
    Teaching at Charing Cross Hospital, London

Finley Peter Dunne ('Mr Dooley')
1867–1936
American humorist

I wondher why ye can always read a doctor's bill an' ye niver can read his purscription.
    Mr. Dooley Says 'Drugs'

Baron Guillaume Dupuytren
1777–1835
Chief surgeon Hôtel Dieu, Paris

Read little, see much, do much.
(*Peu lire, beaucoup voir, beaucoup faire*)
    Attributed

Lawrence Durrell 1912–1990
British novelist

Poor honest sex, like dying, should be a private matter.
    Prospero's Cell Ch. 1

Dutch proverbs

Sickness comes on horseback and departs on foot.

Where a man feels pain he lays his hand.

Hermann Ebbinghaus 1850–1909

German psychologist

Psychology has a long past, but only a short history.
Summary of Psychology

Mary Baker Eddy 1821–1910

US religious leader

Then comes the question, how do drugs, hygiene and animal magnetism heal? It may be affirmed that they do not heal, but only relieve suffering temporarily, exchanging one disease for another.
Science and Health with Key to Scriptures

Health is not a condition of matter, but of Mind; nor can the material senses bear reliable testimony on the subject of health.
Science and Health with Key to Scriptures, Ch. VI

Disease is an experience of mortal mind. It is fear made manifest on the body.
Science and Health with Key to Scriptures, Ch. XIV

Thomas Alva Edison 1847–1931

American inventor

Genius is one per cent inspiration and ninety-nine per cent perspiration.
Aphorism

The doctor of the future will give no medicine but will interest his patients in the care of the human frame, in diet and in the cause and prevention of disease.
Aphorism

Jonathan Edwards 1703–58

US theologian

The bodies of those that made such a noise and tumult when alive, when dead, lie as quietly among the graves of their neighbours as any others.
Practical Sermons Sermon XV, Sect. V

Paul Ehrlich 1854–1915

German bacteriologist

Much testing; accuracy and precision in experiment; no guesswork or self-deception.
Quoted by Martha Marquardt in *Paul Ehrlich* Ch. XIII

Albert Einstein 1879–1955

Mathematician and physicist

We should take care not to make the intellect our god; it has, of course, powerful muscles, but no personality.
Out of My Later Life 517

Do not stop to think about the reasons for what you are doing, about why you are questioning. Curiosity has its own reason for existence.
Attributed

George Eliot (Mary Ann Evans Cross) 1819–80

English novelist

It is seldom a medical man has true religious views—there is too much pride of intellect.
Middlemarch Ch. 21

Many of us looking back through life would say that the kindest man we have ever known has been a medical man, or perhaps that surgeon whose fine tact, directed by deeply-informed perception, has come to us in our need with a more sublime beneficience than that of miracle-workers.
Middlemarch Ch. 66

A man deep-wounded may feel too much pain to feel much anger.
Spanish Gypsy Bk 1

T. S. Eliot (Thomas Stearns Eliot) 1888–1965

US-born writer and poet

I grow old...I grow old
I shall wear the bottoms of my trousers rolled.
Shall I part my hair behind?
Do I dare to eat a peach?
I shall wear white flannel trousers, and walk upon
    the beach.
I have heard the mermaids singing, each
    to each.
I do not think that they will sing to me.
The Love Song of J. Alfred Prufock (1917)

The wounded surgeon plies the steel
That questions the distempered part;
Beneath the bleeding hands we feel
The sharp compassion of the healer's art
Resolving the enigma of the fever chart.
Four Quartets 1944, 'EastCoker' IV

The years between fifty and seventy are the hardest. You are always being asked to do more, and you are not yet decrepit enough to turn them down.
Time 23 October (1950)

Birth, copulation and death.
That's all the facts when you come to brass tacks.
Sweeney Agonistes 'Fragment of an Agon'

Havelock Ellis 1859–1939

British psychologist

The place where optimism most flourishes is the lunatic asylum.
The Dance of Life Ch. 3

Had there been a Lunatic Asylum in the suburbs of Jerusalem, Jesus Christ would infallibly have been shut up in it at the outset of his public career.
Impressions and Comments 5 January (1922)

Pain and death are part of life. To reject them is to reject life itself.
On Life and Sex: Essays of Love and Virtue 2

Men have expended infinite ingenuity in establishing the remote rhythms of the solar system and the periodicity of the comet. They have disdained to trouble about the simpler task of proving or unproving the cycles of their own organisms.
Body Time Gay Gaer Luce., Paladin, Frogmore, UK (1973)

Haven Emerson 1874–1957
US physician and epidemiologist

Nature heals, under the auspices of the medical profession.
Lecture

The social cost of sickness is incalculable. The prevention of disease is for the most part a matter of education, the cost is moderate, the results certain and easily demonstrated.
The Social Cost of Sickness

Ralph Waldo Emerson 1803–82
US essayist and poet

The poisons are our principal medicines, which kill the disease and save the life.
The Conduct of Life Ch. 7

The multitude of the sick shall not make us deny the existence of health.
The Conduct of Life, Worship

Homeopathy is insignificant as an act of healing, but of great value as criticism on the hygeia or medical practice of the time.
Essays (Second series) '*Nominalist and Realist*'

Sanity is very rare: every man almost, and every woman, has a dash of madness.
Journals

All diseases run into one, old age.
Journals

It is dainty to be sick if you have leisure and convenience for it.
Journals Vol. V

Men resemble their contemporaries even more than their progenitors.
Representative Men 'Uses of Great Men'

English proverbs

A bald head is soon shaven.

A deadly disease neither physician nor physic can ease.
James Sanford's *The Garden of Pleasure* (1573)

A dry cough is the trumpeter of death.

A small hurt in the eye is a great one.

A wound heals but the scar remains.

After dinner sit awhile, after supper walk a mile.

Die well that live well.

Feed sparingly and defy the physician.

From the womb to the tomb.
In: Gascoigne's *The Drum of Doomsday* (1576)

Health is better than wealth.

He looks like a tooth-drawer, i.e. very thin and meagre.

He that eats till he is sick must fast till he is well.

He that goes to bed thirsty rises healthy.

Health is not valued till sickness comes.

One doctor makes work for another.
V.S. Lean Collectanea (1902–4)

Never rub your eye but with your elbow.

Physicians' faults are covered with earth, and rich men's with money.

Six hours sleep for a man, seven for a woman, and eight for a fool.

They who would be young when they are old must be old when they are young.

Wash your hands often, your feet seldom, and your head never.

When the head aches, all the body is the worse.

English sailors' proverb

The only cure for sea-sickness is to sit on the shady side of an old brick church in the country.

Ennius 239–169 BC
Roman poet

How like us is that ugly brute, the ape!
On the Nature of the Gods I (Cicero)

Epicurus 341–270 BC
Greek philosoper

So death, the most terrifying of ills, is nothing to us, since so long as we exist, death is not with us; but when death comes, then we do not exist. It does not then concern either the living or the dead, since for the former it is not, and the latter are no more.
Letter to Menoeceus

The magnitude of pleasure reaches its limit in the removal of all pain.
Sovran Maxims 3

Erassistratus c.260 BC
Alexandrian physician

Nature is the great artist who in her care for living beings, has perfected all parts of the body and has organised them purposively.

Erik Erikson
Contemporary

The adolescent mind is essentially a mind of the moratorium, a psychosocial stage between childhood and adulthood, and between the morality learned by the child and the ethics developed by the adult.
Childhood Society. W. W. Norton, New York (1950)

Henri Estienne 1531–98
French scholar

If youth but know,
And old age only could.
Les Prémices (transl. Norbert Guterman)

Euripides 485–406 BC
Greek playwright

Death is a debt we all must pay.
Alcestis 419

In the hour of sorrow or sickness, a wife is a man's greatest blessing.
Antigone, Fragment 164

Bodies devoid of mind are as statues in the market place.
Electra 386

For they which share one father's blood shall oft By many a bodily likeness kinship show.
Electra 522

A weary thing is sickness and its pains!
Hippolytus 176

It is better to be sick than to be a nurse. Sickness poses only one problem for the patient, but for the nurse it involves both mental agony and hard physical work.
Hippolytus

What they say of us (women) is that we have a peaceful time. Living at home, while they do the fighting in war. How wrong they are! I would very much rather stand three times in the front of battle than bear one child.
Medea 248

Sir Grimley Evans 1939–
Professor of Clinical Gerontology, Oxford, England

The aging of an organism is a progressive loss of adaptability as time passes.
Introduction to the *Oxford Textbook of Geriatric Medicine* Oxford University Press Oxford (2000) (2nd edn).

Margaret Jane Evans 1962–
Paediatric pathologist

But pathologists are not butchers. It's an investigation of the dead for the living.
Hospital Doctor 2 August (2001), in response to the reaction to the Alder Hey affair

William M. Evarts 1818–1901
US lawyer and statesman

It was a brilliant affair; water flowed like champagne.
Describing a dinner given by US President Rutherford B. Hayes (1877–81), an advocate of temperance

Noah D. Fabricant 1904–?

Most medical fads are like some women's fashions—frail, fickle and costly.
Amusing Quotations for Doctors and Patients 'Fads'

Joseph Sheridan Le Fanu 1814–73
Irish novelist

Old persons are sometimes as unwilling to die as tired-out children are to say good night and go to bed.

Nathaniel Faxon 1880–1960
US physician, Massachusetts General Hospital

The purpose of a teaching hospital is to, advance knowledge, to train doctors, and to set an example of practice.
Quoted by F. M. R. Walshe in *Teachers of Medicine*

Jean Fernel 1485–1558
Paris trained physician to Catherine de Medici

The physician today seems athirst for blood. Blood-letting, like wine-drinking, is right enough in moderation, but in excess it leads to disaster.
Treatise, 1545 (quoted in The Endeavour of Jean Fernel, Pt 3)

Anatomy is for physiology what geography is for the historian: it describes the scene of action.
A Universal Medicine

Magister Ferrarius 16th century
Salernian physician

Infants do not cry without some legitimate cause.
The Advancement of Child Health (A. V. Neale)

Baron Ernst von Feuchtersleben 1806–94

Half informed physicians are generally sceptics.
Dietetics of the Soul XXII, Entry 27 (transl. G. Pollak)

Henry Fielding 1707–54
English novelist

It hath been often said, that it is not death, by dying, which is terrible.
Amelia Bk III, Ch. 4

It is with jealousy as with the gout. When such distempers are in the blood, there is never any security against their breaking out; and that often on the slightest occasions, and when least suspected.
Tom Jones Bk ii, Ch. 3

He that dies before sixty, of a cold or consumption, dies, in reality, by a violent death.
On the Death of Mr. Robert Levet, a Practiser in Physic

W. C. Fields 1884–1946
US actor and humourist

After two days in hospital I took a turn for the nurse.
Attributed

Lactantius Firmianus *c.* AD 306
African-born Christian apologist

Everyone should bear in mind that the union of the two sexes is given to living beings for procreation, and that these passions are subject to the law that they must beget offspring.
Divine Institutions VI. xxiii

Martin H. Fischer 1879–1962
US physician and writer

Here's good advice for practice: go into partnership with nature; she does more than half the work and asks none of the fee.
Fischerisms Howard Fabing and Ray Marr (1944)

The greatest discoveries of surgery are anaesthesia, asepsis, and roentgenology – and none was made by a surgeon.
Fischerisms Howard Fabing and Ray Marr (1944)

The heart is the only organ that takes no rest.
Fischerisms Howard Fabing and Ray Marr (1944)

Facts are not science, as the dictionary is not literature.
Fischerisms Howard Fabing and Ray Marr (1944)

All the world is a laboratory to the inquiring mind.
Fischerisms Howard Fabing and Ray Marr (1944)

A doctor must work eighteen hours a day and seven days a week. If you cannot console yourself to this, get out of the profession.
Fischerisms Howard Fabing and Ray Marr (1944)

When a man lacks mental balance in pneumonia he is said to be delirious.
When he lacks mental balance without the pneumonia, he is pronounced insane by all smart doctors.
Fischerisms Howard Fabing and Ray Marr (1944)

In the sick room, ten cents worth of human understanding equals ten dollars' worth of medical science.
Fischerisms Howard Fabing and Ray Marr (1944)

An insane man is a sick man. Please don't forget that, gentlemen.
Fischerisms Howard Fabing and Ray Marr (1944)

A man who cannot work without his hypodermic needle is a poor doctor. The amount of narcotic you use is inversely proportional to your skill.
Fischerisms Howard Fabing and Ray Marr (1944)

Diagnosis is not the end, but the beginning of practice.
Fischerisms Howard Fabing and Ray Marr (1944)

Diets were invented of the church, the workhouse and the hospital. They were started for the punishment of the spirit and have ended in the punishment of the body.
Fischerisms Howard Fabing and Ray Marr (1944)

The first rule to proper diet? Ask them what they want and then give it to them. There are few exceptions.
Fischerisms Howard Fabing and Ray Marr (1944)

Whenever ideas fail, men invent words.
Fischerisms Howard Fabing and Ray Marr (1944)

Let your entrance into the sick room decrease, not increase, the irritability of your patient.
Fischerisms Howard Fabing and Ray Marr (1944)

It takes fifty years from the discovery of a principle in medicine to its adoption in practice.
Fischerisms Howard Fabing and Ray Marr (1944)

Geoffrey Fisher 1887–1972
Archbishop of Canterbury

Consultant specialists are a degree more remote (like bishops!); and therefore (again like bishops) they need a double dose of Grace to keep them sensitive to the personal and the pastoral.
Lancet **2**: 775 (1949)

John Fiske 1842–190
US historian, Harvard

All human science is but the increment of the power of the eye, and all human art is the increment of the power of the hand.
The Destiny of Man Ch. VII

Reginald Heber Fitz 1843–1913
US surgeon

One cannot ignore the enormous importance of early detection of an appendix which may burst. In most cases the diagnosis is easy.
Lecture to Boston Medical Society, June (1886)

F. Scott Fitzgerald 1896–1940
US writer

It appears that every man's insomnia is as different from his neighbour's as are their daytime hopes and aspirations.
The Crack-up 'Sleeping and Walking'

Sir Alexander Fleming 1881–1955
British microbiologist

A good gulp of hot whisky at bedtime – it's not very scientific, but it helps.
News Summary 22 March (1954) (quoted when asked about the common cold)

Flemish proverb

Where there is sunshine no doctors are wanted.

Abraham Flexner 1866–1959

The investigator, obviously, observes, experiments and judges; so do the physician and surgeon who practise their art in the modern spirit.
Medical Education, A Comparative Study Ch. I

John Florio 1553–1625

English lexicographer and translator

Patience is the best medicine.
First Frutes

Bernard Le Bovier de Fontanelle 1657–1757

French anatomist

In vain we shall penetrate more and more deeply the secrets of the structure of the human body, we shall not dupe nature; we shall die as usual.
Dialogues des Morts Dialogue V

We anatomists are like the porters in Paris, who are acquainted with the narrowest and most distant streets, but who know nothing of what takes place in the houses.
Attributed

Sir John Forbes 1787–1861

Scottish physician and editor

In a large proportion of cases treated by physicians, the disease is cured by nature, not by them.
Cyclopaedia of Practical Medicine

Henry Ford 1863–1947

US car manufacturer

Exercise is bunk. If you are healthy, you don't need it: if you are sick, you shouldn't take it.
Attributed

The trouble with the human body as compared with the car is that the exhaust is too near the ignition.
Attributed

Nicholas J. Fox

Contemporary Lecturer in Sociology, Department of General Practice, University of Sheffield

Three elements of surgery define it as different from almost all other clinical specialties: the degree of invasiveness, the use of anaesthetic techniques and its emphasis on sterility.
The Social Meaning of Surgery p. 31. Open University Press (1992)

Sir Theodore Fox 1899–1989

Editor of the Lancet

The physician is not the servant of science, or of his race, or even of life. He is the individual servant of his individual patient basing his decisions always on their individual interest.
Lancet **2**: 801–5 (1965)

We shall have to learn to refrain from doing things merely because we know how to do them.
Lancet **2**: 801 (1965)

Johann Peter Frank 1745–1821

German professor of medicine and public health reformer

All persons whether male or female, ascertained to be infected with venereal disease should be restrained from intercourse until this was known to be safe because they had been completely restored to health.
System einer vollständigen medizinischen Polizei Vol ii (1780)

Benjamin Franklin 1706–90

US Statesman and inventor

Be not sick too late, or well too soon.
Poor Richard's Almanack (1734)

A ship under sail and a big-bellied woman,

Are the handsomest two things that can be seen common.
Poor Richard's Almanack (1735)

In general, mankind, since the improvement in cookery, eats twice as much as nature requires.
Poor Richard's Almanack (1760)

Nothing is more fatal to Health, than an over Care of it.
Poor Richard's Almanack (1760)

He's the best physician that knows the worthlessness of the most medicines.
Poor Richard's Almanack (1760)

Be temperate in wine, in eating, girls, and sloth, or the Gout will seize you and plague you both.
Poor Richard's Almanack (1760)

The patient may well be safer with a physician who is naturally wise than with one who is artificially learned.
Poor Richard's Almanack (1760)

He that lives upon hope will die fasting.
The Way to Wealth

Quacks are the greatest liars in the world except their patients.
Attributed

Girolamo Frascastoro 1483–1553

Italian physician, Verona

Mothers and fathers, peasants and rulers, children and greybeards, stood mingled together; all tortured in soul and foul in body, with scabby skin from which matter oozed.
Syphilis, sive Morbus Gallicus Bk III (1530)

Frederick the Great 1712–86

King of Prussia

Every man has a wild beast within him.
Letter to Voltaire (1759)

Men are born with an indelible character
Letter to d'Lembert (1777)

French proverbs

A surgeon should be young, a physician old.
  Also an Italian proverb

A young physician fattens the churchyard.
  C. Holyband's (Desainliens) *The Frenche Littleton* (1576)

Every month, one should get drunk at least once.

He who complains is not hurt.

He who fears to suffer, suffers from fear.

He who is master of his thirst is master of his health.

If you would live ever, you must wash milk from your liver.

L'amour de la médicine fait le savant;
L'amour du malade fait le médicin.
(Love of medicine makes the scholar;
Love of illness makes the doctor)

Short men eat more than tall men.

The doctor is often more to be feared than the disease.

They that are thirsty drink silently.

Philip Freneau 1752–1832
US poet

Tobacco surely was designed
To poison and destroy mankind.
  Poems, 'Tobacco'

Sigmund Freud 1856–1939
Austrian psychoanalyst

The conscious mind may be compared to a fountain playing in the sun and falling back into the great subterranean pool of subconscious from which it rises.
  Bartlett's Unfamiliar Quotations Leonard Louis Levinson

The true believer is in a high degree protected against the danger of certain neurotic afflictions; by accepting the universal neurosis he is spared the task of forming a personal neurosis.
  The Future of an Illusion Ch. 8

Now and then occasions arise in which the physician is bound to take up the position of teacher and mentor, but it must be done with great caution, and the patient should be educated to liberate and to fulfill his own nature and not to resemble ourselves.

The poets and philosophers before me have discovered the unconscious; I have discovered the scientific method with which the unconscious can be studied.
  Letter

Sir Alfred Fripp 1865–1930
British surgeon, Guy's Hospital, London

If we cannot be clever, we can always be kind.
  Emergencies in Medical Practice

Always keep a dying patient's relatives busy.
  Reginald Pound in *Harley Street* p. 122. Michael Joseph, London (1967)

Erich Fromm 1900–80
US psychologist and philosopher

Man always dies before he is fully born.
  Man for himself Ch. 3

The minute study of the process of rationalization is perhaps the most significant contribution of psychoanalysis to human progress.
  Psychoanalysis and Religion Ch. 3

The mother–child relationship is paradoxical and, in a sense, tragic. It requires the most intense love on the mother's side, yet this very love must help the child grow away from the mother and to become fully independent.

Robert Frost 1874–1963
US lyric poet

The brain is a wonderful organ. It starts working the moment you get up in the morning, and does not stop until you get into the office.
  Attributed

James Anthony Froude 1818–94
Professor of History, Oxford, England

Wild animals never kill for sport. Man is the only one to whom the torture and death of his fellow-creatures is amusing in itself.
  Oceana Ch. 5 (1886)

Thomas Fuller 1654–1734
English writer and physician

Commonly physicians, like beer, are best when they are old, and lawyers, like bread, when they are young and new.
  The Holy State and the Profane State Ch. XVI (1642–8)

The tongue is ever turning to the aching tooth.
  Gnomologia No. 4796

J. H. Gaddum 1900–68
British professor of physiology

Patients may recover in spite of drugs or because of them.
  Pharmacology by D. R. Laurence, Churchill Livingstone, Edinburgh (1973), Frontispiece

Gaelic proverb

Every healthy man is king.

J. K. Galbraith 1908–
Canadian-born US economist

Much of the world's work is done by men who do not feel quite well. Marx is a case in point.
  The Age of Uncertainty

Galen AD 130–200
Roman physician

Surgery is the unceasing movement of steady, experienced hands.
Definitiones medicae XXXV

I am of the opinion that the kidneys too are affected in the rare disease which some people call chamber pot dropsy, others again diabetes ('the siphon') or violent thirst.
Quoted by Folke Henschen in *Medical History 1969*, *Wellcome Historical Library* **XIII**, No. 2: 190

That physician will hardly be thought very careful of the health of others who neglects his own.
Of Protecting the Health Bk 5

Most physicians are like athletes who aspire to victory in the Olympic Games without doing anything to deserve it; for they praise Hippocrates as first in the art of healing but make no attempt to resemble him.
Medicus Philosophus

Confidence and hope to do more good than physic.
Attributed

All who drink of this remedy recover in a short time, except those whom it does not help, who all die. Therefore, it is obvious that it fails only in incurable cases.
Attributed

Employment is nature's physician, and is essential to human happiness.
Attributed

We must be daring and search after Truth; even if we do not succeed in finding her, we shall at least come closer than we are at present.
Attributed

Sir Francis Galton 1822–1911
British scientist and explorer

The conditions that direct the order of the whole of the living world around us, are marked by their persistence in improving the birthright of successive generations.
Inquiries Into Human Faculty and Its Development 'The Observed Order of Events'

Mahatma Gandhi 1869–1948
Indian Congress leader

I eat to live, to serve, and also, if it so happens, to enjoy, but I do not eat for the sake of enjoyment.
Attributed

James A. Garfield 1831–81
US President

Suicide is not a remedy.
Inaugural address, 4 March (1881)

Fielding H. Garrison 1870–1935
US physician and medical historian, New York

The future of American medical education is, like all other higher developments, simply in the hands of the only aristocracy we strive for—the aristocracy of an enlightened public opinion.
Introduction to the History of Medicine (2nd edn), Ch. 12

The history of medicine is, in fact, the history of humanity itself, with its up and downs, its brave aspirations after truth and finality, its pathetic failures.
Introduction to the History of Medicine, 2nd edn., Preface

Sir Samuel Garth 1661–1719
English physician and poet

The patient's ears remorseless he assails;
Murder with jargon where his medicine fails.
The Dispensary

Dear gentlemen, let me die a natural death.
Brewer's Dictionary of Phrase and Fable (centenary edition), revised by Ivor Evans (1975)

John Gay 1685–1732
English dramatist

Is there no hope? the sick Man said.
The silent doctor shook his head,
And took his leave, with signs of sorrow,
Despairing of his fee tomorrow.
Fables (Series I), Fable 27

Sir Auckland Geddes 1879–1954
British surgeon and politician

So many come to the sickroom thinking of themselves as men of science fighting disease and not as healers with a little knowledge helping nature to get a sick man well.
The Practitioner

General Medical Council, UK

Patients must be able to trust doctors with their lives and well-being. To justify that trust, we as a profession have a duty to maintain a good standard of practice and care and to show respect for human life.
GMC Good Medical Practice London, UK (1998)

Doctors must keep their knowledge and skills up-to-date throughout their working lives. Doctors should take part regularly in educational activities which develop their competence. In addition, they should respond constructively to appraisals of their competence and performance.
GMC Good Medical Practice London, UK (1998), pp. 3–4, paragraphs 5–7

M. C. Geokas 1930?–
US physician

A ten minute surgical discussion of acute pancreatitis should probably include nine minutes of silence.
Internal Medicine **76**: 105–12 (1972)

William H. George 1918–
US chemical engineer and businessman

Scientific research is not itself a science; it is still an art or craft.
The Scientist in Action Ch. 1

German law

Any person suffering from an hereditary disease may be rendered incapable of procreation by means of a surgical operation if the experience of medical science shows that it is highly probable that his descendants would suffer from some serious physical or mental hereditary defect.

For the Prevention of Hereditarily Diseased Offspring 14 July, (1933)

German proverbs

A half doctor near is better than a whole one far away.

Invalids live longest.

No doctor is better than three.

Old age is a hospital that takes in all diseases.

Sickly body, sickly mind.

When the boy is growing he has a wolf in his belly.

Man without woman is head without body; woman without man is body without head.

Medicines are not meat to live by.

Sauerkraut is good for a cold.

The garden is the poor man's apothecary.

Edward Gibbon 1737–94

English historian

That salutary and lucrative profession.

Describing doctors from Salerno in the twelfth century in The History of the Decline and Fall of the Roman Empire

Kahlil Gibran 1883–1931

Syrian writer and painter

You may give them your love but not your thoughts.

For they have their own thoughts.

You may house their bodies but not their souls,

For their souls dwell in the house of tomorrow, which you cannot visit, not even in your dreams.

The Prophet 'On Children'

André Gide 1869–1951

French writer

True kindness presupposes the faculty of imagining as one's own the suffering and joy of others.

Attributed

W. Gill Wylie 19th century

Harvard-trained US physician

But to extend hospitals any further is to encourage pauperism, idleness, and the breakup of the family. Hospitals tend to weaken the family tie by separating the sick from their homes and their relatives, who are often too ready to relieve themselves of the burden of the sick.

Hospitals: Their History, Organization, and Construction, Appleton New York (1877), pp. 57–66 (quoted in The Social Transformation of American Medicine Paul Starr. Basic Books, New York (1982))

Muriel Gillick

Contemporary, Hebrew Rehabilitation Center, Boston, USA

Doctors cruelly and needlessly prolong the lives of the dying (for reasons) of avarice and passion for technology.

Archives of Internal Medicine **154**: 134–7 (1994)

Sir William S. Gilbert 1836–1911

English author and lyricist

I see no objection to stoutness, in moderation.

Iolanthe Act I

Paul Gill

Contemporary British anthropologist and nurse

Brain death may very well be a distinct, physiological entity but this concept of death is not accepted in many cultures and much anthropological evidence exists to demonstrate this.

Care of the Critically Ill **16**: 219 (2000)

Sir Harold Gillies 1882–1960

Plastic and burn surgeon

It is terrifying to think what will happen when the mystery of organ transference has been solved; it can be as revolutionary as the cleaving of the atom. Anybody would be able to go into his local organ bank and, for a not insurmountable sum, trade in a weak heart or a feeble brain for a better one, or a cirrhotic liver for a healthier one.

In Principles and Art of Plastic Surgery with Ralph Millard (1957)

There is no better training for a surgeon than to be taught observation by a physician.

In Principles and Art of Plastic Surgery with Ralph Millard Vol. I, Ch. 2 (1957)

The great ignominy to the plastic surgeon is his inability to remove a scar without leaving another one.

In Principles and Art of Plastic Surgery with Ralph Millard Vol. I, Ch. 4 (1957)

It is easy to agree to do a beauty operation, but not always quite so easy to be certain it is justified.

In Principles and Art of Plastic Surgery with Ralph Millard Vol. II, Ch. 20 (1957)

Raanan Gillon 1941–

British professor of medical ethics

Meanwhile the medical profession—with our awesome and to some terrifying powers over life and death—must continue to earn that public trust by being absolutely clear that the law as it stands means we must never treat our patients with the intent of accelerating their deaths.

British Medical Journal **318**: 1432 (1999)

Charlotte Perkins Stetson Gilman

1860–1935
US writer on social and economic subjects

Human life consists in mutual service. No grief, pain, misfortune, or 'broken heart', is excuse for cutting off one's life while any power of service remains. But when all usefulness is over, when one is assured of an unavoidable and imminent death, it is the simplest of human rights to choose a quick and easy death in place of a slow and horrible one.

Note written before her suicide, 13 August (1935)

Daniel Coit Gilman 1879–1908

US educator

The medical student is likely to be one son of the family too weak to labour on the farm, too indolent to do any exercise, too stupid for the bar and too immoral for the pulpit.

Attributed

Thomas Gisborne 1758–1846

English cleric and author

There have been physicians, the disgrace of their profession, who seem to have considered themselves, in studying Medicine, as studying not a liberal science, but a mere art for the acquisition of money; and have thence been solicitous to acquire an insight rather into the humours than into the diseases of mankind.

The Duties of Physicians

It is frequently of much importance, not to the comfort only, but to the recovery of the patient, that he should be enabled to look upon his physician as his friend.

The Duties of Physicians

William E. Gladstone 1809–98

British statesman

The disease of an evil conscience is beyond the practice of all the physicians of all the countries of the world.

Speech, Plumstead, UK (1878)

Johann Wolfgang von Goethe

1749–1832
German poet and scientist

The world is so full of simpletons and madmen, that one need not seek them in a madhouse.

Conversations with Goethe Johann Peter Eckermann 17 March (1830).

I have learned much from disease which life could have never taught me anywhere else.

Conversations with Goethe Johann Peter Eckermann 17 March (1830)

Thus I saw that most men only care for science so far as they get a living by it, and that they worship even error when it affords them a subsistence.

Conversations with Goethe 15 October (1825)

Nothing is more terrible than to see ignorance in action.

Maxims and Reflections I

If man thinks about his physical or moral state he usually discovers that he is ill.

Sprüche in Prosa Pt I, Bk II

Medicine absorbs the physician's whole being because it is concerned with the entire human organism.

Attributed

No skill or art is needed to grow old; the trick is to endure it.

Attributed

Science and art belong to the whole world, and the barriers of nationality vanish before them.

Attributed

Oliver St. John Gogarty 1878–1957

Irish politician and author

The Englishman believes that a purgative can fatten or make him thin; he believes that either there is only one kind of ache or that one medicine can cure various kinds.

As I Was Going Down Sackville Street Ch. III (1937)

Oliver Goldsmith 1730–74

Irish-born writer

I am told he makes a very handsome corpse, and becomes his coffin prodigiously.

The Good Natured Man Act I

But the skilful physician distinguishes the symptoms, manures the sterility of nature, or prunes her luxuriance; nor does he depend so much on the efficacy of medicines as on their proper application.

Letter to Revd Thomas Contarine (1753)

Samuel Goldwyn 1882–1974

Polish-born US film producer

Anybody who goes to see a psychiatrist ought to have his head examined.

Attributed

Edward Goodman 1879–?

It is a distinct art to talk medicine in the language of the non-medical man.

Attributed

Mervyn H. Gordon 1872–1953

English bacteriologist, St. Bartholomew's Hospital, London

The object of research is the advancement not of the investigator, but of knowledge.

Attributed

Johannes De Gorter 1689–1762

Medicine discusses diseases which are so rare that one does not encounter them more than once or twice during a lifetime with a thoroughness as if the salvation of the art would depend on it.

De Motu Vitali

Remy de Gourmont 1858–1915
French novelist, poet, and critic

Before undergoing a surgical operation arrange your temporal affairs—you may live.
  Attributed

William Gilbert ('W. G.') Grace
1848–1915
Cricketer and doctor

Medicine is my hobby, cricket is my profession.
  Attributed

Evarts Ambrose Graham 1883–1957
US thoracic surgeon

In many respects surgery is like music, which has its great artists and its great composers. The musical artists are like the great surgeons. They often perform before large audiences with great technical skill, and they have large incomes.
  Attributed

Harvey Graham 1912–
English physician

Venus found herself a goddess
In a world controlled by gods,
So she opened up her bodice
And evened up the odds.
  A Doctor's London Ch. 7

Robert James Graves 1797–1853
Irish physician

He fed fevers.
  Epitaph suggested by Graves himself after emphasizing nutrition in sick patients

From the very commencement the student should set out to witness the progress and effects of sickness and ought to persevere in the daily observation of disease during the whole period of his studies.
  Introductory Lectures (1850)

Greek proverb

A blind man leaned against a wall; 'This is the boundary of the world', he said.

Major Greenwood ?

Do not forget there is a research laboratory greater even than the Cavendish, the streets, the homes, the factories in which common people pass their lives—there is the laboratory of him who adds to our knowledge of social medicine.
  Quoted by J. Pemberton in 'Will Pickles of Wensleydale Bles, London (1970)

Germaine Greer 1939–
Australian-born writer and feminist

The management of fertility is one of the most important functions of adulthood
  Attributed

Alan Gregg 1870–1957
US physician, Rockefeller Institute

Be sparing of criticism, since the habit of trivial comment weakens the force of real protest.
  The Difficult Art of Giving by Wilder Penfield

Our national inclination is to suffer children gladly, prolong adolescence patiently, and deliberately defer maturity.
  Scientific Monthly **58**: 365, (1944)

A good education should leave much to be desired.
  Attributed

James Gregory 1753–1821
Scottish physician

Young men kill their patients; old men let them die.
  Horae Subsecivae 'Locke & Sydenham'

Sir John Grugeon 1928–
Health administrator

Doctors are and should be natural leaders and part of the skill of being a leader is to work with the other leaders in the intricate network of the National Heath Service.
  Hospital Doctor 5 July (1988)

Arthur Guiterman 1871–1943
US poet

Don't tell your friends about your indigestions: 'How are you!' is a greeting, not a question.
  A Poet's Proverbs 'Of Tact'

Sir William Withey Gull 1816–90
British physician, Guy's Hospital, London

The jejunum is more exempt from morbid conditions than any other portion of the alimentary canal.
  St. Bartholomew's Hospital Reports **52**: 45 (1916)

Diseases are but parts of a course of natural history.
  British Medical Journal **2**: 425 (1874)

The road to medical knowledge is through the pathological museum and not through an apothecary's shop.
  Attributed

Never forget that it is not a pneumonia, but a pneumonic man who is your patient.
  Attributed

Nursing, sometimes a trade, sometimes a profession, ought to be a religion.
  Attributed

Savages explain, science investigates.
  Attributed

I do not say no drugs are useful, but there is not enough discrimination in their use.
  Attributed

Robert Marcus Gunn 1850–1909
Scottish-born ophthalmologist, Moorfield's Hospital, London

In my experience it is most exceptional to see an old case of albuminuric retinitis; this latter affection seems to occur at a late stage of the general disease, so that death supervenes before the retinal changes have existed for very long.

Dictionary of Medical Eponyms, (2nd edn), p. 255. Firkin and Whitworth, The Parthenon. Carnforth, Lancs (1996).

Thomas Guthrie 1803–73
Scottish social reformer

If you want to keep a dead man, put him in whisky; if you want to kill a live man put whisky in him.

Attributed

Ernst Haeckel 1834–1919
German professor of zoology

The cell never acts; it reacts.

Generelle Morphologie

Heinrich Haeser 1811–84

Medicine is as old as the human race, as old as the necessity for the removal of disease.

Lehrbruch der Geschichte der Medizin Erste Periode

Christian Friedrich Samuel Hahnemann 1755–1843
German physician and founder of homeopathy

As in a disease where no manifest or exciting cause presents itself for removal, we can perceive nothing but the symptoms then must these symptoms alone guide the physician in the choice of a fit remedy to combat the disease.

Organon of Homeopathic Medicine (3rd American edn), p. 14–18. William Radde, New York (1849)

Similar diseases are cured by similar things.

J. B. S. Haldane 1892–1964
British geneticist and author

I wish I had the voice of Homer
To sing of rectal carcinoma,
Which kills a lot more chaps, in fact,
Than were bumped off when Troy was sacked.

Written when mortally ill with cancer, JBS (Ronald Clark)

Science is vastly more stimulating to the imagination than are the classics.

Daedalus

There are a few honest antivivisectionists. I have not met any of them, but I am quite prepared to believe that they exist.

Possible Worlds 'Some Enemies of Science'

Early diagnosis of disease is the business of the general public even more than of the medical profession.

Possible Worlds 'The Time Factor in Medicine'

I am quite sure that our views on evolution would be very different had biologists studied genetics and natural selection before and not after most of them were convinced that evolution had occurred.

Attributed

The progress of biology in the next century will lead to a recognition of the innate inequality of man. This is today most obviously visible in the United States.

Attributed

Sir Peter Hall 1930–
British theatre director

We do not necessarily improve with age; for better or worse we become more like ourselves.

The Observer 'Sayings of the Week', 24 January (1988)

John Halle 1529–68
English surgeon

A surgeon should have three diverse properties in his person. That is to say, a heart as the heart of a lion, his eyes like the eyes of a hawk, and his hands the hands of a woman.

Epistle to the Reader in the translation of Lanfranchi's *Chirurgia Parva*

But chiefly the anatomy
Ye ought to understand;
If ye will cure well any thing,
That ye do take in hand.

An Historical Expostulation

William Stewart Halsted 1852–1922
US surgeon

The intern suffers not only from inexperience, but also from over-experience.

Bulletin of the Johns Hopkins Hospital **15**: 267 (1904)

The only weapon with which the unconscious patient can immediately retaliate upon the incompetent surgeon is haemorrhage.

Bulletin of the Johns Hopkins Hospital **23**: 191 (1912)

Alexander Hamilton 1740–1810
Professor of Midwifery, Edinburgh

It is particularly observed in surgical wards that there is such a state of the air sometimes as produces almost in every wound symptoms of erysipelas and even, mortification ... when such a state of the air was present puerperal fever raged violently.

The Age of Agony p. 48 Guy Williams. Constable and Co. Ltd, London (1975)

Walton H. Hamilton 1881–1958
US physician

The art of medicine is intricate; the relation of the treatment of the sick to results obtained cannot be appraised by a layman; in medicine, almost more certainly than anywhere else, the patient has not the knowledge requisite for judgment.

Dissenting Opinion on the Report of the Committee on American Medicine (1932)

Hammurabi 1728–1686 BC
Babylonian king

If a man has knocked out the teeth of a man of the same rank, his own teeth shall be knocked out.
Number 200 statement from the 282 provisions to the fees due to Medical Practitioners in the Code of Hammurabi

If a doctor has treated a man with a metal knife for a severe wound, and has caused the man to die, or has opened a man's tumour with a metal knife and destroyed the man's eye, his hand shall be cut off.
Number 200 statement from the 282 provisions to the fees due to Medical Practitioners in the Code of Hammurabi

Garrett Hardin 1968–

Certainly pregnancy is a form of servitude if continued to term it results in parenthood, which is also a kind of servitude to be endured for the best years of a woman's life.

George Harley 1829–96
Scottish physician

True science is the key to wise practice.
Diseases of the Liver, Title page (1870)

George T. Harrell 1908–

The physician's continuing education, whether he is a scientist practising in a medical school or a general practitioner practicing in some rural area, is largely a process within himself, one he pursues on his own.
Journal of Medical Education **33**: 217 (1958)

William Harvey 1578–1657
English physician

Everything from an egg.
De Generatione Animalium, Frontispiece

...the blood passes through the heart and lungs by means of the heart's force and is sent out to all parts of the body where it enters the veins and the pores of the flesh.
Exercitatio Anatomica de Motu Cordis et Sanguinis in Animalibus

The heart of animals is the foundation of their life, the sovereign of everything within them, the sum of their microcosm, that upon which all their growth. depends, from which all power proceeds.
Exercitatio Anatomica de Motu Cordis et Sanguinis in Animalibus

If any part of the after-burden be left sticking to the uterus the after-purgings will flow forth evil-scented, green and as if they proceeded from a dead body: and sometimes the courage and strength of the womb being quite vanquished, a

suddaine Gangrene doth induce a certain death.
Writing in 1651 on puerperal sickness, Age of Agony p. 45, Guy Williams. Constable and Co. Ltd, London (1975)

For the honour of the Profession to continue to mutual love and affection among themselves without which neither the dignity of the College can be preserved nor yet particular men receive benefit by their admission into the College which else they might expect, ever remembering that 'Concordia res parvae crescunt, Discordia magnae dilabunture.'
Trust Deed to the Royal College of Physicians 21 June (1656)

Lady Flora Hastings 1806–39
British poet

Grieve not that I die young. Is it not well
To pass away ere life hath lost its brightness?
Swan Song

Lord Havers 1923–
British lawyer and politician

I am also satisfied that a person who has a duty of care may be guilty of murder by omitting to fulfill that duty, as much as by committing any positive act.
High Court Judgment (1982)

Nathaniel Hawthorne 1804–64
US novelist

A bodily disease, may after all, be but a symptom of some ailment in the spiritual part.
The Scarlet Letter Ch. 10

Sir John Hawton 1904–82
British politician

The British Government have announced that they intend to establish a comprehensive Health Service for everyone in the country.
Statement in 1944

William Hay 1695–1755

A man, that cannot shine in his Person, will have recourse to his Understanding.
Essay on Deformity

William Hazlitt 1778–1830
British writer

Death is the greatest evil, because it cuts off hope.
Characteristics 35

No young man believes he shall ever die.
The Monthly Magazine March (1827)

The most rational cure after all for the inordinate fear of death is to set a just value on life.
Table Talk 'On the Fear of Death'

When a thing ceases to be a subject of controversy, it ceases to be a subject of interest.
The Atlas 31 January, (1830) 'The Spirit of Controversy'

Ali ibn-Hazm 994–1064
Arab theologian of Persian descent

No one is moved to act, or resolves to speak a single word, who does not hope by means of this action or word to release anxiety from his spirit.
Epistle on the to Apply to Souls Sect. 1

R. J. ('Bill') Heald 1936–
Professor of Colorectal Surgery, Basingstoke, UK

There can be little doubt that the ongoing laparoscopic revolution remains the largest stimulus to the refinement of surgical instrumentation the world has yet experienced.
Foreword to *Laparoscopic Colorectal Surgery* S. Wexner (ed). Wiley-Liss, New York (1999)

William Heberden 1710–1801
English physician, London

There is one ailment in the chest which has difficult and peculiar symptoms. It should be heeded, as it is neither free of danger nor particularly uncommon. Its localisation, the patient's feeling of suffocation, and the anguish accompanying it, give reason for calling it angina pectoris.
Lecture at the Royal College of Physicians 'Some Account of a Disorder of the Breast' July (1768)

The love of life, or fear of death, makes most men unwilling to allow that their constitution is breaking; and for this reason they are ready to impute to any other cause what in reality are the signs of approaching and unavoidable decay.
Commentaries on the History and Cure of Diseases Ch. 9 (1802)

The signs of a stone in the bladder are, great and frequent irritations to make water, a stoppage in the middle of making it and a pain with heat just after it is made.
Commentaries on the History and Cure of Diseases Ch. 16 (1802)

The hemicrania, or pain of one half of the head, was very early distinguished by medical writers from the other species of headaches: but we have not yet advanced much in knowing how this differs from other pains of the head.
Commentaries on the History and Cure of Diseases Ch. 17 (1802)

A violent itching of the skin without any eruption is familiar to the jaundice, and adds sometimes to the discomforts of old age.
Commentaries on the History and Cure of Diseases Ch. 23 (1802)

The epilepsy may be called the reproach of physicians as well as the gout; for it was well known before the writing of the most ancient medical books, and yet no certain method of cure has been discovered.
Commentaries on the History and Cure of Diseases Ch. 33 (1802)

A bad state of health is often joined with a fistula in ano, and the mischief, after the cure of the ulcer, has many times fallen upon other parts, and particularly the lungs, and has brought on asthmas, spittings of blood, and consumptions.
Commentaries on the History and Cure of Diseases Ch. 40 (1802)

Consumptive women readily conceive, and during their pregnancy the progress of the consumption seems to be suspended.
Commentaries on the History and Cure of Diseases Ch. 43 (1802)

Women during the state of pregnancy, and just after the menses have finally left them, are peculiarly subject to the piles.
Commentaries on the History and Cure of Diseases Ch. 44 (1802)

In affections of the liver, haemorrhoidal bleedings are very common.
Commentaries on the History and Cure of Diseases (1802)

Swellings of the ankles or legs towards evening, which vanish, or are greatly lessened in the morning, are very common in women while they are breeding, and in hot weather.
Commentaries on the History and Cure of Diseases Ch. 48 (1802)

The globus hystericus in the throat is scarcely ever heard of among men, but is one of the most familiar symptoms with hysteric women.
Commentaries on the History and Cure of Diseases Ch. 49 (1802)

The rheumatism is a common name for many aches and pains, which have yet got no peculiar appellation, though owing to very different causes.
Commentaries on the History and Cure of Diseases Ch. 79 (1802)

Hebrew proverbs

Adultery brings on early old age.

Do not dwell in a city whose governor is a physician.

Honour a physician before thou has need of him.

'Ben Hecht 1894–1964
US Jewish writer

Despite all our toil and progress, the art of medicine still falls somewhere between trout casting and spook writing.
Miracle of the Fifteen Murderers

Doctors have a sense for things unseen and complications unstated.
Miracle of the Fifteen Murderers

The talent for secrecy is highly developed among doctors who, even with nothing to conceal, are often as close mouthed as old-fashioned bomb throwers on their way to a rendezvous.
Miracle of the Fifteen Murderers

Lorenz Heister 1683–1758
German professor of surgery

In every surgical intervention, one should prefer the method which can be used with few and simple instruments, over that which requires a big apparatus difficult to work with: most tools have been invented out of pomposity rather than utility.
Chirurgerie 1752

Hermann von Helmholtz 1821–94
German physicist and physician

I have make a discovery during my lectures on the Physiology of the Sense-organs, which may be of the utmost importance in ophthalmology.
Letter to his father, 17 December (1850)

The great joy of being the first to see a living human retina.
Helmholtz reporting his discovery

Burton Jesse Hendrick 1870–1949
US writer

The consultant's first obligation is to his patient, not his brother physician.

John Hendy 1948–
English barrister

I noticed early on that our National Health Service seemed to spend inordinate time and resources in displaying a standard and style of industrial relations which were quite unique in their inept insensitivity and arrogant incompetence.
Foreword to *Whistleblowing in the Health Service* Geoffrey Hunt (ed.). Edward Arnold, London (1995)

William Ernest Henley 1849–1903
English poet and playwright

And lo, The Hospital, grey, quiet, old, Where Life and Death like friendly chafferers meet.
In Hospital 'Enter Patient'

Henry IV 1553–1610
King of France

Great eaters and great sleepers are incapable of anything else that is great.
Attributed

O. Henry (William Sydney Porter)
1862–1910
US writer

Life is made up of sobs, sniffles, and smiles, with sniffles predominating.
The Gifts of the Magi

Sir Alan Patrick Herbert (AP)
1890–1971
English writer, barrister, and politician
I love the doctors, they are dears,
But must they spend such years and years
Investigating such a lot

Of illnesses that no one's got?
Doctors in Science and Society: Essays of a Clinical Scientist p. 316, Christopher C. Booth. British Medical Journal Publications (1987)

George Herbert 1593–1633
English clergyman and poet

A good digestion turneth all to health.
The Temple 'The Church Porch' (1633)

Oliver Herford 1863–1935
English writer and illustrator

A hair in the head is worth two in the brush.
Attributed

Herodotus 484–424 BC
Greek historian

They have no physicians, but when a man is ill they lay him in the public square, and the passersby come up to him, and if they have ever had his disease themselves or have known anyone who has suffered from it, they give him advice, recommending to do whatever they found good in their own case, or in the case known to them. And no-one is allowed to pass the sick man in silence without asking him what his ailment is.
Attributed

Medicine with them is distributed in the following way; every physician is for one disease and not for several, and the whole country is full of physicians of the eyes; others of the head; others of the teeth; others of the belly; and others of obscure diseases.
On Egyptian Medicine

Dreams in general originate from those incidents which have most occupied the thoughts during the day.
Histories VII. 16 (transl. William Beloe)

Death is a delightful hiding place for weary men.
Histories VII. 46

Don Herold 1889–1966
US writer and cartoonist

Doctors think a lot of patients are cured who have simply quit in disgust.
Penguin Dictionary of Modern Humorous Quotations p. 84, Fred Metcalf. Penguin Books, London (2001)

Herophilus c.280 BC
Alexandrian physician and philosopher

Wisdom and art, strength and wealth, are of no avail if health be lacking.
Sextus Empiricus in Adversus Ethicus XI.50

The best physician is he who can distinguish the possible from the impossible.
Sextus Empiricus in Adversus Ethicus XI.50

Charles Judson Herrick 1868–1960
US anatomist and comparative neurologist

You don't grow old; when you cease to grow, you are old.

James B. Herrick 1861–1954
US Professor of Medicine, Chicago

The doctor may also learn more about the illness from the way the patient tells the story than from the story itself.
Memoirs of Eighty Years Ch. VIII

A study of past American history should cause the medical profession of today to fear the politicians even though they offer gifts.
Memoirs of Eighty Years Ch. VIII

Robert Herrick 1591–1674
English poet

Against diseases here the strongest fence
Is the defensive vertue, abstinence.
Hesperides 'Abstinence'

'Tis the Surgeons praise, and height of Art,
Not to cut off, but cure the vicious part.
Hesperides 'Lenitie'

Christian A. Herter 1865–1910
US neurologist, New York

I like to think of medicine in our day as an ever broadening and deepening river, fed by the limpid streams of pure science.
Address to the College of Physicians and Surgeons, Columbia University (1909)

Sir Austin Bradford Hill 1895–1991
British epidemiologist and statistician

Why did you start, what did you do, what answer did you get, and what does it mean anyway? That is a logical order for a scientific paper.
Attributed

Wayne Hill
Contemporary English journalist

Hospitals are always touted as designed for our superior care, but they actually exist for the convenience of doctors.
Shakespeare's Insults for Doctors p. 21. Ebury Press (1996)

If art outruns science at any point in medical practice, diagnosis is where it happens.
Shakespeare's Insults for Doctors p.39. Ebury Press (1996)

Specialisation is proof of how far medicine has skidded off the path.
Shakespeare's Insults for Doctors p. 57 Ebury Press (1996)

It lets them abandon heaps of medical expertise to sluggish ignorance in the way farmers dump excess production to keep prices up. That is the genius of specialisation; an ability to claim general non-knowledge.
Shakespeare's Insults for Doctors p. 21 Ebury Press (1996)

William Hillary 1697–1763
English physician, clinical scientist, and traveller

It is by this method of reasoning from data, founded upon observations and real facts, that the healing art must be improved and brought to a state of perfection.
Doctors in Science and Society, Essays of a Clinical Scientist p. 80. Christopher C. Booth. British Medical Journal Publications (1987)

Hindu proverbs

Ask the patient not the doctor where the pain is.

Even nectar is poison if taken to excess.

In illness the physician is a father; in convalescence, a friend; when health is restored, he is a guardian.

Walking makes for a long life.

John M. Hinton 1935–
British gastroenterologist

The dissatisfied dead cannot noise abroad the negligence they have received.
The physical and mental distress of the dying. *Quarterly Journal of Medicine* **32**: 21 (1963)

Hippocrates 460–357 BC
Greek physician

Life is short, the art long, opportunity fleeting, experience treacherous, judgement difficult.
Aphorisms I

Extreme remedies are most appropriate for extreme diseases.
Aphorisms I

When sleep puts an end to delirium, it is a good symptom.
Aphorisms II.2

Drinking strong wine cures hunger.
Aphorisms II.21 (transl. Francis Adams)

It is better that a fever succeed to a convulsion, than a convulsion to a fever.
Aphorisms II.26

When a person who is recovering from a disease has a good appetite, but his body does not improve in conditions, it is a bad symptom.
Aphorisms II.31 (transl. Francis Adams)

Sleep and watchfulness, both of them, when immoderate, constitute disease.
Aphorisms II

Old people, on the whole, have fewer complaints than young; but those chronic diseases which do befall them generally never leave them.
Aphorisms II.39

Persons who have had frequent and severe attacks of swooning, without any manifest cause, die suddenly.
Aphorisms II.41

Persons who are naturally very fat are apt to die earlier than those who are slender.
Aphorisms II.44

Sneezing coming on, in the case of a person afflicted with hiccup, removes the hiccup.
Aphorisms VI.13

Opposites are cures for opposites.
Breaths I

Science is the father of knowledge, but opinion breeds ignorance.
The Canon Law IV

In order to prognosticate correctly who will recover and who will die, in whom the days will be long, in whom short, one must know all the symptoms, and must weigh their relative value.
Corpus Hippocraticum

He who desires to practice surgery must go to war.
Corpus Hippocraticum

A great part, I believe, of the Art is to be able to observe.
Corpus Hippocraticum

Leave nothing to chance, overlook nothing; combine contradictory observations and allow yourself enough time.
Corpus Hippocraticum

I will not use the knife, not even on the sufferers from stone, but will withdraw in favour of such men as are engaged in this work.
Corpus Hippocraticum

As to diseases, make a habit of two things; to help or at least not to harm.
Corpus Hippocraticum

A physician who is a lover of wisdom is the equal to a god.
Decorum, V

Foolish the doctor who despises the knowledge acquired by the ancients.
Entering the world (M. Odent)

Use strengthens, disuse debilitates.
In the Surgery XX (transl. E. T. Witherington)

And whatsoever I shall see or hear in the course of my profession, as well as outside my profession in my intercourse with men, if it be what should not be published abroad, I will never divulge holding such things to be holy secret.
The Hippocratic Oath

Declare the past, diagnose the present, foretell the future.
Epidemics

The art has three factors, the disease, the patient, and the physician. The physician is the servant of the art. The patient must co-operate with the physician in combating the disease.
Epidemics I

Natural forces are the healers of disease.
Epidemics VI

The wasting of the brain which leads to baldness.
Epidemics VI.iii.1

What drugs fail to cure, that the knife cures not, that the fire cures; this must be called incurable.
The Oath (transl. Edelstein)

I will neither give a deadly drug to anybody if asked for it, nor will I make a suggestion to this effect.
The Oath

Healing is a matter of time, but it is sometimes a matter of opportunity.
Precepts I

So do not concentrate your attention on fixing what your fee is to be. A worry of this nature is likely to harm the patient, particularly if the disease be an acute one. Hold fast to reputation rather than profit.
Precepts I

Whenever therefore a man suffers from an ill which is too strong for the means at the disposal of medicine, he surely must not even expect that it can be overcome by medicine.
The Art VIII

Sometimes give your services for nothing. And if there be an opportunity of serving one who is a stranger in financial straits, give full assistance to all such. For where there is love of man, there is also love of the art.
The Art VI

Physicians who meet in consultation must never quarrel, or jeer at one another.
The Art VIII

Fat people who want to reduce should take their exercise on an empty stomach and sit down to their food out of breath...Thin people who want to get fat should do exactly the opposite and never take exercise on an empty stomach.
A Regimen for Health IV (transl. John Chadwick and W.N. Mann)

A wise man ought to realise that health is his most valuable possession.
A Regimen for Health IX (transl. John Chadwick and W.N. Mann)

The physician must have a worthy appearance; he should look healthy and be well-nourished, appropriate to his physique; for most people are of the opinion that those physicians who are not tidy in their own persons cannot look after others well.
Attributed

The natural healing force within us is the greatest force in getting well.
Attributed

To teach them this Art, if they shall wish to learn it, without fee or stipulation, and that by precept, lecture, and every other mode of instruction, I will impart a knowledge of the Art.
Attributed

Russell Hoban 1925–

US writer and illustrator

When you suffer an attack of nerves you're being attacked by the nervous system. What chance has a man got against a system?
The Lion of Boaz-Jachin and Jachin-Boaz Ch. 13

Eric Hodgins 1899–1971
US writer and editor

A miracle drug is any drug that will do what the label says it will do.
> *Episode*

Stanley O. Hoerr 1909–

It is difficult to make the asymptomatic patient feel better.
> *American Journal of Surgery* **103**: 411 (1962)

The surgeon is a man of action. By temperament and by training he prefers to serve the sick by operating on them, and he inwardly commiserates with a patient so unfortunate as to have a disease not suited to surgical treatment.
> *American Journal of Surgery* **103**: 411 (1962)

Samuel Goodman Hoffenstein
1890–1947
Lithuanian-born US humorous poet and writer

Babies haven't any hair:
Old men's heads are just as bare;
From the cradle to the grave
Lies a haircut and a shave.
> *Poems in Praise of Practically Nothing* 'Songs of Faith in the Year after Next' (1928)

Friederich Hoffman 1660–1742
German physician

Many severe diseases result from a hereditary disposition.
> *Fundamenta medicinae* (1695)

Any climate and any age, and each sex, has its special diseases.
> *Fundamenta medicinae* (1695)

Oliver Wendell Holmes 1809–94
US humorist and physician

The truth is, that medicine, professedly found on observation, is as sensitive to outside influences, political, religious, philosophical, imaginative, as is the barometer to the changes of atmospheric density.
> *Medical Essays* 'Current and Counter-Currents in Medical Science'

The solemn scepticism of science has replaced the sneering doubts of witty philosophers.
> *Medical Essays* 'Current and Counter-Currents in Medical Science'

No families take so little medicine as those of doctors, except those of apothecaries.
> *Medical Essays* 'Current and Counter-Currents in Medical Science'

Homeopathy . . . a mingled mass of perverse ingenuity, of tinsel erudition, of imbecile credulity, and artful misrepresentation.
> *Medical Essays* 'Homeopathy and its Kindred Delusions'

So long as the body is affected through the mind, no audacious device, even of the most manifestly dishonest character, can fail of producing occasional good to those who yield it an implicit or even a partial faith.
> *Medical Essays* 'Homeopathy and its Kindred Delusions'

A man of very moderate ability may be a good physician, if he devotes himself faithfully to his work.
> *Medical Essays* 'Scholastic and Bedside Teaching'

The most essential part of a student's instruction is obtained, as I believe, not in the lecture room, but at the bedside.
> *Medical Essays* 'Scholastic and Bedside Teaching'

I would never use a long word where a short one would answer the purpose. I know there are professors in this country who 'ligate' arteries. Other surgeons only tie them, and it stops the bleeding just as well.
> *Medical Essays* 'Scholastic and Bedside Teaching'

The best a physician can give is never too good for the patient.
> *Medical Essays* 'Scholastic and Bedside Teaching'

The bedside is always the true centre of medical teaching.
> *Medical Essays* 'Scholastic and Bedside Teaching'

Three natural anaesthetics . . . sleep, fainting, death.
> *Medical Essays* 'The Medical Profession in Massachussets'

What I call a good patient is one who, having found a good physician, sticks to him till he dies.
> *Medical Essays* 'The Young Practitioner'

Let me recommend you, as far as possible, to keep your doubts to yourself, and give the patient the benefit of your decision.
> *Medical Essays* 'The Young Practitioner'

The lawyers are the cleverest men, the ministers are the most learned, and the doctors are the most sensible.
> *The Poet at the Breakfast Table* Sect. V

Truth is the breath of life to human society. It is the food of the immortal spirit. Yet a single word of it may kill a man as suddenly as a drop of prussic acid.
> Valedictory Address, Harvard Commencement, 10 March (1858)

To be seventy years young is sometimes far more cheerful and hopeful than to be forty years old.
> Letter to Julia Ward Howe on her 70th birthday, 27 May (1889)

Doctors are the best-natured people in the world, except when they get fighting each other.
> Attributed

God gave his creatures light and air and water
  open to the skies;
Man locks him in a stifling lair and wonders why
  his brother dies.
> Attributed

It is better for all the world if instead of waiting to execute degenerate offspring for crime or to let them starve for their imbecility, society can prevent those who are manifestly unfit from continuing their kind. The principle that sustains compulsory vaccination is broad enough to cover cutting the Fallopian tubes.

Journal of Heredity **18**: 495 (1927)

Specialised knowledge will do a man no harm if he also has common sense, but if he lacks this, it can only make him more dangerous to his patients.

John Homans 1836–1903
US professor of surgery

I prefer to be called a fool for asking the question, rather than to remain in ignorance.

Boston Medical and Surgical Journal **87**: 1 (1872)

Homer c.850 BC
Greek writer

He hath the flower of youth, wherein is the fullness of strength.

Iliad XIII.484

Sleep and Death, who are twin brothers.

Iliad XVI.681

All deaths are hateful to miserable mortals, but the most pitiable death of all is to starve.

Odyssey VII.215

Earnest Albert Hooton 1887–1954
US anthropologist

Medical science must cease to regard its function as primarily curative and preventive. It must rid itself of its obsession that its chief responsibility is to the individual rather than society.

Apes, Men and Morons Ch. 18 (1937)

James Hope 1801–41
UK physician and cardiologist

In the first place, never keep a patient sick when you can do something for him. In the second place, never take a higher fee than what you truly feel you are entitled to. In the third place, always pray for your patients.

Attributed

Johns Hopkins 1795–1873
Baltimore grocer and founder of a hospital

The indigent sick of this city and its environs, without regard to sex, age or colour, who may require surgical or medical treatment, and who can be received into the Hospital without peril to the other inmates, and the poor of this city and State.

Letter to the first Trustees of the Johns Hopkins Hospital, March (1873)

Horace 65–8 BC
Roman poet

To save a man's life against his will is the same as killing him.

Ars Poetica

Anger is short-lived madness.

Epistles I.ii.62

Remember you must die whether you sit about moping all day long or whether on feast days you stretch out in a green field, happy with a bottle of Falernian (wine) from you innermost cellar.

Odes II.3

Lord Horder 1871–1955
British physician, St. Bartholomews Hospital, London

It is the duty of a doctor to prolong life. It is not his duty to prolong the act of dying.

Speech in House of Lords (1936)

The clinician who relaxes in punctilious attendance at post-mortems . . . is departing from the bed-rock of medicine itself. What he says at the bedside may or not be the truth; what he sees in the post-mortem room is the truth.

Lancet **1**: 178–82 (1936)

Our weakness was partly responsible for the fact that the National Service Act was born in dishonour. Put not your faith in politicians, they come and go, but medicine goes on for ever.

Harley Street p. 182, Reginald Pound. Michael Joseph, London (1967)

Pio de Rio Hortega 1882–1945
Spanish neuroanatomist

Histology is an odd-tasting dish, repulsive as a medicament to students, who must be examined in it, and little liked by physicians who consider their schooling finished. Taken in large quantities under compulsion it is not absorbed, but if tasted in little sips it finally becomes a delight to the palate, and even a cause for addiction.

Article for his students

Russel John Howard 1875–1942
British surgeon, Royal London Hospital, London

The only competent observer is yourself.

Quoted by F. G. St. Clair Strange in *The Hip* Ch. 1

More mistakes are made from want of a proper examination than for any other reason.

Quoted by F. G. St. Clair Strange in *The Hip* Ch. 5

Speed in operating should be the achievement, not the aim, of every surgeon.

Quoted by F. G. St. Clair Strange in *The Hip* Ch. 9

Ed Howe 1853–1937
US writer

After a man is fifty you can fool him by saying he is smart, but you can't fool him by saying he is pretty.

Country Town Sayings

Huai-nan Tze (Liu An) died 122 BC

Doctors cannot cure their own complaints.
  Attributed

Huang Ti c.2600 BC
Yellow Emperor

I have heard that in ancient times the people lived to be over a hundred years old, and yet they remained active and did not become decrepit in their activities.
  Dialogues between the Yellow Emperor (China) and his Prime Minister

All the blood is under control of the heart.
The blood current flows continuously in a circle and never stops.
  Nei Ching Su Wên

The kidneys are like the officials who do energetic work, and they excel through their ability and cleverness.
  Nei Ching Su Wên Bk 3, Sect. 8

The heart is the root of life and causes the versatility of the spiritual faculties.

The heart influences the face and fills the pulse with blood.
  Nei Ching Su Wên Bk 3, Sect. 10

The treatment with poison medicines comes from the West.
  Nei Ching Su Wên BK 3, Sect. 10

Poor medical workmanship is neglectful and careless and must therefore be combatted, because a disease that is not completely cured can easily breed new disease or there can be a relapse of the old disease.
  Nei Ching Su Wên Bk 4, Sect. 13

The most important requirement of the art of healing is that no mistakes or neglect occurs.
  Nei Ching Su Wên Bk 4, Sect. 13

Elbert G. Hubbard 1859–1915
US author and editor

Little minds are interested in the extraordinary; great minds in the commonplace.
  Roycroft Dictionary and Book of Epigrams

Insomnia never comes to a man who has to get up exactly at six o'clock.
Insomnia troubles only those who can sleep any time.
  The Philistine, 'In Re Muldoon'

A merry heart doeth good like a medicine: but a broken spirit drieth the bones.
  Proverbs 17: 22

Frank (Kin) Hubbard 1868–1930
US humorist and journalist

Some people are so sensitive they feel snubbed if an epidemic overlooks them.
  Abe Martin's Broadcast

Henry Huchard 1844–1910
Parisian physician

Gout is to the arteries what rheumatism is to the heart.
  Lancet **1**: 164 (1967) (quoted by D. Evan Bedford)

Christoph Wilhelm Hufeland 1762–1836
German professor of medicine

Someone may be perfectly rational, yet commit manslaughter, adultery, theft: he will easily find a physician who testifies that the action must be credited to temporary insanity.
  Neue Auswahl kleiner medizinischen Schriften I (1834)

The physician must generalise the disease, and individualise the patient.
  Quoted by Oliver Wendell Holmes in *Medical Essays* 'Border Lines in Medical Science'

Patricia Hughes
Contemporary British psychiatrist and educationalist

While we need to maintain diversity of skills and personality, there are some characteristics which we demand in any doctor. Enough intellectual ability to do the job, plus honesty, integrity and conscientiousness, must be at the heart of good practice.
  Journal of the Royal Society of Medicine **95**: 18–20 (2002)

Victor Hugo 1802–85
French writer

If we must suffer, let us suffer nobly.
  Contemplations 'Les Malheureux'

Indigestion is charged by God with enforcing morality on the stomach.
  Les Misérables 'Fantine', Bk III, Ch. 7

The misery of a child is interesting to a mother, the misery of a young man is interesting to a young woman, the misery of an old man is interesting to nobody.
  Les Misérables 'Saint Denis'

David Hume 1711–76
Scottish philosopher and political economist

It appears to me that apothecaries bear the same relation to physicians, that priests do to philosophers; the ignorance of the former makes them positive, and dogmatical, and assuming, and enterprising, and pretending, and consequently much more taking with the people.
  Letter to John Clephane, 18 February (1751)

What we call a mind is nothing but a heap or collection of different perceptions, united together by certain relations, and suppos'd, tho' falsely, to be endow'd with a perfect simplicity and identity.
  A Treatise of Human Nature Bk I, Pt IV, Sect. 2

William Humphreys
Contemporary Welsh vascular surgeon

Surgery is an art, and the best way to teach an art is an apprenticeship system. The longer the apprenticeship the better.
Hospital Doctor 14 October (1999)

Sir George Murray Humphry 1820–96
English professor of surgery

In surgery, eyes first and most; fingers next and little; tongue last and least.
Attributed

Hunayn ibd Ishaq AD 808–73
Baghdad physician

I have already told the Ruler of the Faithful that my art must be used only for the good of the people.
The Illustrated History of Surgery Knut Haeger (1988)

Geoffrey Hunt
Contemporary British ethicist

Health care professionals who always took the service ethic and clinical autonomy for granted now find that they have to speak out to defend it in the face of forces which appear to have little to do with any ethic whatsoever.
Introduction to *Whistleblowing in the Health Service* Geoffrey Hunt (ed.). Edward Arnold, London (1995)

James Henry Leigh Hunt 1784–1859
English poet and essayist

The ground-work of all happiness is health.
The Indicator No. XXXI, 'On the Realities of the Imagination'

James M. Hunter 1924–
US physician

Treat the patient, not the Xray.
Address to the American Fracture Association, October (1964)

John Hunter 1728–93
British surgeon and scientist

I believe your solution is right, but why believe? Why not make an experiment?
Letter to Edward Jenner about his new vaccine for smallpox

The stomach is the distinguishing part between an animal and a vegetable; for we do not know any vegetable that has a stomach nor any animal without one.
Principles of Surgery Ch. V

The operation is a silent confession of the surgeon's inadequacy.
Attributed

By an acquaintance with principles we learn the cause of disease. Without this knowledge a man cannot be a surgeon.
Attributed

When I was a boy I wanted to know all about the clouds and the grasses and why the leaves changed colour in the autumn.
Quoted in the Hunterian Museum, Royal College of Surgeons of England

Nothing in nature stands alone.
Quoted in the Hunterian Museum, Royal College of Surgeons of England

The last part of surgery, namely operations, is a reflection of the healing art; it is a tacit acknowledgement of the insufficiency of surgery. It is like an armed savage who attempts to get that by force which a civilised man would by stratagem.
Attributed

William Hunter 1718–83
British surgeon, anatomist, and religious philosopher

Were I to place a man of proper talents, in the most direct road for becoming truly great in his profession, I would choose a good practical Anatomist and put him into a large hospital to attend the sick and dissect the dead.
Last Course of Anatomical Lectures Lect. 2

Most philosophers, most great men, most anatomists, and most other men of eminence lie like the devil.
Attributed

Sir Robert Hutchison 1871–1960
Physician, the London Hospital, UK and President Royal College of Physicians

Vegetarianism is harmless enough though it is apt to fill a man with wind and self-righteousness.
Address to the British Medical Association, Winnipeg (1930)

It is always well, before handing the cup of knowledge to the young, to wait until the froth has settled.
British Medical Journal **1**: 995 (1925)

It is unnecessary—perhaps dangerous—in medicine to be too clever.
Lancet **2**: 61 (1938)

The scientific truth may be put quite briefly; eat moderately, having an ordinary mixed diet, and don't worry.
Newcastle Medical Journal Vol. 12 (1932)

From inability to let well alone; from too much zeal for the new and contempt for what is old; from putting knowledge before wisdom, science before art, and cleverness before common sense, from treating patients as cases, and from making the cure of the disease more grievous than the endurance of the same, Good Lord, deliver us.
British Medical Journal **1**: 671 (1953)

Sir Julian Huxley 1887–1975
British biologist and author

The human race will be the cancer of the planet.
Attributed

Evolution is the most powerful and the most comprehensive idea that has ever arisen on Earth.
Attributed

Thomas Huxley 1825–1925
British biologist

I asserted – and I repeat – that a man has no reason to be ashamed of having an ape for his grandfather.
Speech, 30 June (1860) replying to Bishop Samuel Wilberforce at the Association for the Advancement of Science in Oxford, 30 June (1860)

It is an error to imagine that evolution signifies a constant tendency to increased perfection.
Social Diseases and Worse Remedies 'The Struggle for Existence in Human Society'

If he is to allowed to let his children go unvaccinated, he might as well be allowed to leave strychnine lozenges about in the way of mine.
Method and Results 'Administrative Nihilism'

Irrationally held truths may be more harmful than reasoned errors.
Darwiniana 'The Coming of Age of the Origin of Species'

Félix Martí-Ibáñez 1915–
US microbiologist and medical historian

The physician must have a thorough knowledge of the history of the world and of the society in which he lives, and he must also know the links between the past and his present duties. For without history nothing has a full meaning
Ariel 'The Fabric and Creation of a Dream'

The history of medicine is a study not only of man's health and diseases throughout history but also the history of all human activities connected directly or indirectly with the pursuits of medicine.
Ariel 'The Fabric and Creation of a Dream'

Henrik Ibsen 1828–1906
Norwegian playwright

Oh, one soon makes friends with invalids; and I need so much to have someone to live for.
Hedda Gabler Act IV

Ivan Illich 1926–
Austrian-born social philosopher and activist

The medicalization of early diagnosis not only hampers and discourages preventative health-care but it also trains the patient-to-be to function in the meantime as an acolyte to his doctor. He learns to depend on the physician in sickness and in health. He turns into a life-long patient.
Medical Nemesis

Healthy people need no bureaucratic interference to mate, give birth, share the human condition and die.
Medical Nemesis

To give the lower class greater access to health care would only equalize the delivery of professional illusions and torts.
Medical Nemesis p. 242

The medical establishment has become a major threat to health.
Limits to Medicine (1976)

Indian proverbs

Bathe every day and sickness will avoid you.

Physicians live by rich patients, officials by unlucky princes, princes by litigants, and clever men by fools.

Indian (Kashmiri) proverb

Until a physician has killed one or two he is not a physician.

Indian (Tamil) proverbs

Domestic medicine is preferable to that of a physician.

Hospitality and medicine must be confined to three days.

William Ralph Inge 1860–1954
British churchman

Man as we know him is a poor creature; but he is halfway between an ape and a god and he is travelling in the right direction.
Outspoken Essays: Second Series 'Confessio Fidei'

Robert G. Ingersoll 1833–99
US lawyer, writer, and agnostic

Reason, Observation, and Experience—the Holy Trinity of Science.
The Gods

Many people think they have religion when they are troubled with dyspepsia.
Liberty of Man, Woman and Child Sect. 3

Dwight J. Ingle 1907–

Science cannot be equated to measurement, although many contemporary scientists behave as though it can. For example, the editorial policies of many scientific journals support the publication of data and exclude the communication of ideas.
Principles of Research in Biology and Medicine Ch. 1

Irish Proverbs

A good laugh and a long sleep are the best cures in the doctor's book.

A long disease does not tell a lie; it kills at last.

Death is the poor man's best physician.

Hope is the physician of each misery.

The silliest charm gives more comfort to
thousands in sorrow and pain
Than they will ever get from the knowledge that
proves it foolish and vain.

What butter and whiskey will not cure, there is no
cure for.

St. Isidore of Seville 560–636
Spanish ecclesiastic

The physician ought to know literature, to be able
to understand or to explain what he reads.
   Etymologiae IV

Italian proverbs

Bed is a medicine.

Health without wealth is half a sickness.

If the patient dies, it is the doctor who has killed
him, and if he gets well, it is the saints who have
cured him.

When children are little they make our heads
ache; when grown, our hearts.

With respect to the gout, the physician is but a lout.

Chevalier Jackson 1865–1958
US laryngologist

All that wheezes is not asthma.
   Boston Medical Quarterly 16: 86 (1965)

In teaching the medical student the primary
requisite is to keep him awake.
   The Life of Chevalier Jackson Ch. 16 (1938)

Thomas (Stonewall) Jackson 1824–63
US Statesman

I like liquor – its taste and its effects – and that is
just the reason why I never drink it.
   Quoted by William Jones in *The Life and Letters of Robert
   Edward Lee, Soldier and Man* p. 443

Mary Corinna Puttnam Jacobi
1842–1906
US physician and social reformer, New York

Nature does not kill and does not heal. If there
were consciousness in Nature, she would feel
indifferent about what she is, viz., mere evolution.
   Medical Proverbs by F. H. Garrison, *Bulletin of the New York
   Academy of Medicine* October, 979–1005 (1928)

The magnetic needle of professional rectitude
should, in spite of occasional deviations, always
point in the direction of pity and humanity.
   Medical Proverbs by F. H. Garrison, *Bulletin of the New York
   Academy of Medicine* October, 979–1005 (1928)

Werner Jaeger 1888–1961
German classical scholar

In classical times, more than at any other period
until a few decades ago, the doctor was more
concerned with healthy people than with invalids.
   Paidea Vol. III

James I 1566–1625
King of England and Scotland

A custom loathsome to the eye, hateful to the
nose, harmful to the brain, dangerous to the lungs.
   A Counterblast to Tobacco

William James 1842–1910
US psychologist

I take it that no man is educated who has never
dallied with the thought of suicide.
   Attributed

Pierre Marie Janet 1859–1947
French professor of psychology, Sorbonne, Paris

If a patient is poor he is committed to a public
hospital as 'psychotic'; if he can afford the luxury
of a private sanitarium, he is put there with the
diagnosis of 'neuroasthenia'; if he is wealthy
enough to be isolated in his own home under
constant watch of nurses and physicians he is
simply an indisposed 'eccentric'.
   Strength and Psychological Debility (La Force et la faibless
   psychologiques)

Japanese proverbs

Better go without medicine than call in an
unskilful physician.

Diseases enter by the mouth.

Every man carries a parasite somewhere.

First the man takes a drink, then the drink takes a
drink, then the drink takes the man.

Good medicine always has a bitter taste.

Randall Jarrell 1914–65
US author

One of the most obvious facts about grown-ups to
a child is that they have forgotten what it is like to
be a child.
   Third book of Criticism

DeForest Clinton Jarvis 1881–?

It is a lot harder to keep people well than it is to
just get them over a sickness.
   Atlantic Monthly June (1939)

Karl Jaspers 1883–1969
German philosopher

The anxiety affects the body. In spite of increasing
longevity, the growing feeling of insecurity is
unmistakable.
   Die geistige Situation der Zeit Pt 1, Ch.3

Thomas Jefferson 1743–1826
US president and philosopher

The office of surgeon has been considered as on a footing with that of chaplain, and the administering of medicine to be as inoffensive as giving religious instruction to those with whom we are contending.
Letter to Philip Turpin, 29 July (1783)

If the body be feeble, the mind will not be strong.
Letter to Thomas M. Randolph Jr, 27 August (1786)

Not less than two hours a day should be devoted to bodily exercise.
Letter to Thomas M. Randolph Jr, 27 August (1786)

The art of life is the art of avoiding pain.
Letter to Maria Cosway, 12 October (1786)

Idleness begets ennui, ennui the hypochondriac, and that a diseased body. No laborious person was ever yet hysterical.
Letter to Martha Jefferson, 28 March (1787)

The most uninformed mind with a healthy body, is happier than the wisest valetudinarian.
Letter to Thomas M. Randolph Jr, 6 July (1787)

Health is the first requisite after morality.
Letter to Peter Carr, 10 August (1787)

Yours is the comfortable reflection that mankind can never forget that you have lived. Future nations will know by history only that the loathsome smallpox has existed and by you has been extirpated.
Letter to Dr Edward Jenner, 14 May (1806)

The only sure foundations of medicine are an intimate knowledge of the human body and observation on the effects of medicinal substances on that.
Letter to Dr Caspar Wistar, 21 June (1807)

The natural course of the human mind is certainly from credulity to scepticism.
Letter to Dr Caspar Wistar, 21 June (1807)

The adventurous physician goes on, and substitutes presumption for knowledge.
Letter to Dr Caspar Wistar, 21 June (1807)

I wish to see this beverage (beer) become common instead of the whiskey which kills one-third of our citizens and ruins their families.
Letter to Col. Charles Yancey, 6 January (1816)

Bodily decay is gloomy in prospect, but of all human contemplations the most abhorrent is body without mind.
Letter to John Adams, 1 August (1816)

We never repent of having eaten too little.
Letter to Thomas Jefferson Smith, 21 February (1825)

Edward Jenner 1749–1823
English country physician

The deviation of man from the state in which he was originally placed by nature seems to have proved to him a prolific source of disease.
An Inquiry into the Causes and Effects of the Variolae Vaccinae, or Cow-Pox

To have admitted the truth of a doctrine at once so novel and so unlike anything that ever had appeared in the annals of medicine, without the test of the most rigid scrutiny, would have bordered upon temerity.
An Inquiry into the Causes and Effects of the Variolae Vaccinae, or Cow-Pox

Sir William Jenner 1815–98
English physician and pathologist

Never believe what a patient tells you his doctor has said.
Attributed

Jerome K. Jerome 1859–1927
British humorist

We drink one another's health and spoil our own.
Idle Thoughts of an Idle Fellow, 'On Eating and Drinking'

Love is like the measles, we all have to go through it.
Idle Thoughts of an Idle Fellow, 'On Being in Love'

I never read a patent medicine advertisement without being impelled to the conclusion that I am suffering from the particular disease therein dealt with in its most virulent form.
Three Men in a Boat Ch. 1

William Stanley Jevons 1835–82
English economist and logician

So-called original research is now regarded as a profession, adopted by hundreds of men, and communicated by a system of training.
The Principles of Science Ch. XXVI (1874)

Jewish proverb

God could not be everywhere and therefore he made mothers.

John of Arderne 1307–80
English surgeon and father of colorectal surgery

A bubo is a tumour developing within the anus in the rectum – of great hardness but little aching.
Treatises of Fistula-in-ano D'Arcy Power. Oxford University Press (1910)

I have never seen, nor have I ever heard of anyone who could be cured of the bubo.
Treatises of Fistula-in-ano D'Arcy Power. Oxford University Press, Oxford (1910)

Sir Elton John 1947–
British rock singer

There's nothing wrong with going to bed with somebody of your own sex. People should be very free with sex – they should draw the line at goats.
Attributed

Samuel Johnson 1709–84
English lexicographer and writer

We palliate what we cannot cure.
Dictionary of the English Language (1755)

I know not that by living dissections any discovery has been made by which a single malady is more easily cured.
The Idler No. 17, 5 August (1758)

Those who do not feel pain seldom think that it is felt.
The Rambler No. 48, 1 September (1750)

Hope is necessary in every condition. The miseries of poverty, sickness, of captivity, would, without this comfort, be insupportable
The Rambler No. 67

The last direction is the principal; with an unquiet mind, neither exercise, nor diet, nor physick can be of much use.
Life of Samuel Johnson by James Boswell.

Visitors are no proper companions in the chamber of sickness.
Letter to Mrs Henry Thrale, 27 December (1783)

It is a man's own fault, it is from want of use, if his mind grows turgid in old age.
Attributed

Don't think of retiring from the world until the world will be sorry that you retire.
Attributed

Peter F. Jones 1920–
Professor of Surgery, Aberdeen, Scotland

It is the nature of emergency surgery that however clear the diagnosis may appear to be, one can never be certain of what will be found, or of the correctness of one's decisions, or of one's ability to cope with the unexpected.
Emergency Abdominal Surgery, Introduction. Chapman & Hall, London (1998)

Ben Jonson 1572–1637
English dramatist

When men a dangerous disease did scape,
Of old, they gave a cock to Aesculape.
Epigrammes

Many funerals discredit a physician.
Attributed

Isaac Judaeus *c.* AD 850–950
Baghdad physician

(Abu Ya'qub Is-haq Sulayman al-Israeli) Most illnesses are cured without the physician's help through the aid of Nature. If you can cure the patient by dietary means, do not turn to drugs.
Attributed

D. G. Julian 1925–
Professor of Medicine, Newcastle, UK

Diseases of the heart and circulation predominate as causes of morbidity and death in the developed parts of the world, and are becoming of increasing importance in developing countries.
Preface to *Diseases of the Heart*. Ballière Tindall, London (1989)

C. G. Jung 1875–1961
Austrian psychoanalyst

Show me a sane man and I will cure him for you.
Attributed

The separation of psychology from the premises of biology is purely artificial, because the human psyche lives in indissoluble union with the body.
Factors Determining Human Behaviour

Every form of addiction is bad, no matter whether the narcotic be alcohol or morphine or idealism.
Memories, Dreams, Reflections Ch. 12

It is indeed high time for the clergyman and the psychotherapist to join forces.
Modern Man in Search of a Soul Ch. 1

Ernst Jünger 1895–?
German novelist

Evolution is far more important than living.
The Rebel Ch. 3 (Albert Camus)

Juvenal *c.* AD 60–130
Roman satirist

Your prayer must be for a sound mind in a sound body (Mens sana in corpore sano).
Satires X

Kahun Papyrus 1900 BC

Knowledge of a woman whose back aches, and the inside of her thighs are painful. Say to her, it is the falling of the womb.
Attributed

Harold A. Kaminetzky 1923–
US gynaecologist

There are no really 'safe' biologically active drugs. There are only 'safe' physicians.
Obstetrics and Gynecology **21**: 512 (1963)

Immanuel Kant 1724–1804
German Philosopher

Physicians think they do a lot for a patient when they give his disease a name.
Attributed

But it is wisdom that has the merit of selecting from among the innumerable problems which present themselves, those whose solution is important to mankind.
Attributed

Helen Singer Kaplan
Contemporary US clinical associate professor of psychiatry

Throughout history, until just a few years ago, the human sexual response was seen monistically, as a single event that passed from lust to excitement and was climaxed by orgasm.
Disorders of Sexual Desire. Ballière Tindall, London (1979)

John Keats 1795–1821
English poet

Now more than ever seems it rich to die,
To cease upon the midnight with no pain.
Ode to Nightingale St. 6 (1820)

Harry Keen

Professor of Human Metabolism, Guy's Hospital, London

Medicine has been caught up like all other human activities in the technological revolution of the last hundred years. It has become a restless, critical discipline, trying desperately to encompass an explosive increase in knowledge in the biological sciences.

Preface to *Triumphs in Medicine*. Paul Elek, London and New Hampshire, USA (1976)

John F. Kennedy 1917–63

US president

A medical revolution has extended the life of our elder citizens without providing the dignity and security those later years deserve.

Acceptance speech, Democratic National Convention, Los Angeles, 15 July (1960)

No costs have increased more rapidly in the last decade than the cost of medical care.

Address on the 25th Anniversary of the Social Security Act, 14 August (1960)

The basic resource of a nation is its people. Its strength can be no greater than the health and vitality of its population. Preventable sickness, disability and physical or mental incapacity are matters of both individual and national concern.

Message to Congress on a Health Program, 9 February (1961)

We cannot afford to postpone any longer a reversal in our approach to mental affliction. For too long the shabby treatment of the many millions of the mentally disabled in custodial institutions and many millions more now in communities needing help has been justified on grounds of inadequate funds, further studies and future promises.

Message to Congress on Mental Health, 5 February (1963)

The needs of children should not be made to wait.

Message to Congress on the Nation's Youth, 14 February (1963)

A proud and resourceful nation can no longer ask its older people to live in constant fear of a serious illness for which adequate funds are not available. We owe them the right of dignity in sickness as well as in health.

Message to Congress on Problems of the Aged, 21 February (1963)

Jean Kerr 1923–

US dramatist

The average, healthy, well-adjusted adult gets up at seven-thirty in the morning feeling just plain terrible.

Please Don't Eat the Daisies

Ellen Key 1849–1926

Swedish writer

At every step the child should be allowed to meet the real experiences of life; the thorns should never be plucked from his roses.

The Century of the Child Ch. 3

Rev Martin Luther King 1929–68

US black civil rights leader

We have genuflected before the god of science only to find that it has given us the atomic bomb, producing fears and anxieties that science can never mitigate.

Strength Through Love Ch. 13

Rudyard Kipling 1865–1936

Indian-born British writer and poet

There are only two classes of mankind in the world—doctors and patients.

A Doctor's Work, address to medical students at London's Middlesex Hospital, 1 October (1908)

The world has long ago decided that you (doctors) have no working hours that anybody is bound to respect.

A Doctor's Work, address to medical students at London's Middlesex Hospital, 1 October (1908)

Those people who would limit, and cripple, and hamper research because they fear research may be accompanied by a little pain and suffering.

A Doctor's Work, address to medical students at London's Middlesex Hospital, 1 October (1908)

We are very slightly changed
From the semi-apes who ranged
India's prehistoric clay.

General Summary

A woman is only a woman, but a good cigar is a smoke.

The Betrothed

John H. Knowles 1926–

President, Rockefeller Foundation

The American Medical Association operating from a platform of negative vigilance presents no solutions but busily fights each change and then loudly supports it against the next proposal.

Speech to the Institute on Medical Center Problems, 9 December (1964)

Theodor Kocher 1841–1917

Swiss surgeon

A surgeon is a doctor who can operate and who knows when not to.

Attributed to Kocher, perhaps reflecting his dismay at the effects of total strumectomy (thyroidectomy) on goitre patients

Sergei S. Korsakoff 1853–1900

Russian neuropsychiatrist

The less restraint for the patient, the more restraint for the doctor.

Dictionary of Medical Eponyms, (2nd edn.), p. 217, Firkin and Whitworth. The Parthenon (1996)

Alfred Korzyybski 1879–1950
US philosopher and semanticist, Connecticut

God may forgive you your sins, but your
nervous system won't.
  Attributed

Frederick James Kottke 1920–
Professor of Physical Medicine and Rehabilitation,
University of Minnesota, USA

The highest quality of life attainable for any
normal person is the achievement of optimal
function, resulting in using all of the assets that
each person has.
  Preface to *Krusen's Handbook of Physical Medicine and*
  Rehabilitation. W. B. Saunders (1990)

Karl Kraus 1874–1936
Austrian writer and satirist

Psychoanalysis is the disease it purports to cure.
  Attributed

Psychology is as unnecessary as directions for
using poison.
  Attributed

Jiddhu Krishnamurti 1891–1986
Indian theosophist

Meditation is not a means to an end. It is both the
means and the end.
  The Second Penguin Krishnamurti Reader Ch. 14

Joseph Wood Krutch 1893–1970

It is sometimes easier to head an institute for the
study of child guidance than it is to turn one brat
into a decent human being.
  If You Don't Mind My Saying 'Whom Do We Picket
  Tonight?'

Maggie Kuhn 1905–?
US writer and reformer

The ultimate indignity is to be given a bedpan by a
stranger who calls you by your first name.
  Observer 20 August (1978)

René Laënnec 1781–1826
French physician

I rolled a quire of paper into a kind of cylinder and
applied one end of it to the region of the heart and
the other to my ear, and was not a little surprised
and pleased to find that I could thereby perceive
the action of the heart in a manner much more
clear and distinct than I had ever been able to do
by the immediate application of the ear.
  Auscultation Mediate (transl. John Forbes)

I saw at once that this means might become a
useful method for studying, not only the beating of
the heart, but likewise all movements capable of
producing sound in the thoracic cavity.
  Auscultation Mediate (transl. John Forbes)

Jean de La Fontaine 1621–95
French poet

Rather suffer than die is man's motto.
  Fables I, 'La Mort et le Bûcheron'

Death never takes the wise man by
surprise; He is always ready to go.
  Fables I, 'La Mort et le Mourant'

R. D. Laing 1927–89
Scottish psychiatrist

Schizophrenia is a special strategy that a person
invents in order to live in an unlivable situation.
  The Divided Self

Children do not give up their innate imagination,
curiosity, dreaminess easily. You have to love them
to get them to do that.
  The Politics of Experience Ch. 3

Charles Lamb 1775–1834
British essayist

How sickness enlarges the dimensions of a man's
self to himself.
  Last Essays of Elia 'The Convalescent'

The first water cure was the Flood, and it killed
more than it cured.
  Attributed

William Lamb, Lord Melbourne
1779–1848
British Statesman

English physicians kill you, the French let you die.
  Queen Victoria Ch. 5, by Elizabeth Longford

Guido Lanfranchi c.1260–1315
French-born physician, Milan, Italy

Keep well in mind that nobody can become a good
internist without knowledge of surgery, and
conversely: nobody can become a good surgeon
who knows nothing about medicine.
  Chirurgia Parva (transl. J. J. Walsh)

It is necessary that a surgeon should have a
temperate and moderate disposition . . . He should
be well grounded in natural science, and should
know not only medicine but every part of
philosophy;
  Chirurgia Magna (transl. J. J. Walsh)

Why is there such a great difference between the
physician and the surgeon? The physicians have
abandoned operative procedures to the laity,
either, as some say, because they disdain to
operate with their hands, or because they do not
know how to perform operations.
  Chirurgia Magna (transl. J. J. Walsh)

Andrew Lang 1844–1912
Scottish man of letters

He uses statistics as a drunken man uses lampposts—for support rather than for illumination.
Attributed

Bernard von Langenbeck 1810–87
German surgeon

It is less important to invent new operations and new techniques of operating than to find ways and means to avoid surgery.
First Congress of Surgery, 10 April (1872)

Lâo-tzu 6th century BC
Chinese philosopher and founder of Tâoism

Wind is the cause of a hundred diseases.
In Tâo-te Ching

Ring Lardner Jr 1885–1933
US humorist

The only exercise I get is when I take the studs out of one shirt and put them in another.
Bartlett's Unfamiliar Quotations

Louis Cesare Lasagna 1923–
US pharmacologist, New York

It would seem important to devote more of the energies of man to improving the quality of life, so that it may be joyous, or noble, or creative.
The Doctor's Dilemmas Epilogue. Gollancz, New York (1962)

Peter Mere Latham 1789–1875
US poet and essayist

The practice of physic is jostled by quacks on the one side, and by science on the other.
Collected Works Vol. 1, 'In Memoriam'

The knowledge of the senses is the best knowledge; but delusions of the senses are the worst delusions.
Diseases of the Heart Lect. IV

You cannot be sure of the success of your remedy, while you are still uncertain of the nature of the disease.
Diseases of the Heart Lect. XIV

It would be difficult to overrate the value, as guides to practice, of the signs which declare themselves through the medium of the lungs in every case of unsound heart.
Diseases of the Heart Lect. XXXV

Amid many possibilities of error, it would be strange indeed to be always in the right.
General Remarks on the Practice of Medicine 'The Heart and Its Affection', Ch. IV

Common sense is in medicine the master workman.
General Remarks on the Practice of Medicine 'The Heart and Its Affections', Ch V

In truth, the amount of irremediable disease in the world is enormous.
General Remarks on the Practice of Medicine 'The Heart and Its Affections', Ch. VI

Poisons and medicines are often times the same substances given with different intents.
General Remarks on the Practice of Medicine 'The Heart and Its Affections', Ch. VII

Faith and knowledge lean largely upon each other in the practice of medicine.
General Remarks on the Practice of Medicine 'The Heart and Its Affections', Ch. VII

Perfect health, like perfect beauty, is a rare thing; and so, it seems, is perfect disease.
General Remarks on the Practice of Medicine 'The Heart and Its Affections', Ch. X, Pt. 2

It is safer to appeal to men's perceptions than to their logic.
General Remarks on the Practice of Medicine 'The Heart and Its Affections', Ch. XIV

It is a truth; and it is a truth also that the whole circle of the sciences is required to comprehend a single particle of matter: but the most solemn truth of all is, that the life of man is three-score years and ten.
Lectures on Clinical Medicine Lect. 1

Medicine is a strange mixture of speculation and action. We have to cultivate a science and to exercise an art.
Attributed

Treatment is concerned with the individual patient and leaves his disease to take care of itself.
Aphorisms from Latham p. 60, William 1 B. Bean.

Latin proverbs

Every animal is sad after intercourse.

If you dwell with a lame man you will learn to limp.

No remedies cause so much pain as those which are efficacious.

Pain of mind is worse than pain of body.

There are some remedies worse than the disease.

The sins of youth are paid for in old age.

The fear of death is crueler than death itself.

Who lives medically lives miserably.

Whom fate wishes to ruin she first makes mad.

Desmond Roger Laurence 1922–
Professor of Pharmacology, University College Hospital, London

Drug therapy involves a great deal more than matching the name of the drug to the name of a disease; it requires knowledge, judgement, skill and wisdom, but above all a sense of responsibility.
Clinical Pharmacology by D. R. Lawrence, P. N. Bennett, and M. J. Brown. Churchill Livingstone, Edinburgh (1997)

The choice before doctors is not whether they should experiment on their patients, but whether they should do so in a planned or in a haphazard fashion.
Clinical Pharmacology p. 53, D. R. Lawrence, P. N. Bennett, and M. J. Brown. Churchill Livingstone, Edinburgh (1997)

Antoine Lavoisier 1943–94
French chemist

We must trust to nothing but facts:
These are presented to us by Nature, and cannot deceive.
Elements of Chemistry Preface (transl. Robert Kerr)

Public usefulness and the interests of humanity ennoble the most disgusting work.
Attributed

Nigel Lawson 1932–
Chancellor of the Exchequer

The British have no unifying faith only a belief in the National Health Service.
Attributed

Stephen B. Leacock 1864–1944
Canadian economist and humorist

Any lover of humanity who looks back on the achievements of medical science must feel his heart glow and his right ventricle expand with the percardiac stimulus of a permissible pride.
Literary Lapses 'How to Be a Doctor' (1910)

Chauncey D. Leake 1896–1978
US pharmacologist

Let us remember always that whatever truth we may get by scientific study about ourselves and our environment is always relative, tentative, subject to change and correction, and that there are no final answers.
New York State Journal of Medicine **60**: 1496 (1960)

Fran Lebowitz 1950–
US writer

Food is an important part of a balanced diet.
Metropolitan Life 'Food for Thought and Vice Versa'

Stanislaw Lec 1909–
Polish poet

Wounds heal and become scars. But scars grow with us.
Unkempt thoughts

John le Carré (David John Moore Cornwell) 1931–
British novelist

He is like the surgeon who has grown tired of blood. He is content that others should operate.
The Spy Who Came In from the Cold

W. E. H. Lecky 1838–1903
Irish historian and philosopher

Abortion . . . was probably regarded by the average Roman of the later days of Paganism much as Englishmen in the last century regarded convivial excesses, as certainly wrong, but so venial as scarcely to deserve censure.
History of European Morals Vol. II, Ch. IV

James Le Fanu
Doctor and medical journalist

The map of mental illness, like that of Africa before the Victorian explorers, remains a blank.
The Rise and Fall of Modern Medicine p. 71. Little, Brown and Co., London (1999)

The failure of the two great projects of the last two decades – The New Genetics and The Social Theory—constitutes the fall of modern medicine.
The Rise and Fall of Modern Medicine p. 382. Little, Brown and Co., London (1999)

Legal phrases

A madman has no free will
(Furiosi nulla voluntas est.)

Edwin P. Lehman 1888–1954
US surgeon

It is asking more than human perfection to assume that a surgeon's judgment may not be influenced unconsciously by pressing financial need.
Surgery **28**: 595 (1950)

Baron Gottfried Wilhelm von Leibnitz 1646–1716
I often say a great doctor kills more people than a great general.
Attributed

Nikolai Lenin
US physician

The most important thing in illness is never to lose heart.
Attributed

Vladimir Ilyich Lenin 1870–1924
Russian revolutionary and head of state

Either socialism will defeat the louse, or the louse will defeat socialism.
Attributed in 1919 on the cause of typhus. Quoted by L. Tarassevitch, *Epidemics in Russia since 1914. Report to the Health Committee of the League of Nations*. Epidemiological Intelligence No. 2, March (1922)

René Leriche 1879–1956
French professor of surgery

Every surgeon carries about him a little cemetery, in which from time to time he goes to pray, a cemetery of bitterness and regret, of which he seeks the reason for certain of his failures.
La Philosophie de la Chirurgie Foreword

Alan Jay Lerner 1918–86
US lyricist and playwright

Just think of the American Medical Association coming out *against* living in the past.
On a Clear Day you Can See Forever

Alain René Lesage 1668–1747
French novelist and dramatist

We come into the world with the mark of our descent, and with our characters about us.
The Adventures of Gil Blas de Santillana (1715)

Gotthold Lessing 1729–81
German man of letters

Not the possession of truth but the effort in struggling to attain it brings joy to the researcher.

John Coatley Lettsom 1744–1815
British physician and philanthropist

Medicine is not a lucrative profession. It is a divine one.
Letter to a friend, 6 September (1791)

Sir Thomas Lewis 1881–1945
British physician and clinical scientist

Diagnosis is a system of more or less accurate guessing, in which the endpoint achieved is a name.
Lancet **1**: 619 (1944)

Georg Christoph Lichtenberg 1742–99
German physicist and satirist

How is it that animals do not squint? Is this another prerogative of the human species?
Reflections

Baron Justus von Liebig 1803–73
German chemist

We are too much accustomed to a single cause that which is the product of several, and the majority of our controversies come from that.
Attributed

R. J. Lilford 1950–
Professor of Public Health and Epidemiology, Birmingham, UK

It would be wrong to think that, as medicine loses its professional hegemony, the whole of health care will dissolve into amorphous and harmonious islands of multidisciplinary practice floating in an egalitarian sea.
Medical practice—where next? *Journal of the Royal Society of Medicine* **94**: 560 (2001)

It is intellectual and communication skills which will become the most crucial competency in health care.
Medical practice—where next? *Journal of the Royal Society of Medicine* **94**: 560 (2001)

The basic contract of health care has changed from a private matter between doctors and patients to a more public one between health care providers – epitomized by hospitals – and patients.
Medical practice—where next? *Journal of the Royal Society of Medicine* **94**: 561 (2001)

Chris Lillehei 1920?–
US surgeon

Good judgment comes from experience; Experience comes from bad judgment.
Attributed to him by David Rothenberger at a meeting in Manchester, 4 July (2002)

Abraham Lincoln 1809–65
US President

If I am killed, I can die but once; but to live in constant dread of it, is to die over and over again.
Abraham Lincoln Vol. II, Ch. 13

James Lind 1716–94
Scottish physician

Armies have been supposed to lose more of their men by sickness than by the sword.
A Treatise of the Scurvy Preface

Art Linklater
Contemporary

Skin is like wax paper that holds everything in without dripping.
A Child's Garden of Misinformation (1965)

Lin Yutang 1895–?
Chinese author and philologist

The Chinese do not draw any distinction between food and medicine.
The Importance of Living Ch. IX, Sect. vii

Eventually we have to come to a conception of health and disease by which the two merge into each other.
The Importance of Living Ch. IX, Sect. vii

Happiness for me is largely a matter of digestion.

John Lister 1920–
English physician and medical journalist

The essence of private medical practice lies in the nature of the relationship between patients and their physicians ... characterised by patients making their own choice of doctors, establishing a direct contract with them, and being responsible for their medical fees.
By the London Post, Massachusetts Medical Society (1985), quoting his article in the *New England Journal of Medicine* of 18 October (1984)

Lord Lister 1827–1912
British surgeon and scientist

Since the antiseptic treatment has been brought into full operation my wards, have completely changed their character; so that during the last nine months not a single instance of pyaemia, hospital gangrene or erysipelas has occurred in them.
British Medical Journal **2**: 246 (1867)
On the Antiseptic Principle of the Practice of Surgery

The material which I have employed is carbolic or phenic acid, a volatile organic compound, which appears to exercise a peculiarly destructive influence upon low forms of life, and hence is the most powerful antiseptic with which we are at present acquainted.

British Medical Journal **2**: 246 (1867)
On the Antiseptic Principle of the Practice of Surgery

It is our proud office to tend the fleshy tabernacle of the immortal spirit, and our path, if rightly followed, will be guided by unfettered truth and love unfeigned. In pursuit of this noble and holy calling, I wish you God-speed.

Address University of Edinburgh, August (1876)

The irritation of the wound by antiseptic irrigation and washing may therefore now be avoided, and nature left quite undisturbed to carry out her best methods of repair.

Report of the British Association for the Advancement of Science (1896)

There are people who do not object to eating a mutton chop, yet who consider it something monstrous to introduce under the skin of a guinea pig a little inoculation of some microbe to ascertain its action.

British Medical Journal **1**: 317 (1897)

The profession to which I have the great honour to belong is, I firmly believe, on the average, the most humane of all professions.

British Medical Journal **1**: 317 (1897)

I regard that all worldly distinctions are as nothing in comparison with the hope that I may have been the means of reducing in some degree the sum of human misery.

Address at Edinburgh, June (1898)

Anaesthetics have abolished the need for operative speed and they allow time for careful procedures.

Lord Lister, His Life and Doctrine. E. S. Livingstone, Edinburgh. (1949)

Next to the promulgation of the truth, the best thing I can conceive that a man can do is the public recantation of an error.

Attributed

Robert Liston 1794–1847
Scottish-born surgeon

This Yankee dodge, gentlemen, beats Mesmerism hollow.

University College London, Operating Room 21 December (1846) (after performing the first operation in Europe under ether)

James Little 1836–85
US professor of surgery

The first qualification for a physician is hopefulness.

Liu Kung Cho
Chinese sage

The able doctor acts before sickness comes.

Derek Llewellyn-Jones 1922–
Professor of Gynaecology, Sydney, Australia

Induced abortion, usually in defiance of the law, is the oldest method of birth control and the most common method by which women prevent the birth of unwanted children.

People Populating p. 273. Faber and Faber (1975)

David Lloyd George 1863–1945
British Liberal statesman

When they circumcised Herbert Samuel, they threw away the wrong bit.

Attributed to Lloyd George referring to the Liberal politician

Percy Lockhart Mummery 1875–1957
Coloproctologist at St. Mark's Hospital, London

Probably more reputations have been damaged by the unsuccessful treatment of cases of fistula than by excision of the rectum or gastroenterostomy. Perhaps that is why the largest surgical fee in history was paid for the performance of an operation for fistula.

Presidential Address to the Royal Society of Medicine (1929)

Robert F. Loeb 1895–?

The patient should be managed the way the doctor or a member of his family would wish to be treated if he were that patient in that bed at that time.

Attributed

Oxyrhynchus Logia (Agrapha)
2nd century

A prophet is not acceptable in his own homeland, nor does a physician work cures on those who know him.

Gospel of Thomas, Saying 31 (from the Eleventh Logion)

Warfield Theobald Longcope
1877–1953
US Professor of Medicine, Johns Hopkins

As I grow older, I have less and less sympathy with the conscientious efforts merely to extend life in old age.

Bulletin of the Johns Hopkins Hospital **50**: 4 (1932)

When a cure is impossible, it is the duty of the physician to bring contentment, comfort or even happiness to his patients to lighten their affliction. But this does not mean necessarily that he should limit living to prolong life.

Bulletin of the Johns Hopkins Hospital **50**: 4 (1932)

Each patient ought to feel somewhat the better after the physician's visit, irrespective of the nature of the illness.

Attributed

Tony Lopez 1963–
Paediatrician, Institute of Child Health, Bristol, UK

Our clinical practice is steered by ethical principles. They guide the decisions we make in our clinics and ward rounds, what we tell our patients, and what we omit to tell them; the research we do.

Journal of the Royal Society of Medicine **94**: 603–4 (2001)

Konrad Lorenz 1903–89
Austrian zoologist and ethologist

Man appears to be the missing link between anthropoid apes and human beings.

The New York Times Magazine 11 April (1965) (John Pfeiffer)

It is a good morning exercise for a research scientist to discard a pet hypothesis every day before breakfast.

On Aggression Ch. 2

Professor A. Ross Lorimer 1936–
President of the Royal College of Physicians and Surgeons of Glasgow

If you want to be a doctor, I would encourage you. There is no better job in the world for trying to help people and make them better.

Hospital Doctor 19 April (2001)

Pierre Charles Alexandre Louis 1787–1872
French physician

The results of my researches on the effects of bloodletting in inflammation, are so little in accordance with the general opinion, that it is not without a degree of hesitation I have decided to publish them.

Researches of the Effects of Bloodletting. Hilliard Grey and Co. (1836)

Richard Lower 1631–91
British physician

To alleviate a stone-attack and the usually consequent retention of urine, take snailshells and bees in equal quantities, dry them in a moderately hot oven, and grind them to a very fine powder.

De Corde (1671)

The cause of our life consists in this alone, that the blood in its continuous passage through the whole of the body carries round heat and nutriment to all the organs, and that ever-fresh chyle passes into the blood in due measure and amount.

De Corde V (1671)

Sir John Lubbock, Baron Avebury 1834–1913
English educationalist and reformer

Man ought to be man and master of his fate; but children are at the mercy of those around them.

The Pleasures of Life Pt 1, Ch. 1

Plain living and high thinking will secure health for most of us.

The Use of Life Ch. 3

Lu Chi
Chinese sage

A good doctor is equal to a good premier.

Lucretius c.96–55 BC
Roman poet

In bodily disease a wandering mind
Is often found; devoid of reason then,
The patient raves and roams delirious.

On the Nature of Things III. 464

The mind is begotten along with the body, and grows up with it, and with it grows old.

On the Nature of Things III. 455

The mind like a sick body can be healed and changed by medicine.

On the Nature of Things III. 510

What is one man's meat is another man's rank poison.

On the Nature of Things IV. 637

Emil Ludwig 1881–1948
German author

Nature puts upon no man an unbearable burden; if her limits be exceeded, man responds by suicide. I have always respected suicide as a regulator of nature.

I Believe Clifton Fadiman (ed.)

Martin Luther 1483–1546
German Protestant reformer

Heavy thoughts bring on physical maladies; when the soul is oppressed so is the body.

Table-Talk 'Of Temptation and Tribulation'

Medicine makes sick patients, for doctors imagine diseases, as mathematics makes hypochondriacs and theology makes sinners.

Attributed

The reproduction of mankind is a great marvel and mystery. Had God consulted me in the matter, I should have advised him to continue the generation of the species by fashioning them of clay.

Table Talk 'Of Marriage and Celibacy'

Men have broad and large chests, and small narrow hips, and more understanding than women, who have but small and narrow breasts, and broad hips, to the end they should remain at home, sit still, keep house, and bear and bring up children.

Table Talk 'Of Marriage and Celibacy'

John Lyly 1554–1606
English dramatist and novelist

The broken bone, once set together, is stronger than ever.
> *Euphues*

The wound that bleedeth inward is most dangerous.
> *Euphues*

Douglas MacArthur 1880–1964
US military commander

Worry, doubt, fear and despair are the enemies which slowly bring us down to the ground and turn us to dust before we die.
> Attributed

Thomas Babington, 1st Baron Macaulay 1800–59
Scottish author and historian

Of all people children are the most imaginative.
> Attributed

John L. McClenahan 1915–

It requires a great deal of faith for a man to be cured by his own placebos.
> Aphorism

Sir William MacCormac 1860?–
British military surgeon

A man wounded in the abdomen dies if he is operated on and remains alive if he is left in peace.
> Comment made during the Boer War (1899–1902) observing high death rates after surgery

Thomas McCrae 1870–1935

More is missed by not looking than by not knowing.
> Aphorism

Benjamin McCready 19th Century
New York physician

The population of the United States is beyond that of other countries, an anxious one. All classes are either striving after wealth, or endeavouring to keep up appearances.
> On the influence of trades, professions and occupations in the United States in the production of disease. *Transactions of the Medical Society of the State of New York* 3: 91–150 (1836–37)

One great source of ill-health among labourers and their families, is the confined and miserable appartments in which they are lodged.
> *Transactions of the Medical Society of the State of New York* 3: 91–150 (1836–37)

Edwin Carleton MacDowell 1887–?

Heredity sets limits, environment decides the exact position within these limits.
> Attributed

Ephraim McDowell 1771–1830
US surgeon, Kentucky

I made an incision about three inches from the musculus rectus abdominis, on the left side, continuing the same nine inches in length, parallel with the fibres of the above-named muscle, extending into the cavity of the abdomen.
> *Eclectic Repertory or Analytical Review* Vol. VIII (1817) description of the world's first three laparotomies or ovariotomies

Sir William Macewen 1848–1924
Professor of Surgery, Glasgow

John Hunter never had more than 20 students at his lectures, and at the beginning, when a solitary student presented himself, he had to ask the attendant to bring in the skeleton, so that he might address them as 'Gentlemen'.
> Address to the British Medical Association (1923)

Bernard MacFadden 1868–1955

If you feed a cold, as is often done, you frequently have to starve a fever.
> *Physical Culture* February (1934)

Malcolm McFarlane 1965–
English physician

How many of our continental colleagues can we say truly envy the system we work in? About as many as lust after our beef?
> *British Medical Association News Review* July (1996) (a reference to both the National Health Service and the bovine spongiform encephalopathy crisis)

A. McGehee Harvey
US physician and educator

Each of us should strive to rise above the routines of the daily ward round and to see in every patient an opportunity not only to serve mankind in the best tradition of medical excellence, but to add to the store of medical knowledge.
> *Phar. Alpha Omega Alpha* 36: 122 (1973)

Ernst Mach 1838–1916
Austrian physicist and philosopher

The aim of research is the discovery of the equations which subsist between the elements of phenomena.
> *Popular Scientific Lectures*

Des McHale
Contemporary Irish mathematician

The average human has one breast and one testicle.
> Attributed

Sir James Mackenzie 1853–1925

British physician and pioneer cardiologist

The seeming exactness of a mechanical device appeals much more strongly to certain minds than a process of reasoning.
  Attributed

A man with angina pectoris is like one of those old martyrs, confined in a room the walls of which gradually folded inwards and crushed him.
  Attributed to Mackenzie as he developed angina

Sir Morell Mackenzie 1838–92

English otorhinolaryngologist

British medicine is extremely conservative and hates specialism.
  Conversation with Dr Felix Semon

Henry McMurtie 1793–1865

Boys, don't study medicine. By the time you earn your bread, you will have no teeth left to eat it with.
  The Barnwell Bulletin **18**: 22, October (1940)

Sir Andrew MacPhail 1864–1938

Canadian professor of pathology and medical historian, McGill University

I am well aware that in these days, when a student must be converted into a physiologist, a physicist, a chemist, a biologist, a pharmacologist, and an electrician, there is no time to make a physician of him.
  British Medical Journal **1**: 443 (1933)

Hermann Boerhaave lectured five hours a day; his hospital contained only twelve beds, but by Sydenham's method he made of it the medical centre of Europe.
  British Medical Journal **1**: 443 (1933)

Sir John Royden Maddox 1925–

Medical editor (Nature) and broadcaster

I suspect that a large part of the formal scientific literature is hardly ever read at all.
  Lancet **2**: 1071 (1968)

François Magendie 1783–1855

French physiologist

Medicine is a science in the making.
  Attributed

Bill Maher

Contemporary American commentator

Kids. They're not easy. But there has to be some penalty for sex.
  Attributed

Moses ben Maimon (Maimonides)

1135–204

Spanish-born Jewish philosopher and physician

O God, let my mind be ever clear and enlightened. By the bedside of the patient let no alien thought deflect it. Let everything that experience and scholarship have taught it be present in it and hinder it not in its tranquil work.
  The Morning Prayer of the Physician

Honey and wine are bad for children but salutary for the elderly.
  Mishneh Torah Ch. 4, No. 2

A person should not eat until his stomach is replete but should diminish his intake by approximately one fourth of satiation.
  Mishneh Torah Ch. 4, No. 2

A person should not sleep on his face nor on his back but on his side; at the beginning of the night, on the left side and at the end of the night on the right side.
  Mishneh Torah Ch. 4, No. 5

Excessive eating is like a deadly poison to the body of any man and it is the principal cause of all illnesses. Most diseases that man is afflicted with are due to bad foods or because he fills his abdomen and eats excessively, even of good foods.
  Mishneh Torah Ch. 4, No. 15

Anyone who lives a sedentary life and does not exercise or he who postpones his excretions or he whose intestines are constipated, even if he eats good foods and takes care of himself according to proper medical principles—all his days will be painful ones and his strength will wane.
  Mishneh Torah Ch. 4, No. 5

He who immerses himself in sexual intercourse will be assailed by premature aging, his strength will wane, his eyes will weaken, and a bad odour will emit from his mouth and his armpits, his teeth will fall out and many other maladies will afflict him.
  Mishneh Torah Ch. IV, 19

A person should not cohabit when he is satiated nor when he is hungry but after the food is digested in his intestines.
  Mishneh Torah Ch. IV, 19

One who is ill has not only the right but also the duty to seek medical aid.
  Attributed

Teach thy tongue to say 'I do not know'.
  Attributed

Medical practice is not knitting and weaving and the labour of the hands, but it must be inspired with soul and be filled with understanding and equipped with the gift of keen observation; these together with accurate scientific knowledge are the indispensable requisites for proficient medical practice.
  Attributed

Grant me an opportunity to improve and extend my training, since there is no limit to knowledge. Help me to correct and supplement my educational defects as the scope of science and its horizon widen day by day.
  Mishneh Torah Ch. IV, 19

Ralph Herman Major 1884–1970
US medical historian

One day walking in the court of the Louvre he (Laennec 1781–1826) saw some children, who, with their ears glued to the two ends of some long pieces of wood ... he conceived instantly the thought of applying this to the study of diseases of the heart.

Quoted in *Physical Diagnosis* p. 17. W. B. Saunders, Philadelphia (1937) (relating the story of Laennec's discovery of the stethoscope)

J. D. Malcolm 1857–1937
British surgeon and gynaecologist

Shock is more a part of the phenomena caused by injury, whether surgical or otherwise, than a complication thereof.

The Physiology of Death from Traumatic Fever p. 22. Churchill, London (1893)

Nelson Mandela 1918–
Freedom fighter and President of South Africa

The doctors and nurses treated me in a natural way as though they had been dealing with blacks on a basis of equality all their lives. It reaffirmed my long-held belief that education was the enemy of prejudice. These were men and women of science, and science had no room for racism.

The Long Walk to Freedom p. 492. Little, Brown and Co, London (1994)

Gerald L. Mandell
Contemporary US professor of medicine

Infectious diseases traverse the usual boundaries established by medical specialists. All organ systems may be involved, and all physicians caring for patients may have to deal with infected patients.

Principles and Practice of Infectious Diseases Preface

Margurite Lucy Manfreda
Contemporary US commentator

People turn to God in times of crisis, an illness is among those times when people feel the need for spiritual guidance. Nurses, therefore, are in a unique position to bring spiritual aid to their patients and to the patients' families.

In *Spiritual Care: The Nurse's Role* Ch. 1, p. 19, by Sharon Fish and Judith Allen Shelly. Intervarsity Press, Illinois, USA (1978)

Marcus Manilius 1st century BC
Latin poet

We begin to die at birth; the end flows from the beginning.

Astronomica IV

Thomas Mann 1875–1955
German novelist

All interest in disease and death is only another expression of interest in life.

The Magic Mountain

Disease has nothing refined about it, nothing dignified.

The Magic Mountain Ch. IV 'Necessary purchases'

A man's dying is more the survivors' affair than his own.

The Magic Mountain Ch. VI

Peter Marcello
Contemporary US surgeon, Tufts University School of Medicine

We make all the calculations, the patient takes the risks.

Colorectal symposium Florida, 14 February (2002)

Antoine B. J. Marfan 1858–1942
French paediatrician, Paris

One rarely records pulmonary tuberculosis in people who during their childhood had been attacked by the disease and in whom the lesions have healed before the age of fifteen years.

Marfan's Law of acquired immunity in tuberculosis. Quoted in: *Dictionary of Medical Eponyms* (2nd edn), p. 256, Firkin and Whitworth. The Parthenon (1996)

Observe methodically and vigorously without neglecting any exploratory procedure using all that can be provided by physical examination, chemical studies, bacteriological findings and experiment, one must compare the facts observed during life and the lesions revealed by autopsy.

Quoted in: *Dictionary of Medical Eponyms* (2nd edn), p. 257, Firkin and Whitworth. The Parthenon (1996)

Don Marquis 1878–1937
US writer and New York columnist

A suicide is a person who has considered his own case and decided that he is worthless and who acts as his own judge jury and executioner and he probably knows better than anyone else whether there is justice in the verdict

the lives and times of archy and mehitabel: archy does his part, 'now look at it'

John Marston 1576–1634
English dramatist and satirist

A pitiful surgeon makes a dangerous sore.

The Malcontent Act IV, Sc. ii (1604)

Marcus Valerius Martialis Martial
c. AD 40–104
Spanish-born Latin poet and epigrammist

Life is not living, but living in health.

Epigrams VI. 70 (transl. W. C. Ker, 1919)

The mode of death is sadder than death itself.

Epigrams XI. 91

Accept this saddle for thy hunting nag,
For riding bare-back causes nasty piles.

Epigrams XIV. 86

Everett Dean Martin 1880–1941
US educator, New York

A crowd is a device for indulging ourselves in a kind of temporary insanity by all going crazy together.
The Behavior of Crowds Ch. 2

Louis Martinet 1795–1875
French physician

It is at the bedside of the patient that the observer must study disease; there he will see it in its true character, stripped of those false shades by which it is so frequently disguised in books.
Exposition of the Various Methods of Examination Used in Medicine. *A Manual of Pathology* (1827)

Karl F. H. Marx 1796–1877
German physician and medical historian and scholar

Medicine heals doubts as well as diseases.
Quoted in *Bulletin of the New York Academy of Medicine* **4**: 1001 (1928)

Physicians see many 'diseases' which have no more real existence than an image in a mirror.
Quoted in *Bulletin of the New York Academy of Medicine* **4**: 1001 (1928)

For thousands of years, medicine has united the aims and aspirations of the best and noblest of mankind. To depreciate its treasures is to discount all human endeavour and achievement as naught.
Quoted in *Bulletin of the New York Academy of Medicine* **5**: 156 (1929)

The education of most people ends upon graduation; that of the physician means a lifetime of incessant study.
Quoted in *Bulletin of the New York Academy of Medicine* **5**: 156 (1929)

In nature those who cry out with pain and those who prescribe remedies therefore are different persons; in politics they are one and the same.
Quoted in *Bulletin of the New York Academy of Medicine* **5**: 156 (1929)

If superstition were curable, the remedy for it would long since have been found; were it mortal it would long since have been buried.
Quoted in *Bulletin of the New York Academy of Medicine* **5**: 156 (1929)

Nathan Masor 1913–
US psychiatrist

The tranquiliser of greatest value since the early history of man, and which may never become outdated, is alcohol, when administered in moderation. It possesses the distinct advantage of being especially pleasant to the taste buds.
The New Psychiatry Ch. 7

William H. Masters 1915–
Virginia E. Johnson 1925–
US sexologists

Our culture has been influenced by and has contributed to manifold misconceptions of the functional role of the penis.
Human Sexual Response Ch. 12, Sect. 2

Rudolph Matas 1860–1957
US surgeon

The transition between life and death should be gentle in the winter of life.
The Soul of a Surgeon

To do all this to be all this, the Master Surgeon must be a man of mind, a man of thought, a man who knows his province, the human body, as a whole and not only one of its parts.
Surgical Papers

Henry Maudsley 1835–1918
English mental pathologist

To despise the little things of functional disorder is to fall by little and little into organic disease.
Attributed

As no one can have perfect knowledge of all parts of medicine a simplicity of nomenclature would seem not merely desirable but essential.
Attributed

W. Somerset Maughan 1874–1965
British writer and doctor

When you have loved as she has loved you grow old beautifully.
The Circle

People ask you for criticism, but they only want praise.
Of Human Bondage Ch. I

... only four professions for a gentleman, the Army, the Navy, the Law, and the Church. but ... no one ever considered the doctor a gentleman.
Of Human Bondage Ch. XXXIII

You will have to learn many tedious things which you will forget the moment you have passed your final examination, but in anatomy it is better to have learned and lost than never to have learned at all.
Of Human Bondage Ch. LIV

The medical profession is the only one which a man may enter at any age with some chance of making a living.
Of Human Bondage Ch. LV

She was very anaemic. Her thin lips were pale, and her skin was delicate, of a faint green colour, with out a touch of red even in the cheeks.
Of Human Bondage Ch. LIX (description of anaemic young woman)

The impression was neither of tragedy nor of comedy...there were tears and laughter, happiness and woe; it was tedious and interesting and indifferent; it was as you saw it: it was tumultuous and passionate; it was grave; it was sad and comic; it was trivial; it was simple and complex; joy was there and despair. ...There was neither good nor bad there. There were just facts. It was life.
A description of an outpatient clinic in *Of Human Bondage* Ch. LXXXI

The mystic sees the ineffable, and the psycho-pathologist the unspeakable.
The Moon and Sixpence Ch. 1

What makes old age hard to bear is not the failing of one's faculties, mental and physical but the burden of one's memories.
Points of View Ch. 1

I'll give you my opinion of the human race...Their heart's in the right place, but their head is a thoroughly inefficient organ.
The Summing Up

Dying is a very dull, dreary affair. And my advice to you is to have nothing to do with it.
Attributed

Andre Maurois 1885–1967
French writer

Growing old is a bad habit which a busy man has no time to form.
The Aging American

Yet had Fleming not possessed immense knowledge and an unremitting gift of observation he might not have observed the effect of the hyssop mould.
Life of Alexander Fleming

I knew a man who had been virtually drowned and then revived. He said that his death had not been painful.
Attributed

Gavin Maxwell 1914–69
British writer and naturalist

Then it came again, thunderous, earthshaking, the longest, loudest and most superbly stupendous fart that I have ever heard in my life, a sound of such magnificent and prolonged volume as to appear utterly beyond human capability.
Raven Seek Thy Brother p.38. Longmans, Harlow (1968)

Tom G. Mayer 1943–
US Professor of Othopaedic Surgery, Dallas, Texas

Voluntary, or skeletal, muscle is by far the muscle type of greatest volume in humans. The musculature involved in spinal movement and control is in turn the largest complex of skeletal muscles in the body.
The Spine Ch. 3, p. 89, Rothman and Simone. W. B. Saunders Co. (1992)

Charles H. Mayo 1865–1939
US physician

While medicine is a science, in many particulars it cannot be exact, so baffling are the varying results of varying conditions of human life.
Collected Papers of the Mayo Clinic and Mayo Foundation **1**: 601 (1909)

The prevention of disease today is one of the most important factors in the line of human endeavour.
Collected Papers of the Mayo Clinic and Mayo Foundation **5**: 17 (1913)

The sooner patients can be removed from the depressing influence of general hospital life the more rapid their convalescence.
Lancet **36**: 1 (1916)

Good health is an essential to happiness, and happiness is an essential to good citizenship.
Journal of the American Dental Association **6**: 505 (1919)

The trained nurse has given nursing the human, or shall we say, the divine touch, and made the hospital desirable for patients with serious ailments regardless of their home advantages.
Lancet **13**: 1242 (1921)

While there are several chronic diseases more destructive to life than cancer, none is more feared.
Annals of Surgery **83**: 357 (1926)

There are two objects of medical education: To heal the sick, and to advance the science.
Collected Papers of the Mayo Clinic and Mayo Foundation **18**: 1093 (1926)

The scientist is not content to stop at the obvious.
Collected Papers of the Mayo Clinic and Mayo Foundation **18**: 1093 (1926)

I have never known a man who died from overwork, but many who died from doubt.
Bartlett's Unfamiliar Quotations

The safest thing for a patient is to be in the hands of a man engaged in teaching medicine. In order to be a teacher of medicine the doctor must always be a student.
Proceedings of the Staff Meetings of the Mayo Clinic **2**: 233 (1927)

Medicine is a profession for social service and it developed organisation in response to social need.
Collected Papers of the Mayo Clinic and Mayo Foundation **23**: 1020 (1931)

The object of health education is to change the conduct of individual men, women and children by teaching them to care for their bodies well, and this instruction should be given throughout the entire period of their educational life.
Minnesota Medicine **15**: 40 (1932)

William J. Mayo 1861–1939

US surgeon

The examining physician often hesitates to make the necessary examination because it involves soiling the finger.

Lancet **35**: 339 (1915)

It is poor government that does not realize that the prolonged life, health and happiness of its people are its greatest asset.

Journal of the American Medical Association **73**: 411 (1919)

Experience is the great teacher; unfortunately, experience leaves mental scars, and scar tissue contracts.

Journal of the American Medical Association **77**: 597 (1921)

Medical science aims at the truth and nothing but the truth.

Journal of the Indiana Medical Association **17** (1924)

The aim of medicine is to prevent disease and prolong life, the ideal of medicine is to eliminate the need of a physician.

National Education Association: Proceedings and Addresses **66**: 163 (1928)

. . . he saw some elegant limousines and remarked, 'The surgeons have arrived.' Then he saw some cheaper cars and said, 'The physicians are here, too.' A few scattered model-T Fords led him to infer that there were pathologists present.

The Way of an Investigator Ch. 19 (Walter B. Cannon)

The surgeon is often intolerant and the internist self sufficient.

Surgery, Gynecology and Obstetrics **32**: 97 (1921)

The glory of medicine is that it is constantly moving forward, that there is always more to learn.

National Education Association: Addresses and Proceedings **66**: 163 (1928)

Truth is a constant variable. We seek it, we find it, our viewpoint changes, and the truth changes to meet it.

Annals of Surgery **94**: 799 (1931)

The church and the law deal with the yesterdays of life; medicine deals with the tomorrows.

Collected Papers of the Mayo Clinic and Mayo Foundation **23**: 1001 (1931)

It is better to think and sometimes to think wrong than not to think at all.

Collected Papers of the Mayo Clinic and Mayo Foundation **27**: 1212 (1935)

I think all of us who have worked years in the profession understand that many very skilful operators are not good surgeons.

Surgery, Gynaecology and Obstetrics **67**: 535 (1938)

Begin with an arresting sentence; close with a strong summary; in between speak simply, clearly, and always to the point; and above all be brief.

Quoted in *The Doctors Mayo* (Helen Clapesattle)

John Mayow 1640–79

English chemist

As a rule disease can scarcely keep pace with the itch to scribble about it.

Da Rachitide Pt V

James Howard Means 1885–1967

US physician and thyroid specialist, Massachussetts

The custom of giving patients appointments weeks in advance, during which time their illness may become seriously aggravated, seems to me to fall short of the ideal doctor–patient relationship.

Daedalus **92**: 701 (1963)

The most conspicuous change in the behaviour of the doctor is that nowadays he is usually in such a hurry that he is less accessible and less communicative.

Daedalus **92**: 701 (1963)

So much of the diagnostic process is now done through technological procedures that the doctor has lost some of his apparent omniscience, prestige and mystique.

Daedalus **92**: 701 (1963)

We have, inadvertently, trained our young doctors to consider it a virtue to prolong life for the sole purpose of prolonging it.

Daedalus **92**: 701 (1963)

Sir Peter Medawar 1915–87

British scientist and Nobel laureate

Science without the underpinning of hypotheses is just kitchen arts.

Attributed

He does not realise that, instead of conceiving him, his parents might have conceived any one of a hundred thousand other children, all unlike each other and unlike himself.

Medieval maxim

In the presence of the patient, Latin is the language.

Ed Meese

Contemporary, US Attorney General 1985–88

An expert is someone who is more than fifty miles from home, has no responsibility for implementing the advice he gives, and shows slides.

Penguin Dictionary of Modern Humorous Quotations p. 104, Fred Metcalf. Penguin Books, London (2001)

Samuel J. Meltzer 1851–1921

US physician and researcher

The fact that your patient gets well does not prove that your diagnosis was correct.

Attributed

Giles Ménage 1613–92
French lexicographer

A mild attack of apoplexy may be called death's retaining fee.
Menagiana Pt II

Menander 341–291 BC
Greek dramatist

Whom the gods love dies young.
Dis Exapaton

H. L. Mencken 1880–1956
US journalist

Pathology would remain a lovely science, even if there were no therapeutics, just as seismology is a lovely science, though no one knows how to stop earthquakes.
A Mencken Chrestomathy Ch. XXX

It is now quite lawful for a Catholic woman to avoid pregnancy by a resort to mathematics, though she is still forbidden to resort to physics and chemistry.
Notebooks Minority Report

Hygiene is the corruption of medicine by morality.
Prejudices Types of Men

George Meredith 1828–1909
English novelist and poet

Good wine lights the candelabra of the brain.
Attributed

Ilya Metchnikoff 1845–1916
Russian biologist

Already it is complained that the burden of supporting old people is too heavy, and statesmen are perturbed by the enormous expense which will be entailed by state support of the aged.
The Prolongation of Life Pt 4, Ch. 1 (ed. P. Chalmers Mitchell)

Alan Milburn 1958–
British Secretary of State for Health 1999–2003

Medicine is not a perfect science. Even the best doctors can make the worst mistakes.
Hospital Doctor 5 July (2001)

John Stuart Mill 1806–73
English philosopher and radical reformer

The fact itself of causing the existence of a human being, is one of the most responsible actions in the range of human life.
On Liberty

Perry H. Millard 19th century
US physician and vice-president of the American Medical Association

Practically the only opposition to effective medical legislation in the country comes from the profession itself.
The propriety and necessity of state regulation of medical practice. *Journal of the American Medical Association* 9: 491 (1887)

C. Jeff Miller 1874–1936
US gynaecologist

Body and soul cannot be separated for purposes of treatment, for they are one and indivisible. Sick minds must be healed as well as sick bodies.
Surgery, Gynaecology and Obstetrics 52: 488 (1931)

Spike Milligan 1918–2002
British comedian and writer

Contraceptives should be used on every conceivable occasion.
The Last Goon Show of All

John Milton 1608–74
English poet

Why, in truth, should I not bear gently the deprivation of sight, then I may hope that it is not so much lost as revoked and retracted inwards, for the sharpening rather than the blunting of my mental edge?
The Familiar Letters No. 21

It is not miserable to be blind; it is miserable to be incapable of enduring blindness.
Attributed

But pain is perfect misery, the worst of evils, and excessive, overturns all patience.
Attributed

In Physic, things of melancholic hue and quality are used against melancholy, sour against sour, salt to remove salt humours.
Samson Agonistes Preface

The fever is to the physicians, the eternal reproach.
The Reason of Church Government Preface

'Minerva'
Contemporary British medical columnist

A good physician appreciates the difference between postponing death and prolonging the act of dying.
British Medical Journal Vol. 324, 4 May (2002)

George R. Minot 1885–1950
US physician, haematologist, and Nobel laureate

To solve problems, an active, creative imagination and scientific curiosity are the necessary tools.
Dictionary of Medical Eponyms, (2nd edn), p. 268, Firkin and Whitworth. The Parthenon (1996)

John of Mirfield 1362–1407
Librarian and doctor, St. Bartholomew's Hospital, London

If there is any doubt as to whether a person is or is not dead, apply lightly roasted onion to his nostrils, and if he is alive, he will immediately scratch his nose.
Breviarum Bartholomei 'De Signis Malis'

S. Weir Mitchell 1829–1914
American neurophysician and author

The success of a discovery depends upon the time of its appearance.
Bulletin of the New York Academy of Medicine **4**: 1002 (1928)

Do not think of the dignity of your profession or what it is beneath you to do.
Medical proverbs by F. H. Garrison, Bulletin of the New York Academy of Medicine October: 979–1005 (1928)

Ever since the Crimean War, nurses have been getting into novels.
Medical proverbs by F. H. Garrison, Bulletin of the New York Academy of Medicine October: 979–1005 (1928)

I can remember when older physicians refused to recognise socially a man who devoted himself to the eye alone.
Medical proverbs by F. H. Garrison, Bulletin of the New York Academy of Medicine October: 979–1005 (1928)

The true rate of advance in medicine is not to be tested by the work of single men, but by the practical capacity of the mass.
Medical proverbs by F.H. Garrison, Bulletin of the New York Academy of Medicine October: 979–1005 (1928)

The true test of national medical progress is what the country doctor is.
Medical proverbs by F.H. Garrison, Bulletin of the New York Academy of Medicine October: 979–1005 (1928)

The arctic loneliness of age.
Medical proverbs by F.H. Garrison, Bulletin of the New York Academy of Medicine October: 979–1005 (1928)

Molière 1622–73
French dramatist

No matter what Aristotle and all philosophy may say, there's nothing like tobacco.
Don Juan Act I, Sc. i

The mind has great influence over the body, and maladies often have their origin there.
Love's the Best Doctor III

Most men die of their remedies, and not of their illnesses.
Le Malade imaginaire III.3

Henri de Mondeville 1260–1320
French surgeon

Anyone who believes that anything can be suited to everyone is a great fool, because medicine is practised not on mankind in general, but on every individual in particular.
Chirurgie

Keep up your patient's spirits by music of viols and ten-stringed psaltery, or by forged letters describing the death of his enemies, or by telling him he has been elected to a bishopric, if a churchman.
Chirurgie

Since dim antiquity the people have believed surgeons to be thieves, murderers and the worst kind of tricksters.
Quoted by M-C. Pouchelle in Corps et chirurgie a l'apogee du Moyen-Age. Flammarion, Paris (1983)

Surgery cures diseases that cannot be cured by any other means, not by themselves, not by nature, nor by medicine. Medicine indeed never cures a disease so evidently that one could say that the cure is due to medicine.
Treatise on Surgery

Lady Mary Wortley Montagu 1689–1762
English writer and traveller and importer of smallpox inoculation from the Middle East

The smallpox, so fatal and so general among us, is here rendered entirely harmless by the invention of ingrafting. They take the smallpox here by way of diversion, as they take the waters in other countries.
Letter from Adrianople 1 April (1717)

Michel de Montaigne 1533–92
French Essayist and moralist

It is good to rub and polish our brains against that of others.
Essays Bk 1 (transl. D. M. Frame)

The religion of my doctor or my lawyer cannot matter. That consideration has nothing in common with the functions of the friendship they owe me.
Essays Bk l, Ch. 28 'Of Friendship'

For the most violent diseases the most violent remedies.
Essays Bk II, Ch. 3 'A Custom of the Island of Cea' (transl. Donald M. Frame)

Old age puts more wrinkles in our minds than on our faces.
Essays Bk III, Ch. 12 'Of Physiognomy'

Our mind grows constipated and sluggish as it grows old.
Essays Bk III, Ch. 12 'Of Physiognomy'

If you do not know how to die, do not worry; Nature will tell you what to do on the spot, fully and adequately. She will do this job perfectly for you; do not bother your head about it.
Essays Bk III, Ch. 12 'Of Physiognomy'

Scratching is one of the sweetest gratifications of nature, and as ready at hand as any.
Essays Bk III, Ch. 13 'Of Experience'

Lawyers and physicians are a bad provision for a country.
Essays Bk III, Ch. 13 'Of Experience'

We are more sensible of one little touch of a surgeon's lancet than of twenty wounds with a sword in the heat of fight.
Attributed

Doctor cures, if the sun sees it; but if he kills, the earth hides it.
Florio II.xxxvii, 356

Montenegrin proverb

In a good hand every sword cuts well.

Montesquieu 1689–1755

French philosopher and jurist

That kind of health which can be preserved only by a careful and constant regulation of diet is but a tedious disease.
  Attributed

Young men ought to come well prepared for the study of Medicine, by having their minds enriched with all the aids they can receive from the languages, the liberal arts.
  A Discourse Upon the Institution of Medical Schools in America

Sir Thomas More 1478–1535

Philosopher and Chancellor of England

It is a wise mans part, rather to avoid sicknes, than to wishe for medicines.
  Utopia Bk II, Ch. 6 (transl. R. Robinson)

Jeanne Moreau

There's a certain moment in life when you realise you're born with a deadly disease which is life.
  Attributed

Giovanni Battista Morgagni 1682–1771

Italian pathologic anatomist

For those who have dissected or inspected many, have at least learned to doubt when the others, who are ignorant of anatomy, and do not take the trouble to attend to it, are in no doubt at all.
  De Sedibus et Causis Morborium Vol. I, Bk 2, Letter 16

Barbara Morgan 1940–

South African-born British anaesthetist, Queen Charlotte's Hospital, London

The anaesthetist is there to look after the mother; the paediatrician is there to look after the baby; the obstetrician is there to look after himself.
  Quoted in *The Anaesthetic Aide Memoire* p. 3 (ed. John Urquhart)

Maldwyn Morgan 1938–

Anaesthetist, Hammersmith Hospital, London

If the surgeon cuts a vessel and knows the name of that vessel, the situation is serious; if the anaesthetist knows the name of that vessel, the situation is irretrievable.
  The Anaesthetic Aide Memoire p. I (ed. John Urquhart)

M. J. Moroney 20th century

A statistical analysis, properly conducted, is a delicate dissection of uncertainties, a surgery of suppositions.
  Facts from Figures Ch. I

Desmond Morris 1928–

British zoologist and writer

He is proud that he has the biggest brain of all the primates, but attempts to conceal the fact that he also has the biggest penis.
  The Naked Ape Introduction

Sir Peter Morris 1937–

President of the Royal College of Surgeons of England

There is a danger that trust hospitals may be overwhelmed with inspections and directives such that there is little time left to look after patients.
  Bulletin of the Annals of the Royal College of Surgeons
  7 *January* (2002), commenting on the new bureaucracy

Robert Tuttle Morris 1857–1945

US surgeon

It is the patient rather than the case which requires treatment.
  Doctors versus Folks Ch. 2

It is the human touch after all that counts for most in our relation with our patients.
  Doctors versus Folks Ch. 3

The number of quacks in a locality is an index to the character of the regular medical profession in that locality.
  Doctors versus Folks Ch. 4

Rutherford Morrison 1853–1939

British surgeon

In men nine out of ten abdominal tumours are malignant; in women nine out of ten abdominal swellings are the pregnant uterus.
  The Practitioner October (1965)

Never neglect the history of a missed menstrual period.
  The Practitioner October (1965)

Beware of the diagnosis of hysteria, neurosis or neuralgia, unless organic disease can be excluded with certainty.
  The Practitioner October (1965)

The functional form of impotence fills the coffers of the quacks, and swells the list of suicides.
  The Practitioner October (1965)

William T. Morton 1819–68

Founder of anaesthesia in US

Your patient is ready, Sir!
  Remark to John Collins Warren 16 October (1846)
  ('Ether Day')

William Moss 18th century

Liverpool surgeon

Bleeding is a remedy much to be depended on when the symptoms of heat, fever, drowsiness and startings are urgent: it is commonly done to children by means of leeches, which may be applied to the foot or heel, and may be repeated.
  Essay on the Management and Nursing of Children in the Earlier Periods of Infancy (1781)

Mother Theresa 1905–1998

Founder of Catholic order and hospital administrator, Calcutta, India

There can be fewer luckier people in the world than the surgeons of India who have the opportunity to treat not only the rich but also the poor and destitute.
  Speech to the International College of Surgeons, Calcutta (1988)

Sir Frederick Walker Mott 1853–1926
British neurologist, psychiatrist, and sociologist

We now recognise the brain as the seat of the psyche, but the functions of the mind are dependent upon the whole body and the harmonious interaction of all its parts.

Quoted by W. S. Dawson in *Aids to Psychiatry* Introduction

T. J. Mott 1936–
British oncologist, Ipswich, Suffolk

Recent over-use of computers by (medical) management is like primitive tribesmen using a motorcycle to cross the road.

Nurses' League Journal **65** (1997)

Sir Berkeley Moynihan 1865–1936
British surgeon, Leeds, UK

As art surgery is incomparable in the beauty of its medium, in the supreme mastery required for its perfect accomplishment, and in the issues of life, suffering, and death which it so powerfully controls.

Addresses on Surgical Subjects 'The Approach to Surgery'

No training of the surgeon can be too arduous, no discipline too stern, and none of us may measure our devotion to our cause. For us an operation is an incident in the day's work, but for our patients it may be, and no doubt it often is, the sternest and most dreaded of all trials, for the mysteries of life and death surround it, and it must be faced alone.

Addresses on Surgical Subjects 'The Approach to Surgery'

On the roll of honour which, in letters of gold, bears the names of the saviours of mankind, no man is more worthy of remembrance than Lister.

Addresses on Surgical Subjects 'Lister as Surgeon'

A discovery is rarely, if ever, a sudden achievement, nor is it the work of one man; a long series of observations, each in turn received in doubt and discussed in hostility, are familiarised by time, and lead at last to the gradual disclosure of truth.

Surgery, Gynecology and Obstetrics **31**:549 (1920)

The operation itself is but one incident, no doubt the most dramatic, yet still only one in the long series of events which must stretch between illness and recovery.

Lancet **2**: 789 (1926)

Every operation is an experiment in bacteriology.

Attributed

Malcolm Muggeridge 1903–89
British journalist

The orgasm has replaced the Cross as the focus of longing and the image of fulfilment.

The Most of Malcolm Muggeridge 'Down with Sex'

I will lift mine eyes unto the pills. Almost everyone takes them, from the humble aspirin to the multi-coloured, king-sized three deckers, which put you to sleep, wake you up, stimulate and soothe you all in one. It is an age of pills.

The New Statesman 'London Diary' 3 August (1962)

Johannes Müller 1801–58
Professor of Medicine and Physiology, University of Berlin

What does not come under the knife, counts for nothing.

Referring to anatomical dissection in *Handbuch der Physiologie des Menschen*

John Benjamin Murphy 1857–1916
Professor of Surgery, Chicago, USA

The patient is the centre of the medical universe around which all our works revolve and towards which all our efforts trend.

Attributed

Vladimir Nabokov 1899–1977
Russian-born US novelist

Life is a great surprise. I do not see why death should not be an even greater one.

Pale Fire 'Commentary'

Napoleon I (Bonarparte)
1769–1821
French general and emperor

The greatest proof of madness is the disproportion of one's designs to one's means.

Maxims

You medical people will have more lives to answer for in the other world than even we generals.

Napoleon in Exile (Barry O'Meara)

A physician and a priest ought not to belong to any particular nation, and be divested of all political opinions.

Napoleon in Exile (Barry O'Meara) 16 October (1817)

Medicine is a collection of uncertain prescriptions, the results of which, taken collectively, are more fatal than useful to mankind. Water, air, and cleanliness are the chief articles in my pharmacopoeia.

Napoleon in Exile (Barry O'Meara)

I do not want two diseases – one nature-made, one doctor-made.

Quoted in *Clinical Pharmacology* by D. R. Laurence, Frontispiece. Churchill Livingstone, Edinburgh (1973)

Ogden Nash 1902–71
US poet

Senescence begins
And middle age ends,
The day your descendants
Outnumber your friends.

A cough is something that you yourself can't help, but everybody else does on purpose just to torment you.

You can't get there from here

Henry Needler 1685–1760
English musician

Who formed the curious texture of the eye
And cloath'd it with the various tunicles,
And texture exquisite; with chrystal juice
Supply'd it, to transmit the rays of light?
A Poem to Prove the Certainty of a God

Horatio, Lord Nelson 1758–1805
English admiral and victor of Trafalgar

I have only one eye – I have a right to be blind
sometimes.
Quoted in Robert Southey's *Life of Nelson* Ch. 7, describing
Nelson putting the telescope up to his blind eye at
Copenhagen.

John Henry, Cardinal Newman
1801–90
British ecclesiastic and philosopher

It is a matter of primary importance in the
cultivation of those sciences that the investigator
should be free, independent, unshackled in his
movements.
Christianity and Scientific Investigation

To discover and to teach are distinct functions;
they are also distinct gifts, and are not commonly
found united in the same person.
On the Scope and Nature of University Education Preface

Frank Nicholson 1937–
US film actor

I'd prefer to have a full bottle in front of me than
a full frontal lobotomy.
Attributed

Sir Harold Nicholson 1886–1968
English writer

One of the minor pleasures in life is to be slightly ill.
Observer (1950)

Delbert H. Nickson 1890–1951

The patient suffered from chronic remunerative
appendicitis.
Attributed

Friedrich Nietzsche 1844–1900
German philosopher and poet

Insanity in individuals is something rare – but in
groups, parties, nations and epochs it is the rule.
Beyond Good and Evil Ch. 4

There is a justice according to which we may
deprive a man of life, but none that permits us to
deprive him of death: that is merely cruelty.
Human, All Too Human Ch. II, Sect. 88 (transl. Alexander
Harvey)

The most dangerous physicians are those who can
act in perfect mimicry of the born physicians.
Human, All Too Human Pt II

The sick are the greatest danger for the healthy; it
is not from the strongest that harm comes to the
strong, but from the weakest.
Genealogy of Morals Essay 3

Idleness is the parent of all psychology.
The Twilight of the Idols

The sick man is a parasite of society. In certain
cases it is indecent to go on living.
The Twilight of the Idols

Two great European narcotics, alcohol and
Christianity
The Twilight of the Idols

One should die proudly when it is no longer
possible to live proudly.
The Twilight of the Idols

The thought of suicide is a great consolation: with
the help of it one has got through many a
bad night.
Attributed

Florence Nightingale 1820–1910
British nurse pioneer

It may seem a strange principle to enunciate as
the very first requirement in a Hospital that it
should do the sick no harm.
Notes on Hospitals Preface

Never be afraid of open windows. People do not
catch cold in bed. This is a popular fallacy.
Notes on Nursing

The nurse should never neglect to attend to the
patient's bodily hygiene on the pretext that such
measures do little good and are not urgent.
Notes on Nursing

My life now is as unlike my Hospital life when
I was concerned with the souls and bodies of men
as reading a cookery book is unlike a good dinner.
Letter to Revd Mother Bermondsey (1864)

The first possibility of rural cleanliness lies in
water supply.
Letter to Medical Officer of Health, November (1891)

The care and government of the *sick* poor is a
thing totally different from the government of
paupers.
Quoted in C. Woodham-Smith's *Florence Nightingale* p. 353.
Reprint Society (1952)

It makes me mad to hear people talk about
unemployed women . . . we can't find the women.
They won't come.
Quoted in C. Woodham-Smith's *Florence Nightingale* p. 360.
Reprint Society (1952)

Carl Wilhelm Hermann Nothnagel
1841–1905
German-born Viennese professor of medicine

Only a good man can be a great physician.
Attributed

Wilfrid G. Oakley 1905–

British physician, King's College Hospital, London

Man may be the captain of his fate, but his also the victim of his blood sugar.

Transactions of the Medical Society of London **78**: 16 (1962)

Julien Offray de la Mettrie 1709–51

French philosopher and army surgeon

The brain has muscles for thinking as the legs have muscles for walking.

L'Homme machine

The human body is a machine which winds its own springs: the living image of perpetual movement.

L'Homme machine

Sir Heneage Ogilvie 1887–1971

Consulting Surgeon, Guy's Hospital, London

A misleading symptom is misleading only to one able to be misled.

Surgery, Orthodox and Heterodox Ch. 11

Joe Orton 1933–67

British dramatist

It's all any reasonable child can expect if the dad is present at the conception.

Entertaining Mr. Sloane III

George Orwell (Eric Blair) 1903–50

British novelist

The essence of being human is that one does not seek perfection.

Shooting an Elephant 'Reflections on Gandhi'

Sir William Osler 1849–1920

Canadian physician and Oxford professor of medicine

There are only two sorts of doctors: those who practise with their brains, and those who practise with their tongues.

Aequanimitas, with Other Addresses 'Teaching and Thinking'

To prevent disease, to relieve suffering and to heal the sick—this is our work.

Aequanimitas, with Other Addresses 'Chauvinism in Medicine'

In the records of no other profession is there to be found so large a number of men who have combined intellectual pre-eminence with nobility of character.

Aequanimitas, with Other Addresses 'Chauvinism in Medicine'

In no profession does culture count for so much as in medicine, and no man needs it more than the general practitioner.

Aequanimitas, with Other Addresses 'Chauvinism in Medicine'

It is astonishing with how little reading a doctor can practise medicine, but it is not astonishing how badly he may do it.

Aequanimitas, with Other Addresses 'Books and Men'

In the mortality bills, pneumonia is an easy second, to tuberculosis; indeed, in many cities the death-rate is now higher and it has become, to use the phrase of Bunyan, 'the Captain of the men of death.'

Aequanimitas, with Other Addresses 'Medicine in the Nineteenth Century'

I desire no other epitaph (*than*) that I taught medical students in the wards, as I regard this as by far the most useful and important work I have been called upon to do.

Aequanimitas, with Other Addresses 'The Fixed Period'

The trained nurse has become one of the great blessings of humanity, taking a place beside the physician and the priest, and not inferior to either in her mission.

Aequanimitas, with Other Addresses 'Nurse and Patient'

Medicine is the only worldwide profession, following everywhere the same methods, actuated by the same ambitions, and pursuing the same ends.

Aequanimitas, with Other Addresses 'Unity, Peace, and Concord'

Errors in judgment must occur in the practice of an art which consists largely in balancing probabilities.

Aequanimitas, with Other Addresses 'Teacher and Student'

The first figure of a physician to stand out clearly from the mists of antiquity.

Writing of 'Imhotep', an Egyptian healing divinity

A physician who treats himself has a fool for a patient.

Sir William Osler: Aphorisms Ch. 1 (William B. Bean)

One of the first duties of the physician is to educate the masses not to take medicine.

Sir William Osler: Aphorisms Ch. 3

Patients should have rest, food, fresh air, and exercise – the quadrangle of health.

Sir William Osler: Aphorisms Ch. 3

Jaundice is the disease that your friends diagnose.

Sir William Osler: Aphorisms Ch. 5

Soap and water and common sense are the best disinfectants.

Sir William Osler: Aphorisms Ch. 5

Adhesions are the refuge of the diagnostically destitute.

Sir William Osler: Aphorisms Ch. 5

A desire to take medicine is, perhaps, the great feature which distinguishes man from other animals.

Science **17**: 170 (1891)

Dysentery has been more fatal to armies than powder and shot.

The Principles and Practice of Medicine p. 130. Appleton, New York (1892)

Varicose veins are the result of an improper selection of grandparents.

The Principles and Practice of Medicine p. 130. Appleton, New York (1892)

Humanity has but three great enemies; Fever, famine and war; of these by far the greatest, by far the most terrible, is fever.

Journal of the American Medical Association **26**: 999 (1896)

Can anything be more doleful than a procession of four or five doctors into the sick man's room?

Montreal Medical Journal **24**: 518 (1896)

In its more aggravated forms diffuse scleroderma is one of the most terrible of all human ills…one is literally a mummy, encased in an ever shrinking, slowly contracting skin of steel.

Journal of Cutaneous Diseases **16**: 49 (1898)

The natural man has only two primal passions, to get and beget.

Science and Immortality

The great majority gave no signs one way or the other; like birth, their death was a sleep and a forgetting.

Science and Immortality

Specialism, now a necessity, has fragmented the specialties themselves in a way that makes the outlook hazardous. The workers lose all sense of proportion in a maze of minutiae.

Address, Classical Association, Oxford, May (1910)

Patients rarely die of the disease from which they suffer. (Secondary or terminal infections are the real cause of death.)

St. Bartholomew's Hospital Reports **52**: 39 (1916)

We doctors have always been a simple trusting folk. Did we not believe Galen implicitly for 1500 years and Hippocrates more than 2000?

Attributed

Sir Fielding Ould 1710–89

Master of the Lying Hospital, Dublin

Caesarean section is a detestable, barbarous, illegal piece of inhumanity.

Quoted in *The Age of Agony* p. 44, Guy Williams. Constable and Co Ltd, London (1975)

Whether we should destroy the mother to save the child is a deplorable dilemma which should certainly be cleared up by the divines.

Quoted in *The Age of Agony* p. 44, Guy William. Constable and Co Ltd, London (1975)

Ovid 43 BC–117 AD

Roman poet

So he whose belly swells with dropsy, the more he drinks, the thirstier he grows.

Fasti I.215

Medicine sometimes snatches away health, sometimes gives it.

Tristia

I am no better in mind than in body; both alike are sick and I suffer double hurt.

Tristia III.viii.33

Tis not always in a physician's power to cure the sick; at times the disease is stronger than trained art.

Pontic Epistles I.iii.17

Sleep, rest of things, O pleasing Deity,
Peace of the soul, which cares dost crucify,
Weary bodies refresh and mollify.

Attributed

Robert Owen 1771–1838

Welsh social reformer

God and the Doctor we alike adore
But only when in danger, not before;
The danger o'er, both are alike requited,
God is forgotten, and the Doctor slighted.

Epigram Cf. 256:27

Frank Kittredge Paddock 1841–1901

A general practitioner can no more become a specialist than an old shoe can become a dancing slipper.

Aphorisms

Sir James Paget 1814–99

English surgeon

As no two persons are exactly alike in health so neither are any two in disease; and no diagnosis is complete or exact which does not include an estimate of the personal character, or the constitution of the patient.

Stephen Paget 1855–1926

English surgeon, writer and reformer

Talk of the patience of Job, said a Hospital nurse, Job was never on night duty.

Confessio Medici Ch. 6

You cannot be a perfect doctor, till you have been a patient.

Confessio Medici Ch. 7

Walter Lincoln Palmer 1896–

Don't refer a patient to a psychiatrist as if you are telling him to go to hell.

Aphorism

Lord Palmerston 1784–1865

British Prime Minister

Die, my dear doctor! That's the last thing I shall do!

Attributed as his last words

Giovanni Papini 1881–1956

Italian author and philosopher

Breathing is the greatest pleasure in life.

Attributed

Paracelsus c.1493–1541
Swiss physician and alchemist

These are the qualifications of a good surgeon:
Regarding his innate temper:
A clear conscience,
Desire to learn and to gather experience,
A gentle heart and a cheerful spirit,
Moral manner of life and sobriety in all things,
Greater interest in being useful to his patient than
    to himself.
Antimedicus (transl. Norbert Guterman in Selected
Writings)

Medicine is not only a science; it is also an art. It
does not consist of compounding pills and plasters;
it deals with the very processes of life, which must
be understood before they may be guided.
Die grosse Wundarznei

The art of healing comes from nature not from
the physician. Therefore the physician must start
from nature, with an open mind.
Seven Defenses Ch. 4

There are two kinds of physician—those who
work for love, and those who work for their own
profit.
Seven Defenses Ch. 5

The physician is only the servant of nature, not
her master. Therefore it behoves medicine to
follow the will of nature.
Three Books on the French Disease Bk III, Ch. XI

He who is happy always gets well.
Attributed

Knowledge makes the physician, not the name or
the school.
Attributed

All things are poisonous and there is nothing that
is harmless. The dose alone decides that
something is no poison.
Attributed

Ambroise Paré 1517–90
French surgeon

Always give the patient hope, even when death
seems at hand.
Attributed

I dressed him and God healed him.
Oeuvres (1585)

There are five duties in surgery: to remove what is
superfluous, to restore was has been dislocated, to
separate what has grown together, to reunite what
has been divided and to redress the defects of
nature.
Attributed

Better a tried remedy than a new-fangled one.
Attributed

When gangrene is pronounced, nothing will help
but the knife.
Attributed

Dorothy Parker 1893–1967
US satirical author

Men seldom make passes
At girls who wear glasses.
Enough Rope 'News Item'

James Parkinson 1755–1824
English general practitioner

I need hardly repeat to you the vulgar observation
that a physician seldom obtains bread by his
profession until he has no teeth to eat it.
The Hospital Pupil, H. D. Symonds (1800)

Involuntary tremulous motion, with lessened
muscular power, in parts not in action and even
when supported; with a propensity to bend the
trunk forward, and to pass from a walking to a
running pace; the senses and intellects being
uninjured.
An Essay on the Shaking Palsy. Sherwood, Neely and Jones,
London (1817)

Samuel Parr 1747–1825
English pedagogue and Latin scholar

Of the three learned professions, in erudition, in
science and in habits of deep and comprehensive
thinking, the pre-eminence must be assigned in
some degree to physicians.
Attributed

Caleb Parry 1755–1822
English physician and researcher

It is as important to know what sort of person has
the disease as to know what sort of disease the
person has.
Attributed

Pashto proverb

Until he gets over smallpox, parents do not count
their child their own.

Boris Pasternak 1890–1960
Russian novelist

At the moment of child-birth, every woman has
the same aura of isolation, as though she were
abandoned, alone.
Doctor Zhivago Ch. 9, Sect. 3

Louis Pasteur 1822–85
French scientist

Science proceeds by successive answers to
questions more and more subtle, coming nearer
and nearer to the very essence of phenomena.
Etudes sur le biere Ch. VI, Sect. vi (transl. Rene J. Dubos)

Wine is the most healthful and most hygienic of
beverages.
Etudes sur le vin Pt 1, Ch. 2, Sect. B

When moving forward toward the discovery of the unknown, the scientist is like a traveler who reaches higher and higher summits from which he sees in the distance new countries to explore.
Quoted by René Dubos in *Louis Pasteur, Free Lance of Science*

To him who devotes his life to science, nothing can give more happiness than increasing the number of discoveries, but his cup of joy is full when the results of his studies immediately find practical applications.
Quoted by René Dubos in *Louis Pasteur, Free Lance of Science*

If you suppress laboratories, physical science will be stricken with barrenness and death.
Some Reflections on Science in France Pt 1

When meditating over a disease, I never think of finding a remedy for it, but, instead, a means of preventing it.
Address to École Centrale des Arts et Manufactures, Paris, 15 May (1884)

One does not ask of one who suffers: What is your country and what is your religion? One merely says: You suffer, this is enough for me: you belong to me and I shall help you.
Speech to the Philanthropic Society, 8 June (1886)

In the field of observation, chance only favours the prepared mind.
Inaugural address as Professor and Dean of the new Faculty of Sciences at Lille, France

I desire judgment and criticism upon all my contributions.
The Germ Theory and its Applications to Medicine and Surgery Ch. 12, Sect. III.

All things are hidden, obscure and debatable if the cause of the phenomena be unknown, but everything is clear if this cause be known.
The Germ Theory and Its Application to Medicine and Surgery Ch. 2

Bachya ben Joseph ibn Pauda 11th century

A sick person who lies to his physician cheats only himself, wastes the physician's efforts and aggravates his sickness.
Duties of the Heart Third Treatise, Ch. 5

Paul of Aegina 615–690
Alexandria-trained physician

All those who have cataract see the light more or less, and by this we distinguish cataract from amaurosis and glaucoma; for persons affected with these complaints do not perceive the light at all.
Works Bk 6 'On Cataracts' (transl. Francis Adams)

Cesare Pavese 1908–50
Italian writer

One stops being a child when one realises that telling one's trouble does not make it better.
The Business of Living: Diaries 1935–1950

No one ever lacks a good reason for suicide.
Attributed

Ivan Pavlov 1849–1936
Russian experimental physiologist

School yourself to demureness and patience. Learn to innure yourself to drudgery in science. Learn, compare, collect the facts.
Bequest to the Academic Youth of Soviet Russia, 27 February (1936)

Experiment alone crowns the efforts of medicine, experiment limited only by the natural range of the powers of the human mind.
Experimental Psychology and Other Essays Pt X, Essay 3 (transl. S. Belsky)

Only by passing through the fire of experiment will medicine as a whole become what it should be, namely a conscious and, hence, always purposefully acting science.
Experimental Psychology and Other Essays Pt X, Essay 3 (transl. S. Belsky)

First of all be systematic, learn to do drudgery, second comes modesty; pride will deprive you of the ability to be objective, and the third thing necessary is passion – be passionate in your work and in your search for truth.
Dictionary of Medical Eponyms (2nd edn), p. 305 Firkin and Whitworth. The Parthenon, Lancashire, UK (1996)

Frank Payne 1840–1910
British medical historian

This basis of medicine is sympathy and the desire to help others, and whatever is done with this end must be called medicine.
English Medicine in the Anglo-SaxonTimes. Clarendon Press, Oxford (1908)

Francis Weld Peabody 1881–1927
US pathologist, haematologist, and author

The treatment of a disease may be entirely impersonal; the care of a patient must be completely personal.
The Care of the Patient

There is no more contradiction between the science of medicine and the art of medicine than between the science of aeronautics and the art of flying.
The Care of the Patient

Disease in man is never exactly the same disease in an experimental animal, for in man the disease at once affects and is affected by what we call the emotional life.
The Care of the Patient

One of the essential qualities of the clinician is interest in humanity, for the secret of the care of the patient is in caring for the patient.
The Care of the Patient

John Pearson 1758–1826
English surgeon, London

He who reduces the province of a Surgeon to the performance of operations, and consequently directs his attention in a transient and careless manner to the less splendid parts of his profession, may learn the art of mutilating his fellow creatures, but will never deserve to be treated as a good Surgeon.
Principles of Surgery Preface

Charles Péguy 1873–1914
French nationalist, publisher and poet

When a man lies dying, he does not die from the disease alone. He dies from his whole life.
Basic Verities 'The Search for Truth'

Wilder Penfield 1891–1976
American-born Canadian neurosurgeon, McGill University

The trouble is not in science but in the uses men make of it. Doctor and layman alike must learn wisdom in their employment of science, whether this applies to atom bombs or blood transfusion.
The Second Career 'A Doctor's Philosophy'

There are times when compassion should prompt us to forego prolonged and costly treatment.
The Second Career 'A Doctor's Philosophy'

It is fair to say that science provides no method of controlling the mind. Scientific work on the brain does not explain the mind—not yet.
Dartmouth Convocation on The Great Issues of Conscience in Modern Medicine (1960)

R. G. Penn 1933–
British clinical pharmacologist, London

The medical herbalist is at fault for clinging to outworn historical authority and for not assessing his drugs in terms of today's knowledge, and the orthodox physician is at fault for a cynical scepticism with regard to any healing discipline other than his own.
Adverse Drug Reaction Bulletin No. 102 (1983)

William Penn 1644–1718
English Quaker and founder of Pennsylvania

Drunkenness spoils health, dismounts the mind, and unmans men.
Fruits of Solitude Maxim 72

Samuel Pepys 1633–1703
English diarist

Thanks be to God, since my leaving drinking of wine, I do find myself much better and do mind my business better, and do spend less money, and less time lost in idle company.
Diary 26 January (1662)

Thomas Percival 1740–1804
English physician and medical ethicist

The invention of an hypothesis is a work of no difficulty to a lively imagination.
Essays Medical, Philosophical, and Experimental Vol. I 'The Empiric'

Meyer A. Perlstein 1902–
If your time hasn't come, not even a doctor can kill you.
Attributed

Persian proverb
When there are two midwives, the baby's head is crooked.

Aulus Flaccus Persius AD 34–62
Roman satirist

Confront disease at its first stage.
Satires III

Jo Peters 1945–
British surgeon

Laparoscopic surgery—up a steep learning curve to a plateau of ignorance.
Personal communication

John Punnett Peters 1887–1955
US physician and clinical biochemist

Too much attention has been paid to the excretory offices of the kidney to the neglect of its conservative services.
Yale Journal of Biology and Medicine **26**: 179 (1953)

Petrarch 1304–74
Italian poet and scholar

It is by poultices, not by words, that pain is ended, although pain is by words both eased and diminished.
Letter to Guido Sette (1359)

Arbiter Petronius 1st century AD
Roman satirist

After all, a doctor is just to put your mind at rest.
Satyricon 42

Vita vinum est (wine is life).
Satyricon 42

Heinrich von Pfolspeundt 15th century
German war surgeon

A wound should be bound with clean white bandages, else there be harmful effects. He should wash his hands before treating anyone.
Buch der Bundth-Erntznei

Thomas Phaer 1510?–60

Sleep is the nourishment and food of a sucking child.

The Book of Children

Philemon ?361–263 BC

There is not a doctor who desires the health of his friends; not a soldier who desires the peace of his country.

Fabulae Incertae Fragment 46 (in Florilegium, CII.5)

Only physicians and advocates can kill without being killed.

Florilegium CII.6 (by Stobaeus)

Melanie Phillips

Contemporary British journalist

Behind many of the most agonising dilemmas in modern medicine, behind the emotional and bitter arguments that accompany them, lies the assumption that human life is sacred.

Doctor's Dilemmas p. 21. Harvester Press (1985)

Medical ethics are a bargain that has to be struck between doctors and society.

Doctor's Dilemmas p. 171. Harvester Press (1985)

S. F. Phillips

Contemporary US gastroenterologist and professor of medicine

Far too long the enteric sciences, basic and clinical, have ignored the large bowel.

Introduction to The Large Intestine, Physiology, Pathophysiology and Disease. Raven Press, New York (1991)

Ludwig Pick 1868–1944

German pathologist, Berlin, and describer of Niemann–Pick disease

Love is an acute psychosis that may always be given a good prognosis.

Dictionary of Medical Eponyms (2nd edn), p. 283, Firkin and Whitworth. The Parthenon, Lancashire, UK (1996)

Sir George Pickering 1904–80

Professor of Medicine and Cardiology, Oxford, UK

Medicine is not yet liberated from the medieval idea that disease is the result of sin and must be expiated by mortification of the flesh.

Resident Physician II (No. 9): 71 (1965)

Pien Ch'iao c.225 BC

Men worry over the great number of diseases, while doctors worry over the scarcity of effective remedies.

Quoted in *History of Chinese Medicine* Bk 1, Ch. 5

Pindar 522–443 BC

Greek poet

The best of healers is good cheer.

Nemean Ode IV.i

Dear Soul, do not strive for immortal life, but exhaust the resources of the feasible.

Pythian Ode

Phillipe Pinel 1755–1826

French Professor of Internal Pathology at Ecole de Médecine, Paris

Every illness has its natural course, with which it behoves the doctor to become acquainted.

Nosographie philosophique, ou la méthode de l'analyse appliquée à la médecine (1798)

Hester Lynch Piozzi (Mrs Henry Thrale) 1741–1821

Poet and friend of Dr Samuel Johnson

A physician can sometimes parry the scythe of death, but has no power over the sand in the hourglass.

Letter to Fanny Burney, 22 November (1781)

Walter B. Pitkin 1878–1953

US writer

Many people are better off with grave handicaps than with trifling ones. The grave handicaps release copious energies.

Life Begins at Forty

A country doctor needs more brains to do his work passably than the fifty greatest industrialists in the world require.

The Twilight of the American Mind Ch. 10

Plato c.429–347 BC

Greek philosopher

Medicine is an art, and attends to the nature and constitution of the patient, and has principles of action and reason in each case.

Gorgias

This is the great error of our day in the treatment of the human body, that the physicians separate the soul from the body.

Charmides

Mind is ever the ruler of the universe.

Philebus

The doctors will treat those of your citizens whose physical and psychological constitution is good: as for the others, they will leave the unhealthy to die and those whose psychological constitution is incurably warped they will be put to death.

Republic

No physician, in so far as he is a physician, considers his own good in what he prescribes, but the good of his patient; for the true physician is also a ruler having the human body as a subject, and is not a mere moneymaker.

Republic I.342.D

They do certainly give very strange and new-fangled names to diseases.

Republic III.405.D

Attention to health is the greatest hindrance to life.

Attributed

Sir Harry Platt 1897–1986
Professor of Orthopaedics, Manchester, and President Royal College of Surgeons of England

A physician should not be a servant of any government local or central, but of all the people and available at all times to those seeking his service.

Quoted in *By the London Post* (Dr John Lister), *New England Journal of Medicine* 29 January (1976)

If you cannot make a diagnosis at least make a decision.

Attributed

Lord Platt 1900–78
Professor of Medicine, Manchester, UK

A conclusion based upon a badly conceived experiment is usually further from the truth than one based on clinical observation.

Universities Quarterly **17**: 327 (1963)

The human lessons which medical practice teaches are great and should be passed on to our pupils.

Republic

There is a side to human behaviour in health and disease which is not a thing of the intellect, which is irrational and emotional but important. It is the main spring of most of what we do and a great deal of what we think. It is being explored by psychiatry but is in danger of being neglected by clinical science.

Republic

Future generations, paying tribute to the medical advances of our time, will say: 'Strange that they never seemed to realize that the real causes of ill-health were to be found largely in the mind.'

British Medical Journal **2**: 551 (1965)

Titus Maccius Plautus 254–184 BC
Roman comic poet

'Tis a portentous sign
When a man sweats,
and at the time shivers.

Asinaria II.ii.289

Whom the Gods love die young.

Bacchides IV.vii.18

Pliny the elder AD 23–79
Roman soldier and author

And there is no doubt that they all busy themselves with our lives, in order by discovery of some new thing or another to win reputations for themselves.

Historia Naturalis 'Greek Physicians'

There is alas no law against incompetency; no striking example is made. They learn by our bodily jeopardy and make experiments until the death of the patients, and the doctor is the only person not punished for murder.

Historia Naturalis 'Greek Physicians'

The Roman people for more than six hundred years were not without medical art but were without physicians.

Historia Naturalis 'Greek Physicians'

There is nothing encourageth a woman sooner to be barren than hard travail in child bearing.

Historia Naturalis 'Greek Physicians'

Amid the sufferings of life on earth, suicide is God's best gift to man.

Natural History II

In sickness the mind reflects upon itself.

Natural History VII

The brain is the highest of the organs in position, and it is protected by the vault of the head; it has no flesh or blood or refuse. It is the citadel of sense-perception.

Natural History XI.49

Pliny the younger AD 62–113
Roman orator, author and politician

The body must be repaired and supported, if we would preserve the mind in all its vigour.

Epistles I, 9

Plutarch C. AD 46–120
Greek essayist

Medicine, to produce health, has to examine disease.

Lives 'Demetrius' I

A man ought to handle his body like the sail of a ship, and neither lower and reduce it much when no cloud is in sight, or be slack and careless in managing it when he comes to suspect something is wrong.

Moralia 'Advice about Keeping Well'

It is contrary to nature for children to come into the world with feet first.

Moralia 'Advice about Keeping Well'

Of all drinks, wine is the most profitable of medicines, most pleasant, and of charity stands most harmless; provided always that it will be well tempered with opportunity of the time.

Moralia 'Advice about Keeping Well'

It is said that no woman ever produced a child without the cooperation of a man.

Moralia 'Advice to Bride and Groom'

Edgar Allan Poe 1809–49
US poet and writer

The boundaries which divide life from death are, at best, shadowy and vague. Who shall say where one ends and where the other begins?

Attributed (1844)

Michael Polanyi 1891–1976
Hungarian chemist and social philosopher

Genius seems to consist in the power of applying
the originality of youth to the experience of
maturity.
  The Study of Man Ch. 1

Polish proverbs

A beggar does not hate another beggar as much as
one doctor hates another.

Every Czech is a musician; every Italian a doctor;
every German a merchant; every Pole a
nobleman.

The doctor demands his fees whether he has killed
the illness or the patient.

The poor are cured by work, the rich by the doctor.

Allyson M. Pollock 1953?–
Professor of Public Health, University College, London

We work in teams, but are blamed as individuals.
  Comment in *GMC News* 10 February (2002)

Alexander Pope 1688–1744
English poet

Know thyself, presume no God to scan,
The proper study of mankind is man.
  An Essay on Man

The more you drink, the more you crave.
Who shall decide when doctors disagree.
  Moral Essays Ep. III, 1.1

Physicians are in general the most amiable
companions and the best friends, as well as the
most learned men I know.
  Letter to Ralph Allen, 13 September (1743)

Hans Popper 1910–
German born US hepatopathologist

I will begin my lecture today in the international
language of medicine—broken English.
  Introduction to a lecture on receiving the Friedenwald
  Medal in New York in 1980 (as related by C. B. Williams)

Karl R. Popper 1902–?
Austrian-born British philosopher

It is not his possession of knowledge of irrefutable
truth that makes the man of science, but his
persistent and recklessly critical quest for truth.
  The Logic of Scientific Discovery Ch. 10

Roy Porter 1946–2002
Professor of Social History, Wellcome Institute, London

The irony is that the healthier Western society
becomes, the more medicine it craves.
  The Greatest Benefit to Mankind. Harper Collins, London
  (1998)

Sir Percivall Pott 1714–88
Surgeon, St. Bartholomews Hospital, London

Surgery has undergone many great
transformations during the past fifty years, and
many are to be thanked for their contributions—
yet when we think of how many remain to be
made, it should rather stimulate our inventiveness
than fuel our vanity.
  Chirurgical Observations (1775)

When the mischief seems to be of such nature as
that gangrene and mortification are most likely to
ensue, no time can be spared . . . a very few hours
make all the difference between probable safety
and destruction.
  Chirurgical Works p. 476. Johnson, London (1779)

Anthony Powell 1905–?
British author

Growing old is like being increasingly penalized for
a crime you haven't committed.
  Temporary Kings Ch. 1 (1973)

Sir Douglas Powell 1860?–
Respiratory physician, London, UK

We hear it often said of the medical profession
that new discoveries are met by captious criticism
and ungenerous mistrust.
  Harveian Oration *c.*1914, quoted in *Harley Street* p. 53,
  Reginald Pound. Michael Joseph, London (1967)

Simon Powis 1940–
British surgeon, Northampton, England

However well trained and highly motivated a
doctor is, it is impossible to respond safely and
efficiently to increasing demands if the
infrastructure is absent.
  The Times 25 February (2001)

Winthrop Mackworth Praed
1802–39
English man of letters

Of science and logic he chatters,
As fine and as fast as he can;
Though I am no judge of such matters,
I'm sure he's a talented man.
  Poems of Life and Manners 'The Talented Man'

William Hickling Prescott
1796–1859
US historian

It is the characteristic of true science to discern
the impassable but not very obvious limits which
divide the province of reason from that of
speculation.
  History of the Conquest of Mexico Bk I, Ch. 4

Matthew Prior 1664–1721
English poet and diplomatist

You tell your doctor, that ye're ill;
And what does he, but write a bill,
Of which you need not read one letter;
The worse the scrawl, the dose the better,
For if you knew but what you take,
Tho' you recover he must break.
Alma Canto III

Cured yesterday of my disease,
I died last night of my physician.
The Remedy is Worse than the Disease

Henry S. Pritchett 1857–1939
US physician

By professional patriotism amongst medical men
I mean that sort of regard for the honour of the
profession and that sense of responsibility for its
efficiency which will enable a member of that
profession to rise above the consideration of
personal or professional gain.
Introduction to Abraham Flexner's *Medical Education in the United States and Canada* (1910)

Marcel Proust 1871–1922
French writer

Happiness is beneficial for the body, but it is grief
that develops the powers of the mind.
A la recherche du temps perdu: Le Temps retrouvé Vol. 2, Ch. 3

The mistakes made by doctors are innumerable.
They err habitually on the side of optimism as to
treatment, of pessimism as to the outcome.
A la recherche du temps perdu: Le Temps retrouvé Vol. 2, Ch. 3

Neurosis has an absolute genius for malingering.
There is no illness which it cannot counterfeit
perfectly . . . If it is capable of deceiving the doctor,
how should it fail to deceive the patient?
Le Côté de Guermantes Pt I

Everything great in the world comes from
neurotics. They alone have founded our religions
and composed our masterpieces.
Le Côté de Guermantes Pt I

Illness is the doctor to whom we pay most heed; to
kindness, to knowledge, we make promise only,
pain we obey.
Cities of the Plain Pt I, Ch. 1, 'My Social Life'

Proverbs

An apple a day keeps the doctor away.

A disease known is half cured.

Age breeds aches.

An ill man is worst when he appeareth good.

All would live long but none would be old.

A man has often more trouble to digest food than
to get it.

Among the blind, the one-eyed man is king.

A surgeon should be young, a physician old.

Bacchus has drowned more men than Neptune.

Blood is thicker than water.

Drunkenness turns a man out of himself, and
leaves a beast in his room.

Experience is the mother of science.

First do no harm. It is a good remedy sometimes to
do nothing.

Get your money when the patient is in pain.

God heals and the doctor takes the fee.

Health is the poor man's riches and the rich man's
bliss.

He lives long that lives till all are weary of him.

He that is uneasy at every little pain is never
without some ache.

He who physics himself poisons a fool.

Late children, early orphans.

Meddlesome midwifery is bad.

More die by food than famine.

Nature, time and patience are the three great
physicians.

Old age, though despised, is coveted by all men.

Patience is a plaster for all sores.

Physicians are costly visitors.

Scratching is bad because it begins with pleasure
and ends with pain.

Sickness is better than sadness.

Sickness is felt, but health not at all.

Temperance is the best physic.

The best smell is bread, the savour salt, the best
love that of children.

The best surgeon is he that has been well hacked
himself.

The choleric drinks, the melancholic eats, the
phlegmatic sleeps.

The eye is bigger than the belly.

The first breath is the beginning of death.

The presence of the doctor is the beginning of the
cure.

There are none so blind as those that cannot see.

There is a remedy for everything, could men find it.

The tongue is ever turning to the aching tooth.

Those whom the Gods wish to destroy they first
drive mad.

We are usually the best men when in the worst
health.

We are born crying, live complaining, and die
disappointed.

James J. Putnam 1846–1918

No argument is needed to show what transforming power the mind can exert.

Boston Medical and Surgical Journal **141**: 53 (1899)

'The man' is above all else, the mind of the man, and not only the mind as an organ of conscious thought but the mind as an organ of bodily nutrition, and the mind as a vast theatre for the interplay of contending forces that do not always recognise the personal consciousness as their ruler.

Boston Medical and Surgical Journal **141**: 53 (1899)

Françis Quarles 1592–1644

English poet

Man is Heaven's masterpiece.

Emblems Bk II

Physicians of all men are the most happy; what success soever they have, the world proclaimeth, and what fault they commit, the earth covereth.

Hieroglyphics of the Life of Man IV

Quintilian AD 35–c. 96

Roman teacher

Medicine for the dead is too late.

François Rabelais 1494–1553

French physician and satirist

'Appetite comes as you eat', said Bishop Hanges Mans; but thirst vanishes as you drink!

Gargantua Bk 1, Ch. 5 (transl. Jacques Le Clercq)

Without health life is not life; it is unlivable. Without health, life spells but languor and an image of death.

Pantagruel Bk IV, Prologue

Bernardino Ramazzini 1633–1714

When you come to a patient's house, you should ask him what sort of pains he has, what caused them, how many days he has been ill, whether the bowels are working and what sort of food he eats . . . I may venture to add one more question: what occupation does he follow?

Diseases of Workers, Preface (transl. W. C. Wright)

Dr Virginia Ramirez de Barquero

Costa Rica health official

We trust the drug companies. They wouldn't lie to us.

Quoted in *The Drugging of the Americas* M. Silverman. University of California Press, Berkeley (1976)

Santiago Ramón y Cajal 1852–1934

Spanish physician, professor of histology, and Nobel Prize winner

It is idle to dispute with old men. Their opinions, like their cranial sutures, are ossified.

Charlas de Cafe

As long as our brain is a mystery, the universe, the reflection of the structure of the brain, will also be a mystery.

Charlas de Cafe

It is best to attenuate the virulence of our adversaries with the chloroform of courtesy and flattery, much as bacteriologists disarm a pathogen by converting it into a vaccine.

Charlas de Cafe

Like an earthquake, true senility announces itself by trembling and stammering.

Charlas de Cafe

That which enters the mind through reason can be corrected. That which is admitted through faith, hardly ever.

Charlas de Cafe

It is notorious that the desire to live increases as life itself shortens.

Charlas de Cafe

Physical pain is easily forgotten, but a moral chagrin lasts indefinitely.

Charlas de Cafe

Svend Ranulf 1894–?

Statistical evidence shows that the greater the intellectual freedom, and the higher the general average of intelligence in a community, the greater is also the number of suicides.

The Jealousy of the Gods, and Criminal Law at Athens Ch. II

Louis-Antoine Ranvier 1835–1922

French professor of histology

It is necessary in a word to make histology experimental. Such is the supreme goal of our research, such is the basis of future medicine.

Quoted in *Dictionary of Medical Eponyms* (2nd edn), p. 325, Firkin and Whitworth. The Parthenon, Lancashire, UK (1996)

Isidor S. Ravdin 1894–1980

Professor of Surgery, University of Pennsylvania

In the surgery of the future the individualist will be left by the roadside, for after all surgery is part of that broader field of experimental pathology to which all the medical sciences belong.

Annals of Surgery **127**: 666 (1948)

John Ray 1627–1705

English naturalist

Diseases are the tax on pleasures.

English Proverbs

Theodor Reik 1888–1969

German psychoanalyst

Work and love—these are the basics. Without them there is neurosis.

Attributed

Paul Reznikoff 1896–?

Conflict between science and religion should never exist. Their aims are entirely different—science tries to find out how, religion deals with why.
Attributed

Rhazes (abu-Bakr Muhammed ibn-Zakariya al Razi) 850–923

Persian physician (Baghdad school)

When the disease is stronger than the patient, the physician will not be able to help him at all, and if the strength of the patient is greater than the strength of the disease, he does not need a physician at all.
The Preservation of Youth

The patient who consults a great many physicians is likely to have a very confused state of mind.
Attributed

All that is written in books is worth much less than the experience of a wise doctor.
Attributed

At the beginning of a disease choose such remedies as will not lessen the patient's strength.
Attributed

Jonathan E. Rhoads

US paediatrician, University of North Carolina

Nurses and doctors who accompany patients on their final journey out of this life observe many ways of dying and many mechanisms of death. Some of these we understand to a greater extent than others.
Foreword in *Atlas of Nutritional Support Techniques*. Little, Brown and Co., Boston (1989)

One of the common mechanisms has been the accumulation of nutritional deficits leading very often to a loss of resistance to infection and the occurrence of an acute infection, such as pneumonia as the immediate prelude to death.
Foreword in *Atlas of Nutritional Support Techniques*. Little, Brown and Co.. Boston (1989)

Dickinson W. Richards 1895–1973

US Professor of Cardiac Surgery, Columbia University, and Nobel laureate

In order for the stethoscope to function, two things have to happen. There has to be, by God, a sick man at one end of it and a doctor at the other! The doctor has to be within thirty inches of the patient.
Transactions of the Association of American Physicians **75**: 1 (1962)

Jean Paul Richter 1713–68

German humorist and prose writer

Sleep, riches, and health are only truly enjoyed after they have been interrupted.
Flower, Fruit and Thorn Pieces Ch. 8 (1796)

David Riesman 1867–1940

US physician

If you want to get out of medicine the fullest enjoyment, be students all your lives.
Attributed

Sydney Ringer 1835–1910

British physician and physiologist

A man is a fool who holds two hospital appointments.
Quoted in *Dictionary of Medical Eponyms* (2nd edn), p. 339, Firkin and Whitworth. The Parthenon, Lancashire, UK (1996)

Isabel P. Robinault

Contemporary US sexologist

Sex is not an antidote for loneliness, feelings of inadequacy, fear of aging, hostility, or an inability to form warm friendships.
Sex, Society and the Disabled, ICD Rehabilitation and Research Unit, New York (Harper and Row, Maryland USA) (1978)

Duc François de la Rochefoucauld 1613–80

French humanist and satirist

Everyone complains of his memory, none of his judgment.
Maxims 89

There are certain situations, as there are maladies, which the accepted remedies serve only to aggravate at times; a truly clever man will know when it is dangerous to apply them.
Maxims 288 (transl. Constantine FitzGibbon)

To preserve one's health by too strict a regime is in itself a tedious malady.
Maxims 623

There are two things which Man cannot look at directly without flinching: the sun and death.
Maxims 623

Few people know how to be old.
Maxims 623

Wilhelm Conrad Roentgen 1845–1923

German physicist and discoverer of X-rays, Professor at Munich

For brevity's sake I shall use the expression 'rays' and to distinguish them from others of this name, I shall call them 'x-rays'.
On a New Kind of Rays

Apparatuses are cleverer than men and anyone who mishandles an apparatus is my enemy.
Quoted in *Dictionary of Medical Eponyms* (2nd edn), p. 334, Firkin and Whitworth. The Parthenon Lancashire, UK (1996)

Roger of Salerno 1031–101

Who from now on, wishes to practise medicine, has to present himself before our officials and examiners, in order to pass their judgment.
Chirugia magistri Rogeri

Karl von Rokitansky 1804–78
Viennese pathologist

The axiom of medicine is that natural science is its mother.
Handbook of Pathological Anatomy

Widespread experience in the field of pathological anatomy must be the foundation, unless the whole procedure is to eventuate in deception.
Handbuch der Pathologischen Anatomie (1842)

Humphrey Rolleston 1862–1944
British physician

Medicine is a noble profession but a damn bad business.
Attributed

James Harvey Robinson 1863–1936
US historian and educator

There are four historical layers underlying the minds of civilized men—the animal mind, the child mind, the savage mind, and the traditional civilized mind.
The Mind in the Making Ch. III, Sect. 6 (1921)

Jules Romains 1885–1972
French writer

Every man who feels well is a sick man neglecting himself.
Knock, ou le triomphe de la médicine.

Romanian proverb

If you wish to die soon, make your physician your heir.

Franklin D. Roosevelt 1882–1945
US President

Nothing can be more important to a State than its public health; the State's paramount concern should be the health of its people.
Report of the Special Health Commission, transmitted to the New York Legislature, 19 February (1931)

It is common sense to take a method and try it. If it fails, admit it frankly and try another. But above all, try something.
Address at Oglethorpe University, 22 May (1932)

Eucharius Roslin 1480–1520
German apothecary and obstretrician

When the birth cometh not naturally, then must the midwife do all her diligence and pain to turn the birth tenderly and with her annointed hands, so that it may be reduced again to a natural birth.
The Birth of Mankind (transl. Thomas Raynalde) (1540)

As concerning the bringing up, nourishment and giving of suckle to the child, it shall be best that the mother give her child suck herself, for the mother's milk is more convenient and agreeable to the infant than any other woman's.
The Birth of Mankind (transl. Thomas Raynalde) (1540)

George G. Ross 1834–92

Any fool can cut off a leg—it takes a surgeon to save one.
Attributed

Sir Ronald Ross 1857–1932
British professor of tropical medicine and discoverer of the cause of malaria

I was tired, and what was the use? I must have examined the stomachs of a thousand mosquitoes by this time. But the Angel of Fate fortunately laid his hand on my head.
Memoirs Ch. 13, words written on 20 August (1897)

Dante Gabriel Rossetti 1828–82
English poet and painter

My doctor's issued his decree
That too much wine is killing me
And furthermore his ban he hurls
Against my touching naked girls.
How then? Must I no longer share
Good wine or beauties, dark and fair?
Doctor, goodbye, my sail's unfurled,
I'm off to try the other world.
Quoted in *Clinical Pharmacology* by D. R. Lawrence, P. N. Bennett, and M. J. Brown. Churchill Livingstone, Edinburgh (1997)

Francis Peyton Rous 1879–1970
US pathologist and virologist

Tumours destroy man in a unique and appalling way, as flesh of his own flesh, which has somehow been rendered proliferative, rampant, predatory and ungovernable.
Quoted in *Dictionary of Medical Eponyms* (2nd edn), p. 349, Firkin and Whitworth. The Parthenon, Lancashire (1996)

Jean-Jacques Rousseau 1712–78
Geneva-born political philosopher and essayist

In regard to sickness, I shall not repeat the vain and false declamations made against medicine by most men in health.
A Discourse Upon the Origin and the Foundation of the Inequality Among Mankind Pt 1 (1755)

Teach him to live rather than avoid death: life is not breath, but action, the use of our senses, our mind, our faculties, every part of ourselves which makes us conscious of our being.
Émile Bk 1 (1762)

Joseph Roux 1834–86

Science is for those who learn; poetry, for those that know.
Meditations of a Parish Priest Ch. 1, No. LXXI (transl. Isabel Hapgood)

C. W. Rucker
Contemporary US ophthalmologist

The eye is a dark chamber, and its entrance, the pupil, appears black because the eye's dark purple lining absorbs all of the light that reaches it.
A History of the Ophthalmoscope. Whiting, Rochester, Minnesota (1971)

Rufus of Ephesus AD 110–180
Roman physician

I believe it is important to be informed of the nature of the disease in each individual patient, because we are not all formed in the same fashion, but we differ markedly from one another in many respects.
On the Interrogation of the Patient

Benjamin Rush 1745–1813
US politician and physician

Let us show the world that a difference of opinion upon medical subjects is not incompatible with medical friendships; and in so doing, let us throw the whole odium of the hostility of physicians to each other upon their competition for business and money.
Letter to Dr David Hosack, 15 August (1810)

John Ruskin 1819–1900
British art critic, reformer, and writer

They, on the whole, desire to cure the sick; and, if they are good doctors, and the choice were fairly put to them, would rather cure their patient and lose their fee, than kill him, and get it.
The Crown of Wild Olive

The work of science is to substitute facts for appearances, and demonstrations for impressions.
Stones of Venice Vol. III, Ch. II

Dora Russell (née Black) c.1894–1986
Wife of Bertrand Russell

We want far better reasons for having children than not knowing how to prevent them.
Hypatia or Women and Knowledge Ch. 4 (1925)

Bertrand Russell 1872–1970
British philosopher

One of the symptoms of approaching nervous breakdown is the belief that one's work is terribly important. If I were a medical man, I should prescribe a holiday to any patient who considered his work important.
The Autobiography of Bertrand Russell Vol. II, Ch. 5 (1914–44)

The people who are regarded as moral luminaries are those who forego ordinary pleasures themselves and find compensation in interfering with the pleasures of others.
Sceptical Essays

Love as a relation between men and women was ruined by the desire to make sure of the legitimacy of the children.
Marriage and Morals

Drunkenness is temporary suicide: the happiness that it brings is merely negative, a momentary cessation of unhappiness.
Attributed

William Russell 1852–1940
Scottish pathologist and physician, Edinburgh

The diagnosis of appendicitis requires the skilled palpation to which the physician is trained and the surgeon may be capable.
Quoted in Dictionary of Medical Eponyms (2nd edn), p. 351, Firkin and Whitworth. The Parthenon, Lancashire, UK (1996)

Russian proverbs

Drink a glass of wine after your soup and you steal a rouble from the doctor.

A word of kindness is better than a fat pie.

He who scratches a scar is wounded twice.

Simply imagine that it's not your child, but someone else's. Everybody knows how to bring up other people's children.

Ira Rutkow 1948–
US hernia surgeon and medical historian

If God operated on a hernia patient who is being paid to be off work, he would still be unable to work for six weeks or more.
Address at a Hernia Conference, Newport, Wales, May (2000)

John A. Ryle 1889–1950
English professor of medicine

The necessary but too rapid subdivision into specialisms and growing competition in every branch have, it would seem, been good for the technique but bad for the soul of medicine.
Fears May Be Liars Ch. 6

Saadi (Muslih-ud-Din) 1184–1291
Persian poet

When belly with bad pains doth swell,
It matters nought what else goes well.
Gulistan III.9 (transl. E. Arnold)

Saki (H. H. Munro) 1870–1916
British novelist and short story writer

'When I was younger boys of your age used to be nice and innocent.'
'Now we are only nice. One must specialise these days.'
The Complete Work of Saki p. 14. Penguin Books, London (1982)

School of Salerno 1095–1224

For ointment juice of Onyons is assign'd

To heads whose haire falls faster than it grows.
Regimen Sanitatis Salernitanum (transl. by Sir John Harington as The Englishman's Doctor)

Drink not much wine, sup light, and soon arise.
Regimen Sanitatis Salernitanum (transl. by Sir John Harington as The Englishman's Doctor)

John of Salisbury c.1115–80
English churchman, philosopher, and scholar

The common people say, that physicians are the class of people who kill other men in the most polite and courteous manner.
  Policraticus Bk II, Ch. 29

Robert, Marquis of Salisbury
1830–1903
English statesman and author

Doctors are a social cement.
  Attributed

William T. Salter 1901–52
US physician and pharmacologist

As he picks up his beautiful new tool, however, it is well for the modern biologist to remind himself how subtly and completely a fascination for gadgets can betray sound sense.
  Science **109**: 453 (1949)

H. Sanfey
Contemporary US surgeon, University of Virginia

Today's trainees have different values and demand a more balanced lifestyle than those who believed the only thing wrong with every other night-call was that you missed half the good cases.
  British Journal of Surgery **89**: 132–3 (2002)

George Santayana 1863–1952
Spanish-born US philosopher and poet

Life is not a spectacle or a feast; it is a predicament.
  Articles and Essays

Science is nothing but developed perception, interpreted intent, common sense rounded out and minutely articulated.
  The Life of Reason: Reason in Science, Ch. 11

There is no cure for birth and death save to enjoy the interval.
  Soliloquies in England 24, 'War Shrines'

Santorio Santorio 1561–1636
Italian physician, Capodistria, and inventor of the clinical thermometer

Obviously this method I have discovered is of great importance, since it enables us to ascertain the precise amount of that insensible perspiration interference which, according to Hippocrates and Galen, is the cause of all diseases.
  Quoted in *The Great Doctors—A Biographical History of Medicine*, Henry E. Sigerist. W. W. Norton and Co., New York (1933)

Dame Cicely Saunders 1918–
Pioneering UK palliative care physician

Approaches to death and dying reveal much of the attitude of society as a whole to the individuals who compose it. The development of ideas of what constitutes a good death can even be traced to prehistory.
  Foreword in *The Oxford Textbook of Palliative Medicine*. Oxford University Press, Oxford (1993)

The old acceptance of destiny has gone, and a new sense of outrage that modern advances cannot finally halt the inevitable makes care of the dying and their families demanding and often difficult, but perhaps all the more rewarding.
  Foreword in *The Oxford Textbook of Palliative Medicine*. Oxford University Press, Oxford (1993)

Frederick Saunders 1807–1902
English-born US author and librarian, New York

Empirics and charlatans are the excrescences of the medical profession.
  Salad for the Social 'The Mysteries of Medicine'

The best practitioners give to their patients the least medicine.
  Attributed

The language of the men of medicine is a fearful concoction of sesquipedalian words, numbered by thousands.
  Attributed

Girolamo Savonarola 1452–98
Italian religious and political reformer

The physician that bringeth love and charity to the sick, if he be good and kind and learned and skilful, none can be better than he.
  Attributed

Dorothy L. Sayers 1893–1957
British crime writer

If accidents happen and you are to blame, take steps to avoid repetition of same.
  In the Teeth of the Evidence 'Bitter Almonds'

Earle P. Scarlett 1896–?
Medical historian

Integrity and rectitude in our profession are paramount.
  Archives of Internal Medicine **118**: 603 (1966)

Richard Schatzki 1901–?
German-born US radiologist

The eyes must finish their work before the gray cells take over.
  Clinical Aphorisms from the Harvard Medical School 'Medicine' (1957)

R. Schaus
Contemporary US surgeon

Surgery is the endeavor where intellect and dexterity meet at the highest level in the creation of a peerless human accomplishment.
  Book Review of *Stapling in Surgery*

Béla Schick 1877–1967
Austrian paediatrician

The human body is like a bakery with a thousand windows. We are looking into only one window of the bakery when we are investigating one particular aspect of a disease.
Aphorisms and Facetiae of Béla Schick 'Early Years' (I. J. Wolf)

Children are not simply micro-adults, but have their own specific problems.
Aphorisms and Facetiae of Béla Schick 'Early Years' (I. J. Wolf)

First the patient, second the patient, third the patient, fourth the patient, fifth the patient, and then maybe comes science. We first do everything for the patient; science can wait, research can wait.
Aphorisms and Facetiae of Béla Schick 'Early Years' (I. J. Wolf)

It is too bad that we cannot cut the patient in half in order to compare two regimens of treatment.
Aphorisms and Facetiae of Béla Schick 'Early Years' (I. J. Wolf)

It is very difficult to slow down. The practice of medicine is like heart muscle contraction – it's all or none.
Aphorisms and Facetiae of Béla Schick 'Early Years' (I. J. Wolf)

The physician's best remedy is Tincture of Time!
Aphorisms and Facetiae of Béla Schick 'Early Years' (I. J. Wolf)

Johann Christoph Friedrich von Schiller 1759–1805
German poet, philosopher, and physician

All significant diseases, especially those issuing from a malignancy of the abdomen, are heralded by a greater or lesser upheaval of personality.
Prosaïsche Schriften (Erste Periode)

Johann Lukas Schönlein 1793–1864
German-born Zurich physician

We return to those foundations, to those pillars from which medicine started. The natural sciences are to serve as our guides and to show how observations must be made in order to gather experience and to elaborate this into facts.
Quoted in *The Great Doctors—A Biographical History of Medicine*, Henry E. Sigerist. Dover Publications, New York (1971) (original W. W. Norton and Co. Ltd, 1933)

Charles M. Schulz 1922–
US cartoonist

I love mankind—it's people I can't stand.
Go Fly a Kite, Charlie Brown

Albert Schweitzer 1875–1965
French Protestant theologian and medical missionary

Here, at whatever hour you come, you will find light and help and human kindness.
Inscribed on the lamp outside his jungle hospital at Lambaréné

Pain is a more terrible lord of mankind than even death himself.
On the Edge of the Primeval Forest Ch. 5

The purpose of human life is to serve and to show compassion and the will to help others.
The Schweitzer Album

It is our duty to remember at all times and anew that medicine is not only a science, but also the art of letting our own individuality interact with the individuality of the patient.

Sir Walter Scott 1771–1832
Scottish author

There is no harder worker in all Scotland, and none more poorly requited, than the village doctor, unless perhaps it be his horse.
The Surgeon's Daughter Ch. 1

Scottish proverb

He that eats but one dish seldom needs the doctor.

Roger Scruton 1944–
Professor of philosophy and author

The hunt has run its course, and the fox will die. His death will be quick—quicker by far than the death of a mouse in the paws of a cat, of a rat in the jaws of a terrier or of a human in the hands of his doctor.
On Hunting p. 133. Yellow Jersey Press, London (1998)

Frank Scully

You are not crippled at all unless your mind is in a splint.
Bartlett's Unfamiliar Quotations (Leonard Louis Levinson)

Sir Harry Secombe 1921–2001
Welsh comedian and singer

My advice if you insist on slimming: Eat as much as you like—just don't swallow it.
Attributed

David Seegal 1899–?
US physician and medical educator

Although many members of the medical profession might agree that their chosen discipline often leads to periods of weariness, frustration, or anxiety, the great majority of individuals in active practice would find it difficult to single out a dull day in their way of life.
Yale Scientific Magazine **36**: 31 (1962)

The apprentice in the various trades is not permitted advancement until his special line of duties has been rigorously tested under close inspection. Certainly no lesser criterion should prevail for the medical student.
Journal of the American Medical Association **180**: 476 (1962)

The involved student may thus come to appreciate that work, work, and more work plus a sense of proportion will ease him over the unexpected and man made hurdles during his career in medical school.
Journal of Medical Education **38**: 605 (1963)

The sound clinician attacks the core of the problem and avoids being mousetrapped by tangential data.

The Pharos of Alpha Omega Alpha **26**: 7 (1963)

Many of those who can teach, can do, and do do.

The Pharos of Alpha Omega Alpha **26**: 82 (1963)

The proper study of geriatrics begins with pediatrics.

Journal of Pediatrics **65**: 685 (1963)

Progress in medical science depends chiefly on the uncommon man, possessed of that rare asset, a brain so beautifully integrated with the retina, that when he looks, he perceives.

Journal of Pediatrics **39**: 321 (1964)

An increasing worship of the instrument for its own sake sometimes leads to enslavement by it.

Journal of Pediatrics **39**: 321 (1964)

John Selden 1584–1654

English historian

'Tis not the drinking that is to be blamed, but the excess.

Table Talk

Molly Selvin

Contemporary US historian

Most physicians no longer consider venereal diseases to be shameful, abhorrent evidence of an individual's degraded moral character.

Changing medical and societal attitudes towards sexually transmitted diseases: A historical overview. In: *Sexually Transmitted diseases*. McGraw-Hill (1984)

Richard Selzer 1928–

US surgeon and author, Connecticut

It is to search for some meaning in the ritual of surgery, which is at once murderous, painful, healing and full of love.

Mortal Lessons p. 9. Chatto & Windus, London (1981)

Who can gaze on so much misery and feel no hurt?

Mortal Lessons p. 10. Chatto & Windus, London (1981)

The surgeon knows all the parts of the brain but he does not know his patient's dreams.

Mortal Lessons p. 21. Chatto & Windus, London (1981)

A man does not know whose hands will stroke for him the last bubbles of his life. That alone should make him kinder to strangers.

Mortal Lessons p. 36. Chatto & Windus, London (1981)

Imagine God as tailor. His shelves are lined with rolls of skin, each with its subtleties of texture and hue. Six days a week He cuts lengths with which to wrap those small piles of flesh and bone into the clever parcels we call babies.

Mortal Lessons p. 95. Chatto & Windus, London (1981)

Ignaz Philipp Semmelweis 1818–65

Austrian-born professor of midwifery in Budapest and pioneer of asepsis

It is owing to the doctors that there is so high a mortality in childbed.

Aetiologie, Begriff und Prophylaxis der Kindbettfiebers

I was instantly struck with the close resemblance of the malady from which Kolletschka died to that which I had seen countless numbers of women perish after childbirth.

On the death of his friend the professor of Jurisprudence after being pricked by a needle during a post-mortem. *Aetiologie, Begriff und Prophylaxis der Kindbettfiebers*

Seneca *c.*4 BC–AD 65

Roman writer and statesman

Death is a punishment to some, to some a gift, and to many a favour.

Hercules Oetaeus

Time heals what reason cannot.

Agamemnon 130

At the beginning no one tries extreme remedies.

Agamemnon 153

Nothing hinders a cure so much as frequent changes of medicine.

Epistulae ad Lucilium

Disease is not of the body but of the place.

Epistulae ad Lucilium

It is not manly to fear to sweat.

Epistulae ad Lucilium XXXI.vii.31

A disease also is farther on the road to being cured when its breaks forth from concealment and manifests its power.

Epistulae ad Lucilium LVI

Drunkenness is simply voluntary insanity.

Epistulae ad Lucilium LXXXIII

Old age is a disease which we cannot cure.

Epistulae ad Lucilium LXXXIII

It is medicine not scenery, for which a sick man must go searching.

Epistulae ad Lucilium CIV

Remember that pain has this most excellent quality: if prolonged it cannot be severe, and if severe it cannot be prolonged.

Epistulae ad Lucilium XCIV

No man can have a peaceful life who thinks too much about lengthening it.

Epistulae ad Lucilium IV

Before I became old I tried to live well; now that I am old, I shall try to die well; but dying well means dying gladly.

Epistulae ad Lucilium LXI

Not even medicine can master incurable diseases.

Epistulae ad Lucilium XCIV

The body is not a permanent dwelling, but a sort of inn which is to be left behind when one perceives that one is a burden to the host.

Epistulae ad Lucilium CXX

People pay the doctor for his trouble; for his kindness they still remain in his debt.

Attributed

To desire to be healthy is part of being healthy.

Attributed

Marie de Sévingé 1626–96

French writer of letters

It is sometimes best to slip over thoughts and not go to the bottom of them.

Letter to her daughter

William Shakespeare 1564–1616

English author and playwright

Our remedies oft in ourselves do lie,
Which we ascribe to heaven.

All's Well That Ends Well I.1

A scar nobly got, or a noble scar, is a good liv'ry of honour.

All's Well That Ends Well IV. v. 105

With the help of a surgeon he might yet recover.

A Midsummer Night's Dream V. I. 316

Last scene of all,
That ends this strange eventful history,
Is second childishness and mere oblivion,
Sans teeth, sans eye, sans taste, sans everything.

As You Like It II. 7

By medicine life may be prolonged, yet death will seize the doctor too.

Cymbeline V.5

He that sleeps feels no toothache.

Cymbeline V.5

Though this be madness, yet there is method in it.

Hamlet II.2

To sleep—perchance to dream: ay, there's the rub!
For in that sleep of death what dreams may come
When we have shuffled off this mortal coil,
Must give us pause.

Hamlet III. i. 59

Is it not strange that desire should so many years outlive performance?

Henry IV, Part Two II. 4

If the cook help to make the gluttony, you help make the diseases.

Henry IV, Part Two II. 44–5

You shall digest the venom of your spleen, Though it do split you.

Julius Caesar IV. iii. 47

Your bum is the greatest thing about you.

Macbeth II. i. 214–216

It provokes the desire, but it takes away the performance. Therefore much drink may be said to be an equivocator with lechery.

Macbeth II. 3

When all's done, you look but on a stool.

Macbeth III. 4. 66–67

Macduff was from his mother's womb
Untimely ripp'd.

Macbeth V. viii. 15

The labour we delight in physics pain.

Macbeth V. viii. 15

The miserable have no other medicine.
But only hope.

Measure for Measure III. i. 2

For there was never philosopher
That could endure the toothache patiently.

Much Ado about Nothing V. 1

Eye is the window of the mind.

Richard II 1.iii

He that is stricken blind cannot forget
The precious treasure of his eyesight lost.

Romeo and Juliet I. i. 239

There's no time for a man to recover his hair that grows bald by nature.

The Comedy of Errors II. ii. 73

Thou cold sciatica,
Cripple our senators, that their limbs may halt
As lamely as their manners.

Timon of Athens IV. I. 23

He will be the physician that should be the patient.

Troilus and Cressida

I would there were no age between ten and three-and-twenty, or that youth would sleep out the rest, for there is nothing in the between but getting wenches with child, wronging the ancientry, stealing, fighting.

The Winter's Tale III. iii. 59

George Bernard Shaw

1856–1950

Irish-born playwright

I enjoy convalescence. It is the part that makes the illness worth while.

Back to Methuselah Pt II

Spend all you have before you die: and do not outlive yourself.
Take utmost care to get well born and well brought up.

From his Preface on Doctors published with *The Doctor's Dilemma* (1911)

All professions are conspiracies against the laity.

From his Preface on Doctors published with *The Doctor's Dilemma* (1911)

Medical science is as yet very imperfectly differentiated from common curemongering witchcraft.

From his Preface on Doctors published with *The Doctor's Dilemma* (1911)

Even the fact that doctors themselves die of the very diseases they profess to cure passes unnoticed.

From his Preface on Doctors published with *The Doctor Dilemma* (1911)

The most tragic thing in the world is a sick doctor.

From his Preface on Doctors published with *The Doctor's Dilemma* (1911)

Do not try to live forever. You will not succeed.
From his Preface on Doctors published with *The Doctor's Dilemma* (1911)

To give a surgeon a pecuniary interest in cutting off your leg, is enough to make one despair of political humanity.
From his Preface on Doctors published with *The Doctor's Dilemma* (1911)

He may be hungry, weary, sleepy, run down by several successive nights disturbed by that instrument of torture, the night bell; but who ever thinks of this in the face of sudden sickness or accident? We think no more of the condition of a doctor attending a case than the condition of a fireman at a fire.
From his Preface on Doctors published with *The Doctor's Dilemma* (1911)

If I refuse to allow my leg to be amputated, its mortification and my death may prove that I was wrong; but if I let the leg go, nobody can ever prove that it would not have mortified had I been obstinate. Operation is therefore the safe side for the surgeon as well as the lucrative side.
From his Preface on Doctors published with *The Doctor's Dilemma* (1911)

It does happen exceptionally that a practising doctor makes a contribution to science ... but it happens much oftener that he draws disastrous conclusions from his clinical experience because he has no conception of scientific method, and believes, like any rustic, that the handling of evidence and statistics needs no expertness.
From his Preface on Doctors published with *The Doctor's Dilemma* (1911)

A serious illness or a death advertises the doctor exactly as a hanging advertises the barrister who defended the person hanged.
From his Preface on Doctors published with *The Doctor's Dilemma* (1911)

When men die of disease they are said to die from natural causes. When they recover (and they mostly do) the doctor gets the credit of curing them.
From his Preface on Doctors published with *The Doctor's Dilemma* (1911)

Stimulate the phagocytes!
Sir Bloomfield Bonnington's cry in *The Doctor's Dilemma* (1911)

There is no love sincerer than the love of food.
Man and Superman Act. 1 'Maxims for Revolutionists'

Mens sana in corpore sano is a foolish saying. The sound body is a product of the sound mind.
Man and Superman Act. 1 'Maxims for Revolutionists'

The man with toothache thinks everyone happy whose teeth are sound.
Mans and Superman Act. 1 'Maxims for Revolutionists'

Life levels all men: death reveals the eminent.
Man and Superman Act. 1 'Maxims of Revolutionists'

The secret of being miserable is to have leisure to bother about whether you are happy or not. The cure for it is occupation.
Misalliance Preface, 'Parents and Children'

No man can be a pure specialist without being in the strict sense an idiot.
Attributed

An asylum for the sane would be empty in America.
Attributed

Youth is a wonderful thing. What a crime to waste it on children.
Attributed

Science is always wrong. It never solves a problem without creating ten more.
Attributed

Percy Bysshe Shelley 1792–1822
English poet

There is no disease, bodily or mental, which adoption of vegetable diet and pure water has not infallibly mitigated, wherever the experiment has been fairly tried.
Queen Mab Notes

William Shenstone 1714–63
English poet

Health is beauty, and the most perfect health is the most perfect beauty.
Essays on Men and Manners 'On Taste'

John Shepherd 1913–
British surgeon

Every surgeon should be something of a physician.
A Concise Surgery of the Acute Abdomen. Churchill Livingstone, Edinburgh (1974)

Richard Brinsley Sheridan 1751–1816
Irish-born British dramatist

I had rather follow you to your grave than see you owe your life to any but a regular-bred physician.
St. Patrick's Day Act II, Sc. iv

Charles Scott Sherrington 1857–1952
British physiologist

If it is for mind that we are searching the brain, then we are supposing the brain to be much more than a telephone-exchange. We are supposing it to be a telephone-exchange along with subscribers as well.
Man on his nature

Michael B. Shimkin 1926–
US Professor of Community Medicine and Oncology

Clinical observations, classifications, and theories of cancer extend to the dawn of medical history.
Cancer, Diagnosis, Treatment and Prognosis, Ackerman and del Regato Mosby (1985)

William Shippen Jr 1736–1808

US obstetrician

Experience is the mother of truth; and by experience we learn wisdom.

Quoted by Betsy C. Corner in *William Shippen, Jr.*

Herb Shriner

Contemporary US comic

Our doctor would never really operate unless it was necessary. He was just that way. If he didn't need the money, he wouldn't lay a hand on you.

Attributed

Aloysius Sieffert (*c.*1858)

The care of the human mind is the most noble branch of medicine.

Medical and Surgical Practitioner's Memorandum

Henry E. Sigerist 1891–1957

Swiss-born US medical historian

Hospitals are the temples of medicine. What may not always be possible in private practice must be possible in a hospital.

American Medicine Ch. 7. New York

The task of medicine is to promote health, to prevent disease, to treat the sick when prevention has broken down and to rehabilitate the people after they have been cured. These are highly social functions and we must look at medicine as basically a social science.

Civilisation and Disease Ch. 12. Phoenix Books, New York (1962)

At all times disease isolated its victims socially because their lives are different from those of healthy people.

Civilisation and Disease p. 66. Phoenix Books, New York (1962)

Most dangerous to society was an unskilled surgeon. The damage he could do was immediate and apparent to all.

Civilisation and Disease p. 100. Phoenix Books, New York (1962)

The problem of abortion is serious. In pre-Hitler Germany it was estimated that the country lost more women from septic abortion than from tuberculosis.

Civilisation and Disease p. 103. Phoenix Books, New York (1962)

It is very probable that euthanasia is actually practised by conscientious physicians much more often than we know.

Civilisation and Disease p. 106. Phoenix Books, New York (1962)

Illness, in general, is not a good literary subject.

Civilisation and Disease p. 182. Phoenix Books, New York (1962)

Disease is a dynamic process. It has a beginning – slow or sudden – develops, reaches in many cases an acme, and ends in recovery or death.

Civilisation and Disease p. 196. Phoenix Books, New York (1962)

A determining point in the history of gynecology is to be found in the fact that sex plays a more important part in the life of woman than in that of man, and that she is more burdened by her sex.

American Journals of Obstetrics and Gynecology **42**: 714 (1941)

Health cannot be forced upon the people. It cannot be dispensed to the people. They must want it and be prepared to do their share and to cooperate fully in whatever health program a country develops.

Canadian Journal of Public Health **35**: 253 (1944)

We see the physician as scientist, educator and social worker, ready to cooperate in teamwork, in close touch with the people he disinterestedly serves.

Proceedings of the American Philosophical Society **90**: 275 (1946)

Disease creates poverty and poverty disease. The vicious circle is closed.

Medicine and Human Welfare Ch. 1

Prevention of disease must become the goal of every physician.

Medicine and Human Welfare Ch. 3

The technology of medicine has outrun its sociology.

Medicine and Human Welfare Ch. 3

The very popular hunting for 'Fathers' of every branch of medicine is rather foolish, it is unfair not only to the mothers and ancestors but also to the obstetricians and midwives.

A History of Medicine Vol. 1. Oxford University Press, Oxford (1951)

We must also keep in mind that discoveries are usually not made by one man alone, but that many brains and many hands are needed before a discovery is made for which one man receives the credit.

A History of Medicine Vol. 1. Oxford University Press, Oxford (1951)

Hawi (*c.*2500 BC) attended to both ends of the gastrointestinal tract by being both physician of the teeth and guardian of the anus.

A History of Medicine Vol. 1, Ch. 3. Oxford University Press, Oxford (1951)

No doctors live on in the memory save the exceptional beings who enriched the healing art with new outlooks, who forged new weapons for the fight against disease.

The Great Doctors Preface

Patients must be adjusted socially as well as medically. The physicians must thus also play a social role.

Quoted in *Journal of the History of Medicine and Allied Sciences* **13**: 214 (1958)

Disease has social as well as physical, chemical, and biological causes.

Attributed

Silius Italicus 25?–101
Roman orator and poet

Men leave arms and legs behind, severed by the frost, and the cruel cold cuts off the limbs already broken.

Punica III.552

Milton M. Silverman 1910– (and P. R. Lee)
US pharmacologist

Patients themselves cannot escape the charge that they, by their own attitudes and actions, have contributed in a devastating fashion to the incidence of needless drug use.

Pills, profits, and politics. In: *Cured to Death*, Arabella Melville and Colin Johnson. Secker and Warburg Ltd, London (1982)

Viscount Simon 1873–1954
Lord Chancellor of England

Death, I suppose, may be a process rather than an instantaneous event.

Medicolegal judgment (1945)

James Young Simpson 1811–70
Professor of Midwifery, Edinburgh

From the time at which I first saw ether inhalation successfully practised I have had the conviction impressed upon my mind that we would ultimately find that other therapeutic agents were capable of being introduced with equal rapidity and success into the system, through the same extensive and powerful channel of pulmonary absorption.

On Chloroform. Rushton Clarke and Co, London (1848)

J. Marion Sims 1813–83
British anaesthetist

My hands are then henceforth, washed of chloroform and devoted to ether.

Letter to his wife, 21 November (1861)

Josef Skoda 1805–81
Bohemian-born professor of medicine in Vienna

Whilst a disease can be described and diagnosed, we can dare not to suspect to cure it by any manner of means.

Quoted in: *Dictionary of Medical Eponyms* (2nd edn), p. 374, Firkin and Whitworth. The Parthenon, Lancashire, UK (1996)

Petr Skrabanek 1941–94
Czech-born epidemiologist

Health, like love, beauty or happiness, is a metaphysical concept, which eludes all attempts at objectivisation.

The Death of Humane Medicine (1994)

Managers . . . as true parasites, they share the profits, without producing anything themselves.

The Death of Humane Medicine (1994)

The pursuit of health is a symptom of unhealth. When this pursuit is no longer a personal yearning but part of state ideology, *healthism* for short, it becomes a symptom of political sickness.

The Death of Humane Medicine (1994)

Medicine is not about conquering diseases and death, but about the alleviation of suffering, minimising harm, smoothing the painful journey of man to the grave.

The Death of Humane Medicine (1994)

Slovakian proverb

Pure water is the world's first and foremost medicine.

Adam Smith 1723–90
Scottish economist

Science is the great antidote to the poison of enthusiasm and superstition.

The Wealth of Nations Bk V, Ch. 1

Alexander Smith 1829–67
Scottish poet

To have to die is a distinction of which no man is proud.

Dreamthorp Ch. II (1863)

Anthony Smith 1927–
Science writer and broadcaster

Man is just another bit of biology, and there much of the animal kingdom is entirely relevant to his body, to his mechanism of sperm transfer, to his sex ratio, to his brain, to his sense of smell.

The Body, Introduction p. 17. Allen and Unwin, London (1968)

Italians used to find their mate at a distance, on average, of 600 yards. With the invention of the bicycle this distance leapt up—to 1600 yards.

Quoted in *The Human Pedigree* George Allen and Unwin, London (1975)

David James Smith 1960?–
British journalist

The murders fed Shipman's fascinating, thrilling, addictive need for proximity to death. Death that he had controlled.

Sunday Times 21 July (2002), commenting on the case of Dr Harold Shipman, mass murderer

Homer William Smith 1895–1962
US renal physiologist

Though we name the things we know, we do not necessarily know them because we name them.

Circulation of the Blood Ch. 9

Logan Pearsall Smith 1865–1946
US writer

The denunciation of the young is a necessary part of the hygiene of older people, and greatly assists the circulation of their blood.

All Trivia 'Last Words'

Sydney Smith 1771–1845
British churchman and essayist and wit

I am convinced digestion is the great secret of life.
Letters to Arthur Kinglake

There is only one rule of professional conduct. Do what you think right and take position and emoluments as an accident; all else is labour and sorrow.
A Memoir of the Revd Sydney Smith (quoted by Lady Holland)

Death must be distinguished from dying, with which it is often confounded.
A Memoir of the Revd Sydney Smith Ch. 6 (quoted by Lady Holland)

Oh! when I have the gout, I feel as if I was walking on my eyeballs.
A Memoir of the Revd Sydney Smith Ch. 11 (quoted by Lady Holland)

That sign of old age, extolling the past at the expense of the present.
A Memoir of the Revd Sydney Smith Ch. 6 (quoted by Lady Holland)

If consumption is too powerful for physicians, at least they should not suffer themselves to be outwitted by such little upstart disorders as the hay-fever.
Letter to Dr Holland, June (1835)

One evil in old age is, that as your time is come, you think every little illness is the beginning of the end. When a man expects to be arrested, every knock at the door is an alarm.
Letter to Sir Wilmot-Horton, 8 February (1836)

People of wealth and rank never use ugly names for ugly things. Apoplexy is an affection of the head; paralysis is nervousness; gangrene is pain and inconvenience in the extremities.
Letter to Mrs Holland, January (1844)

What is childhood but a series of happy delusions?
A Memoir of the Revd Sydney Smith Ch. 11 (quoted by Lady Holland)

Theobald Smith 1859–1934
US Professor of Pathology, Harvard

Great discoveries which give a new direction to currents of thought and research are not, as a rule, gained by the accumulation of vast quantities of figures and statistics.
Boston Medical and Surgical Journal **172**: 121 (1915)

Tobias Smollett 1721–71
English novelist and surgeon

A young man, in whose air and countenance appeared all the uncouth gravity and supercilious self-conceit of a physician hot from his studies.
The Adventures of Peregrine Pickle

Facts are stubborn things.
Gil Glas x.i

A Frenchman will sooner part with his religion than with his hair, which indeed, no consideration will induce him to forego.
Travels through France and Italy, 'Letter from Paris, October 12, 1763'

Francis Scott Smyth 1895–?
US paediatrician

To know what kind of a person has a disease is as essential as to know what kind of disease a person has.
Journal of Medical Education **37**: 495 (1962)

John Snow 1813–58
British physician, anaesthetist, and epidemiologist

The communicability of cholera ought not be disguised from the people, under the idea that the knowledge of it would cause panic or occasion the sick to be deserted.
On the Mode of Communication of Cholera

Socrates 469–399 BC
Greek philosopher

Living well and beautifully and justly are all one thing.
Crito (quoted by Plato)

Base men live to eat and drink, and good men eat and drink to live.
Quoted by Plutarch Moralia, 'How the Young Man should Study Poetry' (transl. F. C. Babbit)

Susan Sontag 1933–
US novelist and essayist

Everyone who is born holds dual citizenship in the kingdom of the well and in the kingdom of the sick.
Illness as Metaphor

Sophocles c.496–406 BC
Greek dramatist

Death is not the greatest of ills, it is worse to want to die, and not be able to.
Electra 1007

Sleep is the only medicine that gives ease.
Philoctetes 766 (transl. F. Storr)

Merrill C. Sosman 1890–1959
US physician

One look is worth a thousand listens.
Aphorism referring to X-rays

Samuel Southard
Contemporary US commentator

Illness may precipitate a spiritual crisis. Since illness is man's reaction to disease, it is a time when men are brought face to face with the ultimate concerns of life.
In Spiritual Care: The Nurse's Role Ch. 1, p. 19, Sharon Fish and Judith Allen Shelly. Intervarsity Press, Illinois, USA (1978)

M. Therese Southgate 1928–
US physician and medical historian

Unfortunately, too many authors write as though they will never have another chance—and they are correct.

Journal of the American Medical Association **181**: 1124 (1962)

Lazaro Spallanzani 1729–99
Italian professor of biology

If I set out to prove something, I am no real scientist—I have to learn to follow where the facts lead me—I have to learn to whip my prejudices.

Attributed

Spanish Proverbs

Bleed him and purge him; if he dies, bury him.

He that seeks finds.

In sleep we are all equal.

Science is madness if good sense does not cure it.

Six men give a doctor less to do than one woman.

Time cures the sick man, not the ointment.

Gavin Spence 1971–
British orthopaedic surgeon

Audit, the science of spying on the obvious, is clearly here to stay.

Hospital Doctor 12 November (1999)

Sir James Calvert Spence 1892–1954
Professor of Child Health, Durham, UK

The essential unit of medical practice is the occasion when, in the intimacy of the consulting room or sick room, a person who is ill, or believes himself to be ill, seeks the advice of a doctor whom he trusts.

The Purpose and Practice of Medicine Ch. 18, pp. 273–4. Oxford University Press, London.

Herbert Spencer 1820–1903
British philosopher and biologist

Science is organised knowledge.

Education Ch. 2

A living thing is distinguished from a dead thing by the multiplicity of the changes at any one moment taking place in it.

Principles of Biology Pt I, Ch. 4, Sect. 25

Survival of the fittest.

Principles of Biology Pt III, Ch. 12

Only when genius is married to science can the highest results be produced.

Education Ch. 1

The preservation of health is a duty. Few seem conscious that there is such a thing as physical morality.

Attributed

Willard L. Sperry 1882–1954
US Professor of Theology, Yale

Once a doctor subordinates the claims of an individual patient under his care to the abstract claims of society in general, or the hypothetical claims of some possible alternate patients, he has sold the pass.

The Ethical Basis of Medical Practice Ch. 8 (1950)

Benjamin Spock 1903–98
US paediatrician and psychiatrist

There are only two things a child will share willingly—communicable diseases and his mother's age.

Bartlett's Unfamiliar Quotations (Leonard Louis Levinson)

David Spodick
Contemporary

Physicians cure little or nothing. We alter physiology, arrest inflammation, and remove tissue, with the exception of some infections and some deficiency states there are few if any cures in terms of *restitutio ad integrum*.

American Heart Journal **81**: 149–57 (1971)

Margaret Stacey 1922–
Professor of Sociology, Warwick University, UK

For the past 135 years, British doctors have had privileged arrangements for accounting for themselves; privileged not only among other health care workers but also among all other occupations.

Medical Accountability. In: *Whistleblowing in the Health Service* p. 35, Geoffrey Hunt; Edwin Arnold, London (1995)

There is a strong case for having a well-organised and united medical profession independent of the state, not only in the interests of the profession itself but to speak up for the health of the nation from the point of view of skilled independent knowledge.

Medical Accountability. In: *Whistleblowing in the Health Service* p. 45, Geoffrey Hunt; Edwin Arnold, London (1995)

George Ernst Stahl 1660–1734
Professor of Medicine at Halle, Germany

If nature induces fever and inflammation, the physician must not try to counteract nature's purpose in these matters.

Quoted in *The Great Doctors—A Biographical History of Medicine* p. 184 Henry E. Sigerist; Dover Publications New York (1971) (original W. W. Norton and Co. Ltd, 1933)

Edward Stanley, Earl of Derby 1826–93
British Statesman

Those who think they have not time for bodily exercise will sooner or later have to find time for illness.

The Conduct of Life, Address at Liverpool College, 20 December (1873)

Issac Starr 1895–?

Too much emphasis on standards is a cause of decay; often it is a psychological defense mechanism set up by persons no longer productive.

Journal of Clinical Investigation **19**: 765 (1940)

Paul Starr 1949–

Professor of Sociology, Harvard University

Modern medicine is one of those extraordinary works of reason: an elaborate system of specialised knowledge, technical procedures, and rules of behaviour.

The Social Transformation of American Medicine Introduction, p. 3, Paul Starr. Basic Books, New York (1982)

The medical profession has had an especially persuasive claim to authority. Unlike the law and the clergy, it enjoys close bonds with modern science, and at least for most of the last century, scientific knowledge has held a privileged status in the hierarchy of belief.

The Social Transformation of American Medicine Introduction, p. 4, Paul Starr. Basic Books, New York (1982)

But medicine is also, unmistakably, a world of power where some are more likely to receive the rewards of reason than are the others.

The Social Transformation of American Medicine Introduction, p. 3, Paul Starr. Basic Books, New York (1982)

In America, no one group has held so dominant a position in this new world of rationality and power as has the medical profession.

The Social Transformation of American Medicine Introduction, p. 3, Paul Starr. Basic Books, New York (1982)

If the medical profession were merely a monopolistic guild, its position would be much less secure than it is. The basis of its high income and status, as I have argued all along, is its authority, which arises from lay deference and institutionalized forms of dependence.

The Social Transformation of American Medicine Introduction, p. 144, Paul Starr. Basic Books, New York (1982)

Probably no event in American history testifies more graphically to public acceptance of scientific methods than the voluntary participation of millions of American families in the 1954 trials of the Salk vaccine.

The Social Transformation of American Medicine Introduction, p. 346, Paul Starr. Basic Books, New York (1982)

Professional autonomy has been protected by the institutional autonomy of hospitals. In the multihospital systems, centralized planning, budgeting, and personnel decisions will deprive physicians of much of the influence they are accustomed to exercise over institutional policy.

The Social Transformation of American Medicine Introduction, p. 447, Paul Starr. Basic Books, NewYork (1982)

A corporate sector in health care is also likely to aggravate inequalities in access to health care. Profit-making enterprises are not interested in treating those who cannot pay. The voluntary hospital may not treat the poor the same as the rich, but they do treat them and often treat them well.

The Social Transformation of American Medicine Introduction, p. 448, Paul Starr. Basic Books, New York (1982)

Sir Richard Steele 1672–1729

Irish-born English essayist and dramatist

There are so few who can grow old with a good grace.

The Spectator 263

Gertrude Stein 1874–1946

US author

We, living now, are always to ourselves young men and women.

The Making of Americans Introduction

John Steinbeck 1902–68

US novelist

The medical profession is unconsciously irritated by lay knowledge.

East of Eden Ch. 54 (1952)

Laurence Sterne 1713–68

Irish-born English writer and churchman

There are worse occupations in the world than feeling a woman's pulse.

A Sentimental Journey

I live in a constant endeavour to fence against the infirmities of ill health, and other evils of life, by mirth.

Tristam Shandy Dedication

Imagine to yourself a little, squat, uncourtly figure of a Doctor Slop, of about four feet and a half perpendicular height, with a breadth of back and a sesquipedality of belly, which might have done honour to a serjeant in the horse-guards.

Tristam Shandy Vol. II, Ch. 9

Sciences may be learned by rote, but Wisdom not.

Tristam Shandy

People who are always taking care of their health are like misers, who are hoarding a treasure which they have never spirit enough to enjoy.

Attributed

Robert Louis Stevenson 1850–94

Scottish writer

He sows hurry and reaps indigestion.

An Apology for Idlers

Even if the doctor does not give you a year, even if he hesitates about a month, make one brave push and see what can be accomplished in a week.

Virginibus Puerisque Ch. 5

It is better to lose health like a spendthrift than to waste it like a miser.

Virginibus Puerisque Ch. 5

Johann Stieglitz 1767–1840

I have often thought it would be important to instruct physicians how to behave in cases of incurable disease; not so much to tell them what to do, but rather what not to do.

Letter to Dr Karl F. H. Marx, 15 December (1826)

Andrew T. Still 1828–1917

Rural Missouri doctor and founder of osteopathy

Quit your pills and learn from Osteopathy the principle that governs you. Learn that you are a machine, your heart an engine, your lungs a fanning machine and a sieve, your brain with its two lobes an electric battery.

Quoted in *The Autobiography of AT Still* Kirksville, MO. self-published (1897)

Alfred Stillé 1813–1900

US professor of medicine Philadelphia

To the vulgar apprehension, nothing seems more natural than that women should be physicians, for is not nursing the chief agent in the cure of disease, and who so fit a nurse as woman!

Transactions of the American Medical Association 22: 73 (1871)

Charles R. Stockard 1879–1939

US gynaecologist and researcher

Success in life depends upon the three I's, Integrity, Intelligence and Industry.

Attributed

Walter C. Stolov 1931–

Professor of Rehabilitation Medicine, University of Washington, Seattle

There is no one-to-one correlation between a disease and the spectrum of disability problems that may be associated with it.

Evaluation of the Patient, p. 1 In: *Krusen's Handbook of Physical Medicine and Rehabilitation*. W. B. Saunders, Philadelphia, USA (1990)

Rex Stout 1886–1975

US writer

There are two kinds of statistics, the kind you look up and the kind you make up.

Death of a Doxy Ch. 9

Maurice B. Strauss 1904–74

US Physician

So far as organization exists in every system from that of the atom to the universe, and from that of the single cell to the society of nations, the properties of no system can be wholly deduced from a knowledge of its isolated parts.

New England Journal of Medicine, 262: 805 (1960)

Medicine can never abdicate the obligation to care for the patient and to teach patient care.

Medicine 43: 19 (1964)

If they are not interested in the care of the patient, in the phenomena of disease in the sick, they should not be in the clinical department of medicine, since they cannot teach students clinical medicine.

Medicine 43: 619 (1964)

Samuel Enoch Stumpf 1918–

US philosopher, Tennessee

Some drugs have been appropriately called 'wonder-drugs' inasmuch as one wonders what they will do next.

Annals of Internal Medicine 64: 460 (1966)

Su Wen

Chinese sage

The sage does not treat those who are ill, but those who are well.

Attributed

The heart is in accord with the pulse.

The complexion of a person shows when the heart is in a splendid condition.

Net Ching Su Wen Book 3, Section 10

William Graham Sumner 1840–1910

US economist and sociologist

It used to be believed that the parent had unlimited claims on the child and rights over him. In a truer view of the matter, we are coming to see that the rights are on the side of the child and the duties on the side of the parent.

The Forgotten Man's Almanac 14 October (1919)

Susruta *c.*400 BC–AD 200

Hindu physician

When the doctor states that a man suffers from honey urine, he has also declared him incurable.

From the *Ayur Veda* quoted by R. Muller in 'Die Harnruhr der Alt-Inder' *Arch. Ges. Med.* 25: 1 (1932)

A pupil who is pure, obedient to his preceptor, applies himself steadily to his work, and abandons laziness and excessive sleep, will arrive at the end of the science he has been studying.

Sushruta-Samhita 'Sutrasthanam' Ch. 3

The patient, who may mistrust his own parents, sons and relations, should repose an implicit faith in his own physician, and put his own life into his hands without the least apprehension of danger; hence a physician should protect his patient as his own begotten child.

Sushruta-Samhita 'Sutrasthanam' Ch. 25

That person alone is fit to nurse or to attend the bedside of a patient, who is cool-headed and pleasant in his demeanour, does not speak ill of any body, is strong and attentive to the requirements of the sick, and strictly and indefatigably follows the instructions of the physician.

Sushruta-Samhita 'Sutrasthanam' Ch. 34.

Swahili proverb

The sick man is the garden of the physicians.

Swedish proverb

With a young lawyer you lose your inheritance; with a young doctor your health.

Jonathan Swift 1667–1745

Anglo-Irish priest and writer

No wise man ever wished to be younger.
Thoughts on Various Subjects, Moral and Diverting

Physicians ought not to give their judgment of religion, for the same reason that butchers are not admitted to be jurors upon life and death.
Thoughts on Various Subjects, Moral and Diverting

Thomas Sydenham 1624–89

British physician

This is all very fine, but it won't do—Anatomy—Botany—Nonsense! Sir, I know an old woman in Covent Garden who understands botany better, and as for anatomy, my butcher can dissect a joint full and well; no, young man, all that is stuff; you must go to the bedside, it is there alone you can learn disease.
Quoted by John Comrie in *Life of Thomas Sydenham*

The art of medicine was to be properly learned only from its practice and its exercise.
Medical Observations Dedicatory Epistle

I watched what method Nature might take, with intention of subduing the symptom by treading in her footsteps.
Medical Observations 5, Ch. 2

Nothing in medicine is so insignificant as to merit inattention.
Medical Observations 5, Ch. 2

What matters is that a doctor should come to know diseases, should learn the conditions out of which they arise and should be aware of the means by which they can be cured.
Quoted in *The Great Doctors—A Biographical History of Medicine* p. 179, Henry E. Sigerist. Dover Publications, New York (1971) (original W. W. Norton and Co. Ltd, 1933)

A disease, however much its course may be adverse to the human body, is nothing more than an effort of Nature, who strives with might and main to restore the health of the patient by the elimination of morbific humour.
Attributed

Simply to enumerate all the symptoms of hysteria would take a long day, so many are they.
Attributed

Gout, unlike any other disease, kills more rich men than poor, more wise than simple.
Works 'A Treatise on Gout and Dropsy' (transl. R. G. Latham) (1683)

I confidently affirm that the greater part of those who are supposed to have died of gout, have died of the medicine rather than the disease—a statement in which I am supported by observation.
Works 'A Treatise on Gout and Dropsy' (transl. R. G. Latham) (1683)

A man is as old as his arteries.
Attributed

Sylvius (François De La Bois) 15th century

French Professor of Anatomy, Paris

The aim of treatment must be to maintain the energies of the organism to drive away the illness, to remove the causes and to mitigate the symptoms.
Praxeos medicae idia nova (1671)

Andrew James Symington 1825–?

The medical profession is a noble and pleasant one, though laborious and often full of anxiety.
Attributed

Publilius Syrus 1st century BC

Roman dramatist

The madman thinks the rest of the world crazy.
Moral Sayings 386

They live ill who expect to live always.
Moral Sayings 457

Whom Fortune wishes to destroy she first makes mad.
Moral Sayings 911

Pain of mind is worse than pain of body.
Sententiae

Thomas Szasz 1920–

Hungarian-born US psychiatrist and writer

Masturbation: the primary sexual activity of mankind. In the nineteenth century it was a disease; in the twentieth it's a cure.
The Second Sin

If you talk to God, you are praying; if God talks to you, you have schizophrenia.
The Second Sin

Psychiatrists classify a person as neurotic if he suffers from his problems in living, and a psychotic if he makes others suffer.
The Second Sin

There is no psychology; there is only biography and autobiography.
The Second Sin

Tacitus c. AD 55–120

Roman historian

The physician is superfluous amongst the healthy.
Dialogus de Oratoribus

Rabindranath Tagore 1861–1941
Bengali poet and mystic

Even so, in death the same unknown will appear as ever known to me. And because I love this life, I know I shall love death as well.
Gitanjali

The fish in the water is silent, the animal on the earth is noisy, the bird in the air is singing.

But Man has in him the silence of the sea, the noise of the earth and the music of the air.
Stray Birds 43

Robert Lawson Tait 1845–99
British surgeon, Birmingham

I advised abdominal section and found the abdomen full of clot. The right Fallopian tube was ruptured and from it a placenta was protruding. I tied the tube and removed it.
Quoted by W.I.S. McKay in *Lawson Tait—His Life and Work*. Balliere Tindall and Cox (1922)

When in doubt, drain.
Quoted in *Archives of Surgery* **89**: 686 (1964)

The Talmud

A dream which is not interpreted is like a letter which is not read.
Berakoth IX.55b (transl. M. Simon)

In eating, a third of the stomach should be filled with food, a third with drink, and the rest left empty.
Gittin

A physician who heals for nothing is worth nothing.
Baba Kamma, VIII.85a

Whoever eats bread without previously washing the hands is as though he had intercourse with a harlot.
Sotah 1.4b

The best of doctors will go to hell.
Kiddushin IV.82a

The house which is not opened for charity will be opened to the physician.
Attributed

Wine is the foremost of all medicines— wherever wine is lacking medicines become necessary.
Attributed

A. J. P. Taylor 1906–90
British historian

The greatest problem about old age is the fear that it may go on too long.
Observer (1981)

Jeremy Taylor 1613–67
English theologian

To preserve a man alive in the midst of so many chances and hostilities, is as great a miracle as to create him.
The Rule and Exercises of Holy Dying Ch. 1, Sect. 1

John Taylor 1694–1761
English dissenting divine and Hebraist

A doctor is a man who writes prescriptions till the patient either dies or is cured by nature.
Attributed

Esaias Tegnér 1782–1846
Swedish Professor of Greek and poet, Lund

Today is my forty-third birthday. I have thus long passed the peak of life where the waters divide.
Letter to F. M. Franzen, November (1825)

William Temple 1881–1944
Archbishop of Canterbury

Science has its being in a perpetual mental restlessness.
Essays and Studies by Members of the English Association Vol. XVII, 'Poetry and Science'

Alfred, Lord Tennyson 1809–92
British poet

Every moment dies a man,
Every moment one is born.
The Vision of Sin Pt IV

Science moves, but slowly slowly,
creeping on from point to point.
Locksley Hall

Terence 185–159 BC (Publius Terentius After)
Carthage-born Roman comic poet

Old age is an illness in itself.
Phormio Act IV (transl. J. Sargeaunt)

Tertullian AD 160–230
Carthaginian father of the Church

To hinder a birth is merely speedier man-killing; nor does it matter whether you take away a life that is born, or destroy one that is coming to the birth. That is a man which is going to be one; you *have* the fruit already in its seed.
Apologiticus IX (transl. S. Thelwall)

Dylan Thomas 1914–53
Welsh poet

An alcoholic is someone you don't like who drinks as much as you do.
Dictionary of 20th Century Quotations quoted by Nigel Rees. Fontana London (1987)

Do not go gentle into that good night,
Old age should burn and rave at close of day;
Rage, rage against the dying of the light.
Do not go gentle into that good night

When I take up assassination, I shall start with the surgeons in this city and work *up* to the gutter.
The Doctor and the Devils 88

Sir Henry Thompson 1820–1904
London surgeon and urologist to royalty

Hence unwittingly these new instruments were absolutely free from any trace of bacterial taint through previous use for other patients.

Attributed to Thompson and quoted in *Harley Street* p. 6, by Reginald Pound. Michael Joseph, London (1967), explaining the absence of infection for the lithotomy on the Belgian king Leopold

Hamish Thomson 1940–
British surgeon, Gloucester

It is one of life's little ironies that surgical disease when not afflicting the unmentionable tends to favour the inaccessible.

Annals of the Royal College of Surgeons of England (College Bulletin) March (2000)

Henry David Thoreau 1817–62
US writer

Decay and disease are often beautiful like the pearly tear of the shellfish and the hectic glow of consumption.

Journal 11 June (1852)

'Tis healthy to be sick sometimes.
Attributed

Jurgen Thorowald 1900?–?
US surgeon

The status and progress of medicine ought always to be judged primarily from the point of view of the suffering patient, and never from the point of view of one who has never been ill.

The Century of the Surgeon. Pantheon, New York (1957)

Count Leo Tolstoy 1828–1910
Russian novelist

All happy families resemble one another, but each unhappy family is unhappy in its own way.

Anna Karenina Pt 1, Ch. 1

This is where the strength of the physician lies, be he a quack, a homeopath or an allopath. He supplies the perennial demand for comfort, the craving for sympathy that every human sufferer feels.

War and Peace Pt 9, Ch. 16

William Whiteman Carlton Topley 1886–1944
British pathologist and immunologist, London

I believe that a research committee can do one useful thing and one only. It can find the workers best fitted to attack a particular problem, bring them together, give them the facilities they need, and leave them to get on with the work.

Authority, Observation and Experiment in Medicine

Jesse Torrey 1787–1834

Coffee, though a useful medicine, if drunk constantly, will at length induce a decay of health, and hectic fever.

The Moral Instructor Pt IV, Sect. II, Ch. 10

Stephen E. Toulmin 1922–
British born US professor of multi-ethnic studies, Southern California

The more we treat the theories of our predecessors as myths, the more inclined we shall be treat our own theories as dogmas.

Journal of the History of Ideas **18**: 206 (1957)

Henri Toulouse-Lautrec 1864–1901
French painter

I can drink without danger, I am so near to the ground.

Comment to Charles Bouget

Arnold Toynbee 1889–1975
British historian

We have been God-like in our planned breeding of our domesticated plants and animals, but we have been rabbit-like in our unplanned breeding of ourselves.

National Observer 10 June (1963)

The twentieth century will be remembered chiefly, not as an age of political conflicts and technical inventions, but as an age in which human society dared to think of the health of the whole human race as a practical objective.

Attributed

Sir Frederick Treves 1853–1923
English surgeon who operated on King Edward VII

The symptoms of disease are marked by purpose, and the purpose is beneficent. The processes of disease aim not at the destruction of life, but at the saving of it.

Address to the Edinburgh Philosophical Institution, 31 October (1905)

Anthony Trollope 1815–82
English novelist

A physician should take his fee without letting his left hand know what his right hand was doing; it should be taken without a thought, without a look, without a move of the facial muscles; the true physician should hardly be aware that the last friendly grasp of the hand had been made precious by the touch of gold.

Doctor Thorne Ch. III

Théodore Tronchin 1709–81
Swiss physician from Geneva and discoverer of lead poisoning

In medicine, sins of commission are mortal, sins of omission venial.

Quoted in *Bulletin of the New York Academy of Medicine* **5**: 155 (1929)

Wilfrid Trotter 1872–1939

British surgeon, University College Hospital, London

Mr. Anaesthetist, if the patient can keep awake, surely you can.

Quoted in the *Lancet* **2**: 1340 (1965)

Disease often tells its secrets in a casual parenthesis.

Collected Papers Sect. 6 'Art and Science in Medicine'

All knowledge comes from noticing resemblances and recurrences in the events that happen around us.

Collected Papers Sect. 6 'Has the Intellect a Function?'

Armand Trousseau 1810–67

French physician

Take care not to fancy that you are physicians as soon as you have mastered scientific facts; they only afford to your understandings an opportunity of bringing forth fruit, and of elevating you to the high position of a man of art.

Clinical Medicine Vol. 1, Introduction

A knowledge of the specific element in disease is the key of medicine.

Clinical Medicine Vol. 1, Introduction

From facts adduced, we must conclude with the physiologist (Brown-Sequard) that the supra-renal capsules are organs essential to life.

Lectures on Clinical Medicine p. 156 (1872), on describing Addison's disease

Medicine consists of science and art in a certain relationship to each other, yet wholly distinct. Science can be learned by anyone, even the mediocre. Art, however, is a gift from heaven.

Attributed

Tung-su Pai

Chinese sage

A dirty cook gives diarrhoea quicker than rhubarb.

Quoted in *Bulletin of the New York Academy of Medicine* **4**: 985 (1928)

Samuel L. Turek 1920–

US orthopedic surgeon, Cook County Hospital

Orthopaedics is a medical and surgical science that continues to encompass an ever expanding spectrum of subsciences each of which appears to endlessly widen its horizons as new principles evolve and formerly held tenets are modified.

Preface to *Orthopaedicas and Their Application*, (4th edn). J.B. Lippincott Co. Philadelphia, USA (1984)

Ivan Turgenev 1818–83

Russian novelist

Illness isn't the only thing that spoils the appetite.

A Month in the Country Act IV (transl. Constance Garnett)

Mark Twain (Samuel L. Clemens) 1835–1910

US writer

Adam and Eve had many advantages, but the principal one was that they escaped teething.

The Tragedy of Pudd'nhead Wilson Ch. 4

Why is it that we rejoice at a birth and grieve at a funeral: It is because we are not the person involved.

The Tragedy of Pudd'nhead Wilson Ch. 9

Surgeons and anatomists see no beautiful women in all their lives, but only a ghastly stack of bones with Latin names to them, and a network of nerves and muscles and tissues inflamed by disease.

Letter to the Alta Californian, San Francisco, 28 May (1867)

If there is one thing that will make a man peculiarly and insufferably self-conceitied, it is to have his stomach behave itself, the first day at sea, when nearly all his comrades are seasick.

The Innocents Abroad Ch. III

The higher animals get their teeth without pain or inconvenience. Man gets his through months and months of cruel torture; he will never get a set which can really be depended on 'till a dentist makes him one.

The Damned Human Race

The reports of my death are greatly exaggerated.

Cable to the Associated Press 2 June (1897), in *Mark Twain, Wit and Wisdom*

To cease smoking is the easiest thing I have ever done. I ought to know because I have done it a thousand times.

Attributed

David Tweedle 1941–

British surgeon

Surgeons have little knowledge of bacteriology and continue to use rituals without scientific evidence. Bacteriologists are out of touch with clinical reality and propose investigative and prophylactic procedures which create havoc in the running of the hospital.

Book review. *British Journal of Surgery* **68**(9): 696 (1981)

Miguel de Unamuno y Jugo 1864–1936

Spanish writer and philosopher

Science says: 'We must live,' and seeks the means of prolonging, increasing, facilitating and amplifying life, of making it tolerable and acceptable; wisdom says: 'We must die,' and seeks how to make us die well.

Essays and Soliloquies 'Arbitrary Reflections'

True science teaches, above all, to doubt and to be ignorant.

The Tragic Sense of Life Ch. V

Maximilianus Urentius 1621–51

Wherein differs the surgeon from the doctor? In this way, that one kills with his drugs, the other with his knife. Both differ from the hangman only in doing slowly what he does quickly.

Attributed

Jerry Vale

Whiskey is the most popular of all the remedies that won't cure a cold.

Bartlett's Unfamiliar Quotations (Leonard Louis Levenson)

Paul Valéry 1871–1945

French writer

The object of psychology is to give us a totally different idea of the things we know best.

Tel Quel

Marcos Varro 1st century BC

Roman physician

In damp places there grow tiny creatures, too small for us to see, which make their way into our bodies through mouth and nose and give rise to grave illnesses.

De re rustica

Thorsten Veblen 1857–1929

US sociologist

The outcome of any serious research can only be to make two questions grow where only one grew before.

The Place of Science in Modern Civilisation

James Venable c.1846

First ether patient

I commenced inhaling the ether before the operation was commenced and continued it until the operation was over. I did not feel the slightest pain from the operation and could not believe the tumor was removed until it was shown to me.

Account by first patient who underwent ether anaesthetic at Massachusetts General, Boston

Venetian proverb

Woollen clothing keeps the skin healthy.

Tobias Venner 1577–1660

English apothecary

Men of lean habit of body are commonly a long time healthy, having good appetites and strong stomachs for digestion.

Via recta ad vitam longam

Queen Victoria 1819–1901

British monarch

Dr. Snow gave that blessed Chloroform and the effect was soothing, quieting and delightful beyond measure.

Journal, describing her labour

Leonardo da Vinci 1452–1519

Italian artist and scientist

Why does the eye see a thing more clearly in dreams than the imagination when awake?

Arundel MSS British Museum (transl. Edward MacCurdy in *The Notebooks of Leonardo da Vinci* Vol. I, Ch. I)

Man and the animals are merely a passage and channel for food, a tomb for other animals, a haven for the dead, giving life by the death of others, a coffer of corruption.

Codice Atlantico 76 in *The Notebooks of Leonardo da Vinci* Vol. I, Ch. I

The common sense is that which judges the things given to it by the other senses.

Codice Atlantico 90

If you are mindful that old age has wisdom for its food, you will so exert yourself in youth, that your old age will not lack sustenance.

Codice Atlantico 112

Iron rusts from disuse; stagnant water loses its purity and in cold weather becomes frozen; even so does inaction sap the vigour of the mind.

Codice Atlantico 289

Life well spent is long.

Codice Trivulziano 63 (transl. Edward MacCurdy in *The Notebooks of Leonardo da Vinci* Vol. I, Ch. I)

As a well-spent day brings happy sleep, so life well used brings happy death.

Codice Trivulziano 281

Veins which by the thickening of their funicles in the old restrict the passage of the blood, and by this lack of nourishment destroy their life without any fever, the old coming to fail little by little in slow death.

Dell' Anatomia Fogli B (transl. Edward MacCurdy in *The Notebooks of Leonardo da Vinci* Vol. I, Ch. III)

The act of procreation and the members employed therein are so repulsive, that if it were not for the beauty of the faces and the adornments of the actors and the pent-up impulse, nature would lose the human species.

Dell' Anatomia Fogli B (transl. Edward MacCurdy in *The Notebooks of Leonardo da Vinci* Vol. I, Ch. III)

All the veins and arteries proceed from the heart; and the reason is that the maximum thickness that is found in these veins and arteries is at the junction that they make with the heart; and the farther away they are from the heart the thinner they become and they are divided into more minute ramifications.

Dell' Anatomia Vol. I, Ch. III

The function of muscle is to pull and not to push except in the case of the genitals and the tongue.

Dell' Anatomia Vol. I, Ch. III

Those who are enamoured of practice without science are like a pilot who goes into a ship without rudder or compass and never has any certainty where he is going.

Practice should always be based upon a sound knowledge of theory.

Dell' Anatomia Vol. II, Ch. 29

The black races in Ethiopia are not the product of the sun; for if black gets black with child in Scythia, the offspring is black; but if a black gets a white woman with child the offspring is grey.

Quaderni d'Anatomia Vol. III (transl. Edward MacCurdy in *The Notebooks of Leonardo da Vinci* Vol. I, Ch. III)

No human investigation can be called true science without passing through mathematical tests.

Treatise on Painting Ch. I (transl. Jean Paul Richter)

Rudolf Virchow 1821–1902
German pathologist

A cell in which every cell is a citizen.
Die Cellularpathologie (1858) Disease, Life and Man p. 142–9 (transl. Lelland J. Rather, Stanford University Press, 1958)

All cells come from other cells.
Die Cellularpathologie (1858) Disease, Life and Man p. 142–9 (transl. Lelland J. Rather, Stanford University Press, 1958)

At that time we attempted to shake off the spell which philosophy, nature-philosophy in particular, had for a long period cast over science. We fought against 'a priori' speculation; we rejected systems, and we relied solely on experience.
Standpoints in Scientific Medicine 142–9 (1877) (transl. Lelland J. Rather, Stanford University Press, 1958)

There can be no scientific dispute with respect to faith, for science and faith exclude one another.
Disease, Life, and Man 'On Man'

The physicians are the natural attorneys of the poor and the social problems should largely be solved by them.
Rudolf Virchow, 'The Doctor' (Ervin H. Ackernecht)

Marriages are not normally made to avoid having children.
Quoted in 'Medical Proverbs' by F. H. Garrison, *Bulletin of the New York Academy of Medicine* October: 979–1005 (1928)

Has not science the noble privilege of carrying on its controversies without personal quarrels?
Quoted in 'Medical Proverbs' by F. H. Garrison, *Bulletin of the New York Academy of Medicine* October: 979–1005 (1928)

The touchstone of science is power of performance, for it is a truism that what can, also will, and thus attains to real existence.
Quoted in 'Medical Proverbs' by F. H. Garrison, *Bulletin of the New York Academy of Medicine* October: 979–1005 (1928)

Should medicine ever fulfill its great ends, it must enter into the large political and social life of our time; it must indicate the barriers which obstruct the normal completion of the life-cycle and remove them.
Quoted in 'Medical Proverbs' by F. H. Garrison, *Bulletin of the New York Academy of Medicine* October: 979–1005 (1928)

Even in the hands of the greatest physicians, the practice of medicine is never identified with scientific (laboratory) medicine, but is only an application of it.
Quoted in 'Medical Proverbs' by F. H. Garrison, *Bulletin of the New York Academy of Medicine* October: 979–1005 (1928)

Medical instruction does not exist to provide individuals with an opportunity of learning how to make a living, but in order to make possible the protection of the health of the public.
Address to medical students in Berlin.

Virgil 70–19 BC
Roman poet

Miseris succurrere disco.
(I learn to relieve the suffering)
Aeneid I.630

That sweet, deep sleep, so close to tranquil death.
Aeneid VI. 522

It was his part to learn the powers of medicine and the practice of healing, and careless of fame, to exercise the quiet art.
Aeneid

Time carries all things, even our wits, away.
Eclogues IX

Karl Vogt 1817–95
German zoologist

The brain secretes thought as the stomach secretes gastric juice, the liver bile and the kidneys urine.
Köhlerglaube and Wissenschaft

Richard Volkmann 1830–89
German professor of surgery, Leipzig

I reject the feeling expressed in England in their preference for colostomy over resection of the rectum.
Beitragen Zur Chirurgie, Leipzig 1875, quoted by Marvin Corman in *Diseases of the Colon and Rectum* **29**: 679–685 (1986)

François Voltaire 1694–1778
French writer and philosopher

Wounds of the soul are a disease wherein the patient must minister to himself.
Letter to a friend (1728)

Men will always be mad and those who think they can cure them are the maddest of all.
Letter (1762)

Men who are occupied in the restoration of health to other men, by the joint exertion of skill and humanity, are above all the great of the earth. They even partake of divinity, since to preserve and renew is almost as noble as to create.
A Philosophical Dictionary 'Physicians' (1764)

Man can have only a certain number of teeth, hair and ideas; there comes a time when he necessarily loses his teeth, hair and ideas.
A Philosophical Dictionary 'Physicians' (1764)

Not that suicide always comes from madness.
Letter to James Marriott (1767)

I know nothing more laughable than a doctor who does not die of old age.
Letter to Charles Feriol 6 November (1767)

Who are the greatest deceivers? The doctors? And the greatest fools? The patients?
Attributed

A physician is one who pours drugs of which he knows little into a body of which he knows less.
Attributed

Peter de Vries 1910–93
US writer

We know the human brain is a device to keep the ears from grating one on another.
Comfort me with Apples Ch. 1

Gluttony is an emotional escape, a sign something is eating us.
Comfort Me with Apples Ch. 15

Johann Wagner 1800–33
German pathologist

The auditory nerves were atrophied. The convolutions of the brain, which was rather soft and oedematous, seemed to be twice as deep and twice as numerous as normal.
Report on post-mortem of Ludwig van Beethoven in *Beethoven Handbuch* Vol. 1 (Hans Waine)

Arthur M. Walker 1896–1955

I would like to remind those responsible for the treatment of tuberculosis that Keats wrote his best poems while dying of this disease. In my opinion he would never have done so under the influence of modern chemotherapy.
Quoted in *Walkerisms* by Julius L. Wilson

Andrew Wall
Contemporary health scientist, University of Birmingham, UK

Health service managers usually work with utilitarian assumptions and may describe their obligation as one of maximising benefits to the greatest number of patients. Doctors and other professionals may find this view at odds with their responsibility to their individual patient.
Quoted in *Whistleblowing in the Health Service* p. 29, Geoffrey Hunt. Edwin Arnold, London (1995)

Patrick David Wall 1925–
Professor of Anatomy, University College, London

The immediate origins of misery and suffering need immediate attention. The old methods of care and caring had to be rediscovered and the best of modern medicine had to be turned to the task of new study and therapy specifically directed at pain.
Pain **25**: 1–4 (1986)

Alfred R. Wallace 1823–1913
British naturalist and traveller

The Darwinian theory, even when carried out to its extreme logical conclusion, not only does not oppose, but lends a decided support to, a belief in the spiritual nature of man.
Darwinisms Ch. 15

W. A. Wallis
British statistician

Statistics may be defined as 'a body of methods for making wise decisions in the face of uncertainty'.
Statistics, A New Approach. Methuen, London (1957)

Horace Walpole 1717–97
English writer

When people will not weed their own minds, they are apt to be overrun with nettles.
Letter to Lady Ailesbury, 10 July (1779)

Sir Francis Martin Rouse Walshe 1888–1973
British clinical neurologist

It is therefore reasonable to think that anyone who has spent a long professional life in medicine must have something to hand on—however small or modest.
Canadian Medical Association Journal **67**: 395 (1952)

Symposia, like hard liquor, should be taken in reasonable measure, at appropriate intervals.
Perspectives in Biology and Medicine **2**: 197 (1959)

Izaak Walton 1593–1683
English writer

Look to your health: and if you have it, praise God, and value it next to a good conscience;
The Compleat Angler Pt 1, Ch. 21

Owen Wangensteen 1898–1980
US surgeon

For the difficult surgery of today, a sturdy pair of legs is also an indispensable necessity!
Surgery, Gynecology and Obstetrics **84**: 567 (1947)

Charles Dudley Warner 1829–1900
US writer

In the minds of the public, there is mystery about the practice of medicine.
Attributed

John Collins Warren 1778–1856
US surgeon

A hospital is an institution absolutely essential to a medical school, and one which would afford relief and comfort to thousands of the sick and miserable.
Fund-raising letter, 20 August (1810)

Well, Sir, your patient is ready!
Gentlemen, this is no humbug!
Attributed to Warren on witnessing the first ether anaesthetic in Boston in 1846

Benjamin Waterhouse 1754–1846

Cannot wisdom devise a plan of social intercourse independent of the stimulus of the bottle?
Cautions to Young Persons Concerning Health

David Waters
Contemporary US cardiac surgeon

When applying a new technique or instrumentation, do not test the waters with both feet at the same time.
Attributed

Sir Reginald Watson-Jones 1902–72
British orthopaedic surgeon

It is worse to sprain an ankle than to break it.
Quoted in *Watson-Jones' Fractures and Joint Injuries* p. 19
(ed. J. N. Wilson)

Evelyn Waugh 1903–66
British satirist and novelist

All this fuss about sleeping together. For physical
pleasure I'd sooner go to my dentist any day.
Vile Bodies (1930)

Warren Weaver 1894–1978
Director, Rockefeller Foundation, New York

And gradually there is coming into being a new
branch of science—molecular biology—which is
beginning to uncover many secrets concerning
the ultimate units of the living cell.
The Natural Sciences (1938)

Sir Alfred Webb-Johnson 1880–1958
British surgeon

The well equipped clinician must possess the
qualities of the artist, the man of science, and the
humanist, but he must exercise them only in so
far as they subserve the getting well of the
individual patient.
Medical Press **216**: 312 (1946)

Lord Robert Webb-Johnstone 1879–?

A neurotic is the man who builds a castle in the
air. A psychotic is the man who lives in it. And a
psychiatrist is the man who collects the rent.
Collected Papers

John Webster 1580–1625
English dramatist

Death hath ten thousand several doors
For men to take their exits.
The Duchess of Malfi Act IV, Sc. ii

Physicians are like kings, they brook no
contradiction.
The Duchess of Malfi Act IV, Sc. ii

Jerome Pierce Webster 1888–?
US plastic surgeon

The plastic surgeon works with living flesh as his
clay, and his work of art is the attempted
achievement of normalcy in appearance and
function.
Foreword to *The Principles and Art of Plastic Surgery*

Otto Weininger 1880–1903

With the woman, thinking and feeling are
identical, for man they are in opposition.
Sex and Character Pt II, Ch. 3

It is not the fear of death which creates the desire
for immortality, but the desire for immortality
which causes the fear of death.
Sex and Character Pt II, Ch. 5

Soma Weiss 1899–1942
Hungarian-born US physician, Boston

A diagnosis is easy as long as you think of it.
Quoted in *Dictionary of Medical Eponyms* (2nd edn), p. 252.
Firkin and Whitworth. The Parthenon, Lancashire, UK
(1996)

William H. Welch 1850–1934
US professor of pathology

Medical education is not completed at the medical
school: it is only begun.
Bulletin of the Harvard Medical School Association **3**: 55 (1892)

Cleanliness and comfort demand that means shall
be taken to render pure the ground on which we
live, the air which we breathe, and the water and
food with which we are supplied, and we must
meet these needs without waiting to learn just
what relation infectious agents bear to the earth,
air, water and food.
Maryland Medical Journal **21**: 201 (1889)

The main cause of this unparalleled progress in
physiology, pathology, medicine and surgery has
been the fruitful application of the experimental
method of research.
Speaking against the Antivivisection Bill in the US Senate
21 February (1900)

H. Gideon Wells 1875–1943
US biochemist

Maternity is a matter of fact—paternity is a
matter of speculation.
Attributed

Welsh proverbs

Disease and sleep keep far apart.

Heaven defend me from a busy doctor.

Thin women live long.

Three things give hardy strength; sleeping on
hairy mattresses, breathing cold air, and eating
dry food.

Karl Frederik Wenckebach 1864–1940
Dutch-born professor of medicine, Vienna

I owe my reputation to the fact that I use digitalis
in doses the text books say are dangerous and in
cases that the text books say are unsuitable.
Lancet **2**: 633 (1937)

Timberlake Wertenberger
Contemporay US playwright

It is possible that human beings have come to the
end of their evolution, but we will never come to
the end of our imagination.
Attributed

John Wesley 1703–91
Evangelist and founder of Methodism

In former times people treated themselves, but the physicians then concocted complicated theories to confuse ordinary people.
Primitive Physic: Or an Easy and Natural Method of Curing Most Diseases London (1791)

Hugh Wheeler 1912–
US writer

To lose a lover or even a husband or two during the course of one's life can be vexing. But to lose one's teeth is a catastrophe.
A Little Night Music

James McNeil Whistler 1834–1903
US painter and wit

The explanation is quite simple. I wished to be near my mother.
Explaining why he had been born in a small unfashionable Massachusetts town and not fashionable New York or London.

E. B. White 1899–1985
US journalist and humorist

The imaginary complaints of indestructible old ladies.
Harper's Magazine November (1941)

In a man's middle years there is scarcely a part of the body he would hesitate to turn over to the proper authorities.
The Second Tree from the Corner 'A Weekend with the Angels'

Raymond Whitehead 1904–65
British pathologist

Medicine is not a field in which sheep may safely graze.
British Medical Journal **2**: 491 (1956)

Katherine Whitehorn 1926–
British journalist

A food is not necessarily essential just because your child hates it.
How to Survive Children

Stop people dying of the illnesses they die of now, and they will die of something else later, and the slower and the costlier.
Observer 3 February (1991)

Arthur Whitfield 1847–1947
English Professor of Dermatology, King's College, London

Always examine your cases thoroughly. Re-examine them. Re-examine your own deductions.
Dictionary of Medical Eponyms (2nd edn), Firkin and Whitworth. The Parthenon, Lancashire, UK (1996)

John Greenleaf Whittier 1807–92
US Quaker poet and abolitionist

It is the special vocation of the doctor to grow familiar with suffering.
Motto on the seal of the New Jersey College

George F. I. Widal 1862–1929
Professor of medicine, Paris

I want to get a job where I can learn something of general medicine; the neurologists just talk and do nothing.
Personal reply to Clovis Vincent, famous neurosurgeon

Samuel Wilberforce 1805–73
British churchman

I would like to ask the gentleman ... whether the ape from which he is descended was on his grandmother's or his grandfather's side of the family.
British Association for the Advancement of Science, Oxford, 30 June (1860)

Aaron Wildavsky
Contemporary US health economist

The marginal value of one or one billion-dollars spent on medical care will be close to zero in improving health.
Doing Better and Feeling Worse, The Political Pathology of Health Policy p. 106. Daedulus Winter (1977)

Oscar Wilde 1854–1900
Irish writer and wit

Illness is hardly a thing to be encouraged in others. Health is the primary duty of life.
The Importance of Being Earnest Act 1

One can survive everything nowadays, except death.
A Woman of No Importance I

Ah well, I suppose I shall have to die beyond my means.
Attributed

Heredity is the last of the fates, and the most terrible.
Attributed

Sir William Wilde 1815–76
ENT surgeon and father of Oscar

There are two kinds of deafness. One is due to wax and is curable; the other is not due to wax and is not curable.
Attributed

Thornton Niven Wilder 1897–?
US author and playwright

Doctors are mostly impostors. The older a doctor is and the more venerated he is, the more he must pretend to know everything. Of course, they grow worse with time. Always look for a doctor who is hated by the best doctors, Always seek out a bright young doctor before he comes down with nonsense.

John Wilkes 1727–97
English politician

The chapter of accidents is the longest chapter in the book.
  Attributed in *The Doctor* (Southey) Vol. IV

Wendell L. Wilkie 1892–1944

The real public health problem, of course, is poverty.
  One World Ch. 2

George Wilkins 17th century
English dramatist

Drinke makes men hungry, or it makes them lie.
  The Miseries of Inforsed Marriage Act II

Christopher Williams 1938–
Gastroenterologist, St. Mark's Hospital, London

Children are not little adults but paediatricians are.
  Quoting a Belgium professor 14 May (2000)

Guy Williams 1930–
English historical writer

Death from the bubonic plague is rated, with crucifixion, among the nastiest human experiences of all.
  The Age of Agony p. 68, Guy Williams. Constable and Co. Ltd, London (1975)

Leonard Williams 1861–1939
Harley Street physician and author

The crime of our civilisation is gluttony.
  Attributed

John Wilson (Christopher North) 1785–1854
Scottish poet, essayist and critic.

Doctors are generally dull dogs.
  Attributed

John Rowan Wilson 1919–
UK surgeon and novelist

I've always said that the most useful equipment for a successful surgeon is a pessimistic pathologist.
  Hall of Mirrors Pt III, Ch. 7

Maxwell Wintrobe 1901–86
US professor of internal medicine and haematologist

The study of blood has a long history.

Humankind probably always has been interested in the blood because it is likely that even primitive peoples realized that loss of blood, if sufficiently great, was associated with death.
  Introduction to *Wintrobe's Clinical Hematology*. Williams and Wilkins, Baltimore, USA (1999)

William Withering 1741–99
English physician and discoverer of digitalis

The foxglove's leaves with caution given,
Another proof of favouring Heav'n
Will happily display;
The rapid pulse it can abate;
The hectic flush can moderate
And, blest by Him whose will is fate,
May give a lengthen'd day.
  Botany

It is much easier to write upon a disease than upon a remedy.
  Attributed

Poisons in small doses are the best medicines; and useful medicines in too large doses are poisonous.
  Attributed

P. G. Wodehouse 1881–1975
British-born US based humorist

There is only one cure for grey hair. It was invented by a Frenchman. It is called the guillotine.
  The Old Reliable

Humbert Wolfe 1885–1940
English poet and critic

The doctors are a frightful race.
I can't see how they have the face
to go on practising their base
profession; but in any case
I mean to put them in their place.
  Cursory Rhymes 'Poems Against Doctors' I

Paul Hamilton Wood 1907–62
British cardiologist, London

The best history taker is he who can best interpret the answer to a leading question.
  Diseases of the Heart and Circulation (1950)

Virginia Woolf 1882–1941
British writer

... strange indeed that illness has not taken its place with love and battle and jealousy among the prime themes of literature.
  The Moment and Other Essays 'On being ill'

I am certain now that I am going mad again. It is just as it was the first time, I am always hearing voices.
  Letter to her sister just before she killed herself in March 1941

World Medical Association

I will maintain the utmost respect for human life from the time of conception.
Declaration of Geneva (1948)

If at all possible, consistent with patient psychology, the doctor should obtain the patient's freely given consent after the patient has been given a full explanation.
Declaration of Helsinki (1964)

Almroth Wright 1861–1947
British immunologist, St. Mary's Hospital, London

Microbial infections are conveniently divided into septicaemias and intoxications. In the case of the former the bacteria multiply freely in the blood and produce their poisons there. In the latter case the micro-organisms do not proliferate in the blood.
British Medical Journal **i:** 227 (1893)

Frank Lloyd Wright 1867–1959
US architect

The physician can bury his mistakes, but the architect can only advise his client to plant vines.
New York Times Magazine 4 October (1953)

Carl August Wunderlich 1815–77
German Professor of Medicine, Leipzig

Latter-day medicine recognises its tasks and its duties as part of the immeasurably extensive and sublime science of nature. We know in addition that genuine facts and trustworthy data are solely attainable by means of the strictest attention to the methods of investigation and through continually bearing in mind the possible sources of fallacy.
Vienna and Paris Concluding paragraphs (1866)

A knowledge of the course of temperature in disease is indispensable to medical practitioners. The temperature can neither be feigned nor falsified.
Preface to *Medical Thermometry and Human Temperature* (1871)

Leon R. Yankwich 1888–1970
US judge

There are no illegitimate children—only illegitimate parents.
Decision in *Zipkin v. Mozon*, California, June (1928)

Yiddish proverb

An imaginary ailment is worse than a disease.

Francis Brett Young 1884–1954
English novelist and physician

Half the patients who get you up in the middle of the night and think they are dying are suffering from wind!
Dr. Bradley Remembers (1935)

It was a son's duty to see his father into the grave.
Far Forest p. 22. Heinemann Ltd. London (1936)

Henry Youngman 1907–98

I was so ugly when I was born, the doctor slapped my mother.
A one liner quoted in the British Press from this contemporary comedian at time of his death

Gaspar Zavala y Zamora ?–1813

The doctor says there is no hope, and as he does the killing he ought to know.
El Triunfo del Amor y de la Amistad II. 8

Zeno of Elea 5th century BC

Nature has given man one tongue, but two ears, that we may hear twice as much as we speak.
Fragments VI

Zeta (Sir (Vincent) Zachary Cope 1884–1974)
Surgeon, St. Mary's Hospital, London

The diagnostic problem of to-day
Has greatly changed—the change has come to stay;
We all have to confess, though with a sigh
On complicated tests we much rely
And use too little hand and ear and eye.
The Acute Abdomen in Rhyme Preface. H. K. Lewis (1949)

Acute abdominal disease
Is sometimes diagnosed with ease
But oft the best attempts will meet
With sad and sorrowful defeat.
The Acute Abdomen in Rhyme p. 4 Preface. H. K. Lewis (1949)

Not every acute abdomen requires
Immediate operation for its cure
And each good surgeon eagerly desires
To make the needs for operation fewer.
The Acute Abdomen in Rhyme p. 88 Preface. H. K. Lewis, London (1949)

Hans Zinsser 1878–1940
US bacteriologist

To the average professional officer, the military doctor is an unwillingly tolerated noncombatant who takes sick call, gives cathartic pills, makes transportation troubles, complicates tactical plans, and causes the water to smell bad.
Rats, Lice and History Ch. 8

Bibliography

The Acute Abdomen in Rhyme Zeta (Zacary Cope). H. K. Lewis, London, 1949.
The Age of Agony Guy Williams. Constable, London, 1975.
The Anaesthetic Aide-Mémoire John Urquhart. Oxford University Press, Oxford, 1996.
Bailery and Bishop's Notable Names in Medicine and Surgery (4th edn). Revised by Harold Ellis. H. K. Lewis, London, 1983.
Familiar Quotations: A collection of passages phrases and proverbs J. Bartlett. London, 1909.
A Bibliography of Medical and Biomedical Biography Leslie T. Morton and Robert J. Moore. Scolar Press, UK, 1989.
A Biographical Dictionary of Scientists T. I. Williams (ed.). A. & C. Black, London, 1969.
Body Time Gay Gaer Luce. Paladin, Frogmore, UK, 1973.
Book of Humorous Medical Anecdotes S. Greenwood. p. 47. Springwood Books, Ascot, Berkshire, UK, 1989.
Bragg Healthy Lifestyle. Health Science, Box 7, Santa Barbara, California 93102 USA.
Brewer's Dictionary of Phrase and Fable, (Centenary edition). Revised by Ivor Evans, Cassell, London, 1975.
The Cambridge Illustrated History of Medicine Roy Porter (ed.). Cambridge University Press, Cambridge, 1996.
Chambers Biographical Dictionary. W. & R. Chambers, Edinburgh, 1974.
Clinical Pharmacology D. R. Lawrence, P. N. Bennett, and M. J. Brown. Churchill Livingstone, Edinburgh, 1997.
Clinical Thinking and Practice H. J. Wright and D. B. Macadam. Churchill Livingstone, Edinburgh, 1979.
The Concise Dictionary of National Biography. Oxford University Press, Oxford, 1965.
Concise Oxford Dictionary of Quotations. Oxford University Press, Oxford, 1994.
Cured to Death Arabella Melville and Colin Johnson. Seeker & Warburg, London, Carnforth, Lancs, 1982.
The Death of Humane Medicine Petr Skrabanek. The Social Affairs Unit, 1994.
Dicken's Doctors David Waldron Smithers. Oxford, Pergamon Press, 1979.
Dictionary of Medical Eponyms (2nd edn). Firkin and Whitworth. The Parthenon, 1996.
Dictionary of 20th Century Quotations Nigel. Rees. Fontana, 1987.
The Doctor's Quotation Book Robert Wilkins. Robert Hale Ltd, London, 1991.
Doctors in Science and Society: Essays of a Clinical Scientist Christopher C. Booth, British Medical Journal Publications, 1987.
Encyclopedia Britannica (15th edn), 1984.
Encyclopedia of Medical History Roderick E. McGrew. MacMillan Press, London, 1985.
Familiar Medical Quotations Maurice B. Strauss (ed.). Little, Brown and Company, Boston, 1968.
Fischerisms (M. H. Fischer) H. Fabing and R. Marr. 1944.
The Garden of Pleasure James Sanford, 1573.
The Great Doctors – A Biographical History of Medicine Henry E. Sigerist. Dover Publications, New York, 1971 (original W. W. Norton & Co. Ltd, 1933).
Harley Street Reginald Pound. Michael Joseph, London, 1967.
A History of Medicine Lester S. King (ed.). Penguin Books, London, 1971.
The Human Pedigree Anthony Smith. George Allen & Unwin, 1975.
The Hutchinson Dictionary of Scientific Biography Roy Porter (ed.). Helicon, Oxford, 1994.
The Illustrated History of Surgery Knut Haeger. Harold Starke (Medical), London, 1989.
International Medical Who's Who. Published by Francis Hodgson, UK, 1980.
James Parkinson—From Apothecary to General Practitioner. RSM Press, London, 1997.
Law, Ethics and Medicine P. D. G. Skegg. Clarendon Press, Oxford, 1984.
The Little Book of Stress Rohan Candappa. Ebury Press, London, 1998.
A Medical Bibliography Leslie T. Morton. Gower Publishing, Aldershot, UK, 1983.
Medically Speaking Carl C. and Alma E. Gaither. Institute of Physics Publishing, Bristol and Philadelphia, 1999.
Medical Proverbs F. H. Garrison, *Bulletin of the New York Academy of Medicine,* October. 1928, 979–1005.
Medical Quotes—A Thematic Dictionary J. Daintith and A. Isaacs (eds.). Market House Books, Oxford, 1989.
Medicine—An Illustrated History Albert S. Lyons and R. J. Petrucelli. Times Mirror Books, New York, 1987.
Mortal Lessons David Selzer. Chatto & Windus, London, 1981.
Morton's Medical Biography Jeremy M. Norman. Scolar Press, Aldershot, UK, 1991.
Oxford Dictionary of English Proverbs William George Smith (3rd edn), F. P. Wilson (ed.). Clarendon Press, Oxford, 1970.

Penguin Dictionary of Modern Humorous Quotations Fred Metcalf. Penguin Books, London, 1986.
Plato of Praed Street—The Life and Times of Almroth Wright Michael Dunnill. RSM Press, London, 2000.
A Sense of Asher Richard Asher, selected by Ruth Holland. BMA, London, 1984.
Seven Star Diary 2001.
Sidelights of Medical History Zachary Cope. The Royal Society of Medicine, London 1957.
Shakespeare's Insults for Doctors Wayne F. Hill and Cynthia J. Öttchen. Ebury Press, London, 1996.
The Social Transformation of American Medicine Paul Starr. Basic Books, New York, 1982.
Thorne's Better Medical Writing Stephen Lock. Pitman Medical, Tunbridge Wells, UK, 1977.
Webster Biographical Dictionary Merriam Co., Springfield, Mass., USA, 1965.
Who Was Who 1897–1990 A. & C. Black, London, 1991.

Index

abdomen

man wounded in the a. dies — MACC:63
extending into the cavity of the a. — MCDO:63
issuing from a malignancy of the a. — SCHIL:88
found the a. full of clot — TAIT:99
Not every acute a. requires — ZETA:108

abdominal

nine out of ten a. tumours — MORR:71
Acute a. disease — ZETA:108

abortion

No woman wants an a. — ANON:4
a. scarcely to deserve censure — LECK:59
a., usually in defiance of the law — LLEW:61
problem of a. is serious — SIGE:92

absent

two of whom are a. — COPEL:25

absent-minded

appear to be in a hurry, and never a. — BILLR:13

abstainer

A., n. A weak person who yields — BIERC:13

abstinence

A. is a good thing — ANON:3
defensive virtue, a. — HERR:46

accidents

you cannot be insured for the a. — COREN:25
If a. happen and you are to blame — SAYE:87
chapter of a. is the longest — WILKE:107

accountability

Most of all it carries a. — BEAT:10

accounting

arrangements for a. for themselves — STAC:95

ache

is never without some a. — PROV:82

aches

Age breeds a. — PROV:82

aching

of great hardness but little a. — JOHN:54

action

provisional formulae for a. — COHEN:23

active

they remained a. — HUANG:50

actors

glory of surgeons is like that of a. — BALZ:8

acute

A. disease must be seen at least once — BRIG:15
Not every a. abdomen requires — ZETA:108

adaptability

progressive loss of a. as time passes — EVANS:34

addiction

Every form of a. is bad   JUNG:55

addictive

a. need for proximity to death   SMITH:93

adhesions

A. are the refuge   OSLER:74

adolescence

prolong a. patiently   GREGG:41

adolescent

a. mind is essentially a mind   ERIK:34

adult

a. is one who has ceased to grow   ANON:3
average, healthy, well-adjusted a.   KERR:56

adultery

stage between infancy and a.   ANON:4
men call gallantry, and gods a.   BYRON:18
A. brings on early old age   HEBR:44

adulthood

stage between childhood and a.   ERIK:34
most important functions of a.   GREER:41

adults

Children are not little a.   WILL:107

advance

ignores any a. originating outside its own BROW:16
true rate of a. in medicine is   MITC:70

advances

from a. made in surgical research   BELL:10

advertise

work like hell and a.   BEYN:12

advice

A. is seldom welcome   CHES:21
they give him a.   HEROD:45

advocates

Only physicians and a. can kill   PHILE:79

Aesculape

Of old, they gave a cock to A.   JONS:55

Aesculapius

true disciple of A.   ABER:1

affluence

half is succumbing to disease of a.   CARRU:19

age

Old a. is but a second childhood   ARIS:6
through indolence than through a.   CHRI:22
true way to render a. vigorous   COLLI:24
a. without decay   DEFOE:28
Each advancing a. period of life   DUBL:31
not necessarily improve with a.   HALL:42
arctic loneliness of a.   MITC:70
A. breeds aches   PROV:82
I would there were no a.   SHAK:90

aged

state support of the a.   METC:69

ages

same for individuals of all a.   ATCH:7

aging

a. of an organism is a progressive   EVANS:34
be assailed by premature a.   MAIM:64
feelings of inadequacy, fear of a.   ROBI:84

AIDS

to stop them catching A.   CURR:27

ailment

imaginary a.   YIDD:108

air

Fresh a. impoverishes the doctor   DANI:27
there is such a state of the a.   HAMI:42

airy

make them a. and well perflated   ARBU:6

albumin

most ready means of detecting a.   BRIG:15

alcohol

and also the drinking of a.   CHUR:22
whether the narcotic be a.   JUNG:55
a when administered in moderation   MASOR:66
narcotics, a. and Christianity   NIET:73

alcoholic

An a. has been lightly defined   BARA:8
treatment for a. doctors   BERN:11
An a. is someone you don't like   THOMA:99

alimentary

in a healthy state of the a. canal   CURL:26
any other portion of the a. canal   GULL:41

alive

It is the mind which is really a.   CHARC:20
Officiously to keep a.   CLOU:23

remains a. if he is left in peace   MACC:63
he is a., he will immediately scratch   MIRF:69

allergists

a hive of a.   ANON:3

alternative medicine

In some aspects of a. we are fighting   DIAM:29

alters

The eye altering a. all   BLAKE:14

amateurs

has been left exclusively to a.   ANON:4

amaurosis

distinguish cataract from a.   PAUL:77

America

In A., no one group has held   STARR:96

American

at least half a million A. lives   COLLI:24
The future of A. medical education   GARR:38
A study of past A. history   HERR:46
no event in A. history testifies more   STARR:96

American Medical Association

The A. operating from a platform   KNOW:56
Just think of the A. coming out   LERN:59

Americans

A. are indeed in a constant state   BOTS:15

amour

L'a. de la médicine fait le savant   FRENC:37

amputated

refuse to allow my leg to be a.   SHAW:91

amputation

a. injures our whole profession   CATH:19

anaemic

She was very a.   MAUG:66

anaesthesia

a., asepsis, and roentgenology   FISC:35

anaesthetics

natural a. . . . sleep, fainting, death   HOLM:48
A. have abolished the need   LISTE:61

anaesthetist

In America there exist professional a. s   BIER:13
The a. is there   MORG:71
a. knows the name of that vessel   MORG:71
Mr. A., if the patient can keep awake   TROT:101

anatomist

I would choose a good practical A.   HUNTE:51

anatomists

We a. are like the porters   FONT:36
most a., and most other men   HUNT:51
a. see no beautiful women   TWAIN:101

anatomy

until he has studied a.   BALZ:8
when he is ignorant of a.   CHAU:21
A. is for physiology what geography   FERN:34
the a. Ye ought to understand   HALL:42
in a. it is better to have learned   MAUG:66
those . . . who are ignorant of a.   MORG:71
a. must be the foundation   ROKI:85
A. – Botany – Nonsense   SYDE:98

ancestors

never look backward to their a.   BURKE:17

angel

Is man an ape or an a.   DISR:30

anger

A. is short-lived madness   HORA:49

angina

reason for calling it a. pectoris   HEBE:44
A man with a. pectoris   MACK:63

animal

from things lifeless to a. life   ARIS:6
between an a. and a vegetable   HUNTE:51
Every a. is sad after intercourse   LATIN:58
same disease in an experimental a.   PEAB:77

animals

Wild a. never kill for sport   FROU:37
distinguishes man from other a.   OSLER:74

ankles

Swellings of the a.   HEBE:44

anorexia nervosa

In my experience of a.   ABRA:1

anthropological

much a. evidence exists   GILL:39

antiquity

stand out clearly from the mists of a.   OSLER:74

antiseptic

Since the a. treatment has been	LISTE:60
hence is the most powerful a.	LISTE:61
The irritation of the wound by a.	LISTE:61

antivivisectionists

There are a few honest a.	HALD:42

anus

An artificial a. in the loin	CURL:26
a tumour developing within the a.	JOHN:54
guardian of the a.	SIGE:92

anxieties

a. that science can never m.	KING:56

anxiety

to release a. from his spirit	HAZM:44
a. affects the body	JASP:53
laborious and often full of a.	SYMI:98

anxious

population of the US an a. one	MCCR:63

aorta

passed my finger between the a.	COOP:25

ape

Is man an a. or an angel	DISR:30
like us is that ugly brute, the a.	ENNI:33
having an a. for his grandfather	HUXL:52
halfway between an a. and a god	INGE:52
the a. from which he is descended	WILB:106

apes

semi-a. who ranged	KIPL:56
anthropoid a. and human beings.	LORE:62

apoplexy

attack of a. may be called death's	MENA:69
A. is an affection of the head	SMITH:94

apothecaries

except those of a.	HOLM:48
a. bear the same relation	HUME:50

apothecary

garden is the poor man's a	GERM:39
not through an a.'s shop	GULL:41

apparatuses

A. are cleverer than men	ROEN:84

appartments

the confined and miserable a.	MCCR:63

appearance

normalcy in a. and function	WEBS:105

appendicitis

There are two kinds of a.	CABOT:18
chronic remunerative a.	NICK:73
diagnosis of a. requires...physician	RUSSE:86

appendix

early detection of an a.	FITZ:35

appetite

The a.s of the belly	CICE:22
has a good a.	HIPP:46
A. comes as you eat	RABE:83
that spoils the a.	TURG:101

apple

An a. a day keeps the doctor away	PROV:82

appointments

The custom of giving patients a.   MEANS:68
fool who holds two hospital a.   RING:84

appraisals

should respond constructively to a.   GENE:38

apprenticeship

way to teach an art is an a. system   HUMP:51

architect

the a. can only advise his client   WRIG:108

arise

sup light, and soon a.   SALE:86

armamentarium

the other a therapeutic a.   CHIN:21

armies

A. have been supposed to lose   LIND:60
more fatal to a. than powder   OSLER:74

art

science and the physician's a.   BILLR:13
The a. of medicine   CELS:20
healing a. enables one to make   CHIN:21
salvation of the a. would depend   DE GO:40
What A. was to the ancient world   DISR:30
it is still an a. or craft   GEOR:38
Science and a.   GOET:40
Wisdom and a., strength and wealth   HEROP:45
If a. outruns science   HILL:46
the A. is to be able to observe   HIPP:47
To teach them this A' if they shall   HIPP:47
requirement of the a. of healing   HUANG:50
a. must be used only for the good   HUNA:51

to exercise an a.   LATH:58
As a. surgery is incomparable   MOYN:72
the a. of medicine   PEAB:77
high position of a man of a.   TROU:101
A., however, is a gift from heaven   TROU:101
to exercise the quiet a.   VIRG:103

arteries

A man is as old as his a.   SYDE:98
a. proceed from the heart   VINCI:102

arthritis

forms of a. or articular inflammation   BELL:10

artist

must possess the qualities of the a.   WEBB:105

arts

Among the a.   BUCKL:17

asepsis

anaesthesia, a., and roentgenology   FISC:35

aspirations

man's insomnia, hopes and a.   FITZG:35

assassination

When I take up a.   THOMA:99

asthma

A. is a disease   ANON:3
All that wheezes is not a.   JACK:53

asylum

most flourishes is the lunatic a.   ELLIS:32

Had there been a Lunatic A.   ELLIS:32
An a. for the sane would be empty   SHAW:91

asymptomatic

make the a. patient feel better   HOER:48

atom

as revolutionary as the cleaving of the a.   GILLI:39

audit

A., the science of spying   SPEN:95

auditory

a. nerves were atrophied   WAGN:104

authority

an especially persuasive claim to a.   STARR:96

authors

a long list of a.' names   ANON:5
Unfortunately, too many a. write   SOUT:95

autobiography

there is only biography and a.   SZASZ:98

autonomy

Professional a. has been protected   STARR:96

autopsy

not without an a.   BOER:14
the lesions revealed by a.   MARF:65

average

The a. human has one breast   MCHA:63

babies

Speeches are like b. easy   ARIST:6
putting milk into b.   CHUR:22
nearly all b. were born   CLAYT:23
B. haven't any hair   HOFFE:48
into the clever parcels we call b.   SELZ:89

baby

When the first b. laughed   BARRI:9
Every b. born into the world   DICKE:29
the b.'s head is crooked   PERS:78

bacteria

the b. multiply freely in the blood   WRIG:108

bacterial

free from any trace of b. taint   THOMP:100

bacteriologists

much as b. disarm a pathogen   RAMN:83
B. are out of touch   TWEE:101

bacteriology

operation is an experiment in b.   MOYN:72
Surgeons have little knowledge of b.   TWEE:101

bald

the hair on a b.-headed man   BENN:10
A b. head is soon shaven   ENGL:33
his hair that grows b. by nature   SHAK:90

baldness

leads to b.   HIPP:47

barren

encourageth a woman sooner to be b.   PLINY:80

bathe

B. every day and sickness will avoid   INDI:52

beauty

It is easy to agree to do a b.   GILLI:39
health is the most perfect b.   SHEN:91

bed

There is no b. shortage   ANON:5
Early to b., early to rise   BEYN:12
Rest in b. will do more for more   CLEN:23
B. is a medicine   ITAL:53

bedpan

to be given a b. by a stranger   KUHN:57

bedside

at the b.   HOLM:48
b. is always the true centre   HOLM:48
It is at the b. of the patient   MART:66
you must go to the b.   SYDE:98

beef

About as many as lust after our b.   MCFAR:63

beggar

A b. does not hate another b.   POLI:81

beginning

At the b. no one tries   SENE:89

behaviour

side to human b. in health   PLATT:80

being

makes us conscious of our b.   ROUSS:85

beings

in her care for living b.   ERAS:33

belief

the foolish b.   ANON:4
privileged status in the hierarchy of b.   STARR:96

believe

in seeing what we b.   ALLB:2

believer

true b. is in a high degree protected   FREUD:37

bellied

sail and a big-b. woman   FRAN:36

belly

he has a wolf in his b.   GERM:39
The eye is bigger than the b.   PROV:82
When b. with bad pains   SAADI:86

benefit

at the same time give b. to others   CHIN:21

better

I am getting b. and b.   COUÉ:26

bicycle

with the invention of the b.   SMITH:93

bill

the size of his b.   DA CO:23
And what does he, but write a.   PRIOR:82

biological

In b. sciences, the role of method   BERN:11
physical, chemical, and b. causes   SIGE:92

biological sciences

increase in knowledge in the b.   KEEN:56

biologist

without whom no b. can live   BRÜC:16
for the modern b. to remind himself   SALT:87

biology

progress of b. in the next century   HALD:42
Man is just another bit of b.   SMITH:93

birth

b.' life and death   BRUY:16
for the nine months preceding his b.   COLER:24
B., copulation and death   ELIOT:32
to mate, give b.   ILLI:52
to die at b.   MANI:65
When the b. cometh not naturally   ROSL:85
There is no cure for b. and death   SANTA:87
to hinder a b.   TERT:99
rejoice at a b. and grieve at a funeral   TWAIN:101

birth control

the oldest method of b.   LLEW:61

birthday

Today is my forty-third b.   TEGN:99

black

if b. gets b. with child in Scythia,   VINCI:102

blame

If accidents happen and you are to b.   SAYE:87

blamed

in teams, but are b. as individuals   POLL:81

bleed

B. him and purge him   SPAN:95

bleedeth

The wound that b. inward   LYLY:63

bleeding

Beneath the b. hands we feel   ELIOT:32
it stops the b. just as well   HOLM:48
B. is a remedy much to be depended   MOSS:71

blind

If the b. lead the b.   BIBLE:12
A b. man leaned against a wall   GREEK:41
I have a right to be b.   NELS:73
Among the b.   PROV:82
There are none so b.   PROV:82
He that is stricken b. cannot forget   SHAK:90

blindness

My b. is my sight   CARY:19
signifies inner b.   DOBIE:30
be incapable of enduring b.   MILT:69

blood

Let out the b., let out the disease   ANON:4
the nose shall bring forth b.   BIBLE:12
In letting of b.   BURT:17
are pouring out b.   CELS:20
When such distempers are in the b.   FIEL:34
the b. passes through the heart   HARV:43
b. is under control   HUANG:50
fills the pulse with b.   HUANG:50
b. in its continuous passage   LOWE:62
no flesh or b. or refuse   PLINY:80
B. is thicker than water   PROV:82
The study of b. has a long history.   WINT:107

blood letting

B., like wine-drinking, is right   FERN:34

blunders

The b. of a doctor   AR-RU:6

bodice

she opened up her b.   GRAH:41

bodies

attenuate our b.   BURT:17
Minds like b. will often fall   DICKE:29
b. of those that made such a noise   EDWA:32
B. devoid of mind are as statues   EURI:34
teaching them to care for their b. well   MAYO:67
be healed as well as sick b.   MILLE:69
with the souls and b. of men   NIGH:73
Weary b. refresh and mollify   OVID:75

body

a sound b. before riches   APOC:5
The b. is most fully developed   ARIS:6
perceived anywhere in his b.   BENT:11
The light of the b. is the eye   BIBLE:12
the failure of the b.   BRAIN:15
The b. is but a pair of pincers   BUTL:18
b. may be healed, but not the mind   CHIN:21
all the members in our b.   CHRY:22
more numerous than those of the b.   CICE:23
as in a disordered b.   CICE:23
B. and mind, like man and wife   COLT:24
all the b. is the worse   ENGL:33
perfected all parts of the b.   ERAS:33
ended in the punishment of the b.   FISC:35
all tortured in soul and foul in b.   FRAS:36
Sickly b., sickly mind   GERM:39
the b. is affected through the mind   HOLM:48
If the b. be feeble   JEFF:54
uniformed mind with a healthy b.   JEFF:54
most abhorrent is b. without mind.   JEFF:54
indissoluble union with the b.   JUNG:55
sound mind in a sound b.   JUVE:55
mind is begotten along with the b.   LUCR:62
The mind like a sick b.   LUCR:62
B. and soul cannot be separated   MILLE:69
mind has great influence over the b.   MOLI:70
I am no better in mind than in b.   OVID:75
the treatment of the human b.   PLATO:79
The b. must be repaired   PLINY:80
A man ought to handle his b.   PLUT:80
Happiness is beneficial for the b.   PROU:82
The human b. is like a bakery   SCHIC:88

The b. is not a permanent dwelling   SENE:89
b. is a product of the sound mind   SHAW:91
Pain of mind is worse than pain of b.   SYRUS:98
scarcely a part of the b.   WHITE:106

Boerhaave

B. lectured five hours a day   MACP:64

bone

The broken b., once set together   LYLY:63

bones

a broken spirit drieth the b.   HUBB:50

books

All that is written in b.   RHAZ:84

born

to die as to be b.   BACON:8
One is not b. a woman   BEAUV:10
We all are b. mad   BECK:10
b. with an indelible character.   FRED:36
before he is fully b.   FROM:37
b. with a deadly disease which is life.   MOREA:71
We are b. crying, live complaining   PROV:82
Take utmost care to get well b.   SHAW:90
Everyone who is b.   SONT:94
Every moment one is b.   TENN:99
I was so ugly when I was b.   YOUN:108

botany

Anatomy – B. – Nonsense   SYDE:98

bottle

a full b. in front of me   NICH:73
the stimulus of the b.   WATE:104

bowel

set or rise on a small b. obstruction   ANON:4
sciences have ignored the large b.   PHILL:79

bowels

the feet warm and the b. open   BOER:14
For colic, get the b. open   CHIN:21

boy

Speak roughly to your little b.   CARRO:19
When I was a b. I wanted to know   HUNTE:51

brain

Impressions arriving at the b.   CABA:18
The b. is a wonderful organ   FROST:37
The wasting of the b.   HIPP:47
the candelabra of the b.   MERE:69
the biggest b. of all the primates   MORR:71
the b. as the seat of the psyche   MOTT:72
The b. has muscles for thinking   OFFR:74
The b. is the highest of the organs   PLINY:80
As long as our b. is a mystery   RAMON:83
a b. so beautifully integrated   SEEG:89
surgeon knows all the parts of the b.   SELZ:89
b. to be much more than a
telephone-exchange   SHERR:91
your b. with its two lobes   STILL:97
The b. secretes thought   VOGT:103
We know the human b.   VRIES:103
The convolutions of the b.   WAGN:104

brain death

B. may very well be a distinct   GILL:39

brains

those who practise with their b.   OSLER:74
polish our b. against that of others   MONTA:70

brave

make one b. push   STEV:96

bravery

The heroic b. of the man   AYER:7

bread

By the time you earn your b.   MCMU:64

break

worse to sprain an ankle than to b. it WATS:105

breasts

have but small and narrow b.   LUTH:62

breath

The first b. is the beginning of death PROV:82

breathing

B. is the greatest pleasure in life   PAPI:75
b. cold air   WELSH:105

breeding

continue b. like rabbits   DUBOS:31
unplanned b. of ourselves.   TOYN:100

brief

above all be b.   MAYO:68

bring up

to b. other people's children   RUSSI:86

British

B. Government have announced   HAWTO:43
The B. have no unifying faith   LAWS:59
B. medicine is extremely   MACK:64
B. doctors have had privileged   STAC:95

British Medical Association

The B. is a club of London physicians   ANON:4

bubo

A b. is a tumour developing   JOHN:54
could be cured of the b.   JOHN:54

bubonic

Death from the b. plague WILL:107

building

The first Care in the b. of Cities ARBU:6

buildings

b. which are positively healing CHARL:21

bum

Your b. is the greatest thing SHAK:90

burden

one is a b. to the host SENE:89

business

nor the efficiency of b. methods BRADF:15
a damn bad b. ROLL:85

busy

Heaven defend me from a b. doctor WELSH:105

butter

What b. and whiskey will not cure IRISH:53

caesarean section

C. is a detestable, barbarous, illegal OULD:75

calculations

We make all the c. MARC:65

California

The C. climate makes the sick AMER:2

calling

In pursuit of this noble and holy c. LISTE:61

camel

Love and pregnancy and riding on a c. ARAB:5

cancer

my father died of c. ACE:1
reeking with hypertension, c. CLEN:23
C. is a word, not a sentence DIAM:29
more destructive to life than c. MAYO:67
theories of c. extend to the dawn SHIM:91

cancers

and many c. will be wiped out ANON:3

carbolic

material which I have employed is c. LISTE:61

carburettor

A man's liver is his c. ANON:3

care

For want of timely c. ARMS:6
a person who has a duty of c. HAVE:43
c. of a patient must be PEAB:77
c. of the dying and their families. SAUN:87
not interested in the c. of the patient STRA:97
the old methods of c. and caring WALL:104

cases

was that you missed half the good c. SANF:87
examine your c. thoroughly WHITF:106

cast

A c. of orthopaedic ANON:3

cataract

All those who have c. see the light PAUL:77

Catholic

for a C. woman to avoid pregnancy MENC:69

cause

too much accustomed to a single c.   LIEB:60
c. of the phenomena be unknown,   PAST:77

cell

The c. never acts   HAEC:42
c. state in which every cell is a citizen   VIRC:103
the ultimate units of the living c.   WEAV:105

cells

composed of countless millions of c.   CHRI:22
before the gray c. take over   SCHAT:87
All c. come from other c.   VIRC:103

centralized

c. planning, budgeting   STARR:96

champagne

water flowed like c.   EVAR:34

chance

Leave nothing to c.   HIPP:47

character

no index of c. so sure as the voice   DISR:30
born with an indelible c.   FRED:36

characters

with our c. about us   LESA:60

charity

house which is not opened for c.   TALM:99

charlatans

c. are the excrescences   SAUN:87

cheeks

c. are rounded and extended   DOWN:30

cheer

The best of healers is good c.   PIND:79

cheerfulness

Health and c. naturally beget   ADDI:1

chemical

short cut from c. laboratory to clinic   ANON:5

chemotherapy

under the influence of modern c.   WALK:104

chest

for detecting diseases of the c.   AUEN:7
A medical c. specialist is long-winded   BIRD:14
There is one ailment in the c.   HEBE:44

child

Either she wants a c.   ANON:4
chronic abdominal pain in a c.   APLEY:5
as soon as she is delivered of the c.   BIBLE:12
If a c. is constantly sick   CHIN:21
the early development of the c.   COCK:23
bowed impotent beside the dying c.   DOCK:30
morality learned by the c.   ERIK:34
than bear one c.   EURI:34
love must help the c. grow   FROMM:37
The misery of a c. is interesting   HUGO:50
facts about grown-ups to a c.   JARR:53
the c. should be allowed   KEY:56
institute for the study of c. guidance   KRUT:57
all any reasonable c. can expect   ORTON:74
destroy the mother to save the c.   OULD:75
parents do not count their c.   PASH:76
One stops being a c.   PAVE:77
nourishment and food of a sucking c.   PHAE:79
no woman ever produced a c.   PLUT:80
giving of suckle to the c.   ROSL:85
Simply imagine that it's not your c.   RUSSI:86
C. are not simply micro-adults   SCHIC:88
only two things a c. will share   SPOCK:95
the rights are on the side of the c.   SUMN:97
just because your c. hates it   WHIT:106

childbearing

hard travail in c.   PLINY:80

childbed

there is so high a mortality in c.   SEMM:89

childbirth

At the moment of c.   PAST:76
numbers of women perish after c.   SEMM:89

childhood

Old age is but a second c.   ARIS:6
stage between c. and adulthood   ERIK:34
during their c. had been attacked   MARF:65
c. but a series of happy delusions   SMITH:94

childishness

Is second c. and mere oblivion   SHAK:90

children

C. are one third of our population   ANON:3
attention is paid to our c.'s minds   ANON:4
In c. may be observed the traces   ARIS:6
fear in c. is increased with tales   BACON:8
thou shalt bring forth c.   BIBLE:12
Give me c. or else I die   BIBLE:12
You can do anything with c.   BISM:14
half of the c. born in Great Britain die   BUCH:17
last people on earth who ought to have c.   BUTL:18
C., in general, are overclothed   CADO:18
about the care of young c.   CATH:20
Dreams, C. of the night   CHUR:22
What we desire our c. to become   COMB:24
the second half by our c.   DARR:28
inclination is to suffer c. gladly   GREGG:41
'On C.'   GIBR:39
When c. are little   ITAL:53
c. should not be made to wait   KENN:56
C. do not give up   LAING:57
prevent the birth of unwanted c.   LLEW:61
c. are at the mercy of those around   LUBB:62
c. are the most imaginative   MACAU:63
honey and wine are bad for c.   MAIM:64
he (Laennec) saw some c.   MAJOR:65
one of a hundred thousand other c.   MEDA:68
done to c. by means of leeches   MOSS:71

It is contrary to nature for c.   PLUT:80
Late c., early orphans   PROV:82
the best love that of c.   PROV:82
better reasons for having c.   RUSSE:86
sure of the legitimacy of the c.   RUSSE:86
to bring up other people's c.   RUSSI:86
made to avoid having c.   VIRC:103
C. are not little adults   WILL:107
There are no illegitimate c.   YANK:108

Chinese

The C. do not draw any distinction   LIN:60

chloroform

washed of c. and devoted to ether   SIMS:93
that blessed C.   VICT:102

cholera

c. twice than that I should have it   COBB:23

choleric

The c. drinks, the melancholic eats   PROV:82

Christ

Jesus C. would infallibly   ELLIS:32

church

will not be buried in the c.   ANON:5
the c. and the law   MAYO:68

churchyard

A young physician fattens the c.   FRENC:37

chyle

ever-fresh c. passes into the blood   LOWE:62

circumcise

Ye shall c. the flesh   BIBLE:12

circumcised

When they c. Herbert Samuel   LLOY:61

citizen

A cell state in which every cell is a c.   VIRC:103

citizenship

health . . . is an essential to good c.   MAYO:67

city

a c. whose governor is a physician   HEBR:44

civilization

each c. has a pattern of disease   DUBOS:31
The crime of our c. is gluttony   WILL:107

class

To give the lower c. greater access   ILLI:52

cleanliness

Water, air, and c.   NAPO:72
c. lies in water supply   NIGH:73
C. and comfort demand   WELCH:105

clergy

Unlike the law and the c.   STARR:96

clergyman

c. and the psychotherapist to join   JUNG:55

clever

If we cannot be c   FRIPP:37
dangerous . . . to be too c.   HUTC:51

climate

Any c. and any age   HOFFM:48

clinical

c. acumen is the most important tool   BROOK:16
the service ethic and c. autonomy   HUNT:51
one based on c. observation   PLATT:80
being neglected by c. science   PLATT:80
cannot teach students c. medicine   STRA:97

clinician

A c. is complex   ADDIS:1
c. who relaxes   HORD:49
One of the essential qualities of the c.   PEAB:77
c. attacks the core of the problem   SEEG:89
The well equipped c. must possess   WEBB:105

clinicians

extremely busy c.s   BOER:14

coarctation

It is with c. surgery as with love   BROM:15

coffee

C., though a useful medicine   TORR:100

coffin

and becomes his c. prodigiously   GOLDS:40

cohabit

A person should not c.   MAIM:64

cold

It leapt straight past the common c.   AYRES:8
Sauerkraut is good for a c.   GERM:39
If you feed a c., as is often done   MACF:63
People do not catch c. in bed   NIGH:73
the cruel c. cuts off the limbs   SILI:93
remedies that won't cure a c.   VALE:102

colic

For c., get the bowels open   CHIN:21

colleagues

friendly criticism by c. BEVE:12

college

the dignity of the C. can be preserved HARV:43

colostomy

preference for c. over resection VOLK:103

comedy

neither of tragedy nor of c. MAUG:67

comfort

from mere excess of c. DICKE:29
Heal the sick and c. the dying DOUG:30
the perennial demand for c. TOLS:100

commission

In medicine, sins of c. are mortal TRON:100

committee

a c. should consist of no more COPE:25
research c. can do one useful thing TOPL:100

common sense

practice of medicine depends on c. CUSH:27
cleverness before c. HUTC:51
C is in medicine the master LATH:58
c. rounded out SANTA:87
The c. is that which judges VINCI:102

communicability

The c. of cholera SNOW:94

communication

It is intellectual and c. skills LILF:60

communicative

less accessible and less c. MEANS:68

community

no finer investment for any c. CHUR:22

compassion

times when c. should prompt us PENF:78
to serve and to show c. SCHW:88

complains

He who c. most is not hurt FRENC:37

complaints

Doctors cannot cure their own c. HUAI:50
The imaginary c. WHITE:106

complexion

The c. of a person shows SU:97

complexity

the immense c. of the phenomena BERN:11

complications

things unseen and c. unstated HECHT:44

comprehension

beyond his c. and . . . control CHUR:22

computers

Recent over-use of c. by management MOTT:72

conceiving

instead of c. him, his parents MEDA:68

conception

if the dad is present at the c.   ORTON:74
human life from the time of c.   WORLD:108

conclusions

general laws or c. may be drawn   DARW:28

confession

Psychoanalysis is c.   CHES:21

confidence

curing people by heightening their c.   CATH:19

confusion

the c. is your own fault   CAST:19

conjecture

correct idea has ever emanated from c.   COOP:25

conscience

Science without c. is the death   ANON:4
value it next to a good c.   WALT:104

conscious

The c. mind may be compared   FREUD:37

consent

obtain the patient's freely given c.   WORLD:108

conservative

British medicine is extremely c.   MACK:64

conspiracies

All professions are c.   SHAW:90

constitution

psychological c. is good   PLATO:79

consultant

A c. is a man sent in after the battle   ANON:3
A c. is a man who knows   DENNI:29
C. specialists are . . . more remote   FISH:35
The c.'s first obligation   HEND:45

consultation

Physicians who meet in c.   HIPP:47

consumption

to take him away was the c.   BUNY:17
in c. do not treat the end   CHIN:21
the c. seems to be suspended   HEBE:44
If c. is too powerful for physicians   SMITH:94
the hectic glow of c.   THORE:100

consumptions

asthmas, spittings of blood, and c.   HEBE:44

consumptive

common fallacy of c. Persons   BROW:16

continental

How many of our c. colleagues   MCFAR:63

contraceptives

C. should be used   MILLI:69

contradiction

they brook no c.   WEBS:105

control

beyond his comprehension and . . . c.   CHUR:22

controversies

the majority of our c. come — LIEB:60

controversy

ceases to be a subject of c. — HAZL:43

convalescence

the more rapid their c. — MAYO:67
I enjoy c. — SHAW:90

conviviality

C. has a levelling — CATH:19

convulsion

man is not strong who takes c.-fits — CARL:19
a fever succeed to a c. — HIPP:46

cookery

since the improvement in c. — FRAN:36

copulation

Birth, c. and death — ELIOT:32

coronary

killers such as c. heart disease — ANON:3

corporate

A c. sector in health care is — STARR:96

corpse

he makes a very handsome c. — GOLDS:40

cost

social c. of sickness is incalculable — EMER:33

costlier

slower and the c. — WHITE:106

costly

Physicians are c. visitors — PROV:82

costs

No c. have increased more rapidly — KENN:56

cough

A dry c. is the trumpeter of death — ENGL:33
A c. is something — NASH:72

coughs

c. and sneezes spread diseases — ANON:3
were less troubled with C. — BROW:16

country

what the c. doctor, is — MITC:70

court

held up in c. in a suit for damages — CATH:19

courtesy

There is no c. in science — CLARK:23

cowardice

Self-destruction is the effect of c. — DEFOE:28

cradle

From the c. to the grave — HOFFE:48

craftsman

part c., part practical scientist — ADDIS:1

create

as great a miracle as to c. him — TAYL:99

creatures

tiny c., too small for us to see — VARRO:102

cricket

c. is my profession — GRACE:41

crime

a c. you haven't committed — POWE:81

Crimean

Ever since the C. War, nurses have — MITC:70

crippled

You are not c. at all — SCUL:88

criticism

Be sparing of c. — GREGG:41
People ask you for c. — MAUG:66
I desire judgment and c. — PAST:77

crowd

A c. is a device for indulging — MART:66

crucifixion

c., among the nastiest human — WILL:107

cultural

reference to social and c. values — DAAR:27

culture

Our c. has been influenced by — MAST:66

cure

To c. safely, swiftly and pleasantly — ASCL:6
C. the disease and kill the patient — BACON:8
man has not found a c. — BARU:9
labour against our own c. — BROW:16
They leave it to Nature to c. — BURG:17
When a disease relapses there is no c. — CHIN:22
consider that the c. is discovered — CICE:23
you will have no patients to c. — COOP:25
If ye will c. well any thing — HALLE:42
Not to cut off, but c. the vicious part — HERR:46
What drugs fail to c. — HIPP:47
Doctors cannot c. their own — HUAI:50
the c. of the disease more grievous — HUTC:51
What butter and whiskey will not c. — IRISH:53
We palliate what we cannot c. — JOHNS:54
I will c. him for you — JUNG:55
first water c. was the Flood — LAMB:57
When a c. is impossible — LONG:61
the beginning of the c. — PROV:82
Nothing hinders a c. — SENE:89
disease which we cannot c. — SENE:89
we can dare not to suspect to c. it — SKODA:93
Physicians c. little or nothing — SPOD:95
those who think they can c. them — VOLT:103
only one c. for grey hair — WODE:107
Immediate operation for its c. — ZETA:108

cured

that means it cannot be c. — CHEK:21
the disease is c. by nature — FORB:36
a disease that is not completely c. — HUANG:50
could be c. of the bubo — JOHN:54
A disease known is half c. — PROV:82
There is no c. for birth and death — SANTA:87
farther on the road to being c. — SENE:89
the means by which they can be c. — SYDE:98

cures

hardly any specific c. — CHAM:20
Medicine c. the man who is fated — CHIN:21
Opposites are c. for opposites — HIPP:47
the best c. in the doctor's book — IRISH:52
Medicine indeed never c. a disease — MOND:70
Doctor c., if the sun sees it — MONTA:70

curing

no c. a sick man — AMIEL:2
the doctor gets the credit of c. them — SHAW:91

custom

A c. loathsome to the eye   JAMES:53

cut

C. well, get well, stay well   DEAV:28
Not to c. off, but cure the vicious part   HERR:46

cuts

In a good hand every sword c. well   MONTE:71

dad

Or a d. from his fond son   BENN:10

dangerous

The most d. physicians are those   NIET:73

Darwinian

The D. theory   WALLA:104

data

journals support the publication of d.   INGLE:52
mousetrapped by tangential d.   SEEG:89

day

Every d., in every way   COUÉ:26

daybreak

well to be up before d.   ARIS:6

days

Man's d. shall be to one hundred   BIBLE:12

DDT

D. went further   DUBOS:31

dead

A place in which the d. are laid   BIERC:13
he is half d.   DAVIS:28
when d., lie as quietly   EDWA:32
investigation of the d. for the living   EVANS:34
If you want to keep a d. man   GUTH:42
to attend the sick and dissect the d.   HUNTE:51
whether a person is or is not d.   MIRF:69
Medicine for the d. is too late   QUIN:83
distinguished from a d. thing   SPEN:95

deafness

There are two kinds of d.   WILDE:106

death

to condemn the patient to a certain d.   ANON:4
Science without conscience is the d.   ANON:4
the suicide braves d.   ARIS:6
D. is a release from the impressions   AURE:7
Men fear D., as children fear to go   BACON:8
come to accept his impending d.   BAIN:8
There is no such thing as a natural d.   BEAUV:10
We have made a covenant with d.   BIBLE:12
functions that resist d.   BICH:12
murder, and from sudden d.   BOOK:14
observations after d.   BRIG:15
d. is the cure of all diseases   BROW:16
only the stroke of d.   BROW:16
birth, life and d.   BRUY:16
The captain of all these men of d.   BUNY:17
D. in anything like luxury   BUTL:18
gives d. to all things   CARL:19
remedy for everything except d.   CERV:20
the same road, the road of d.   CLYN:23
D. a friend that alone can bring   COLLI:24
when one contemplates d.   DAVIS:28
Birth, copulation and d.   ELIOT:32
A dry cough is the trumpeter of d.   ENGL:33
So d., the most terrifying of ills   EPIC:33
D. is a debt we all must pay   EURI:34
not d., but dying, which is terrible   FIEL:34
let me die a natural d.   GARTH:38
this concept of d. is not accepted   GILL:39
to choose a quick and easy d.   GILM:40
d. supervenes before the retinal   GUNN:42
D. is the greatest evil   HAZL:43
the inordinate fear of d.   HAZL:43
The love of life, or fear of d.   HEBE:44
Where, Life and D. . . . . meet   HENL:45
D. is a delightful hiding place   HEROD:45
dissatisfied d. cannot noise abroad   HINT:46

Sleep and D., who are twin brothers — HOMER:49
D. is the poor man's best physician — IRISH:52
D. never takes the wise man — LA FO:36
The fear of d. is crueler than d. — LATIN:58
All interest in disease and d. — MANN:65
The mode of d. is sadder than d. itself — MART:65
The transition between life and d. — MATAS:66
may be called d.'s retaining fee — MÉNA:69
difference between post-poning d. — MINE:69
d. should not be — NABO:72
none that permits us to deprive him of d. — NIET:73
sometimes parry the scythe of d. — PIOZ:79
boundaries which divide life from d. — POE:80
The first breath is the beginning of d. — PROV:82
the immediate prelude to d. — RHOA:84
the sun and d. — ROCH:84
Teach him to live rather than avoid d. — ROUS:85
There is no cure for birth and d. — SANTA:87
ideas of what constitutes a good d. — SAUN:87
than even d. itself — SCHW:88
D. is a punishment to some — SENE:89
For in that sleep of d. what dreams — SHAK:90
d. will seize the doctor too — SHAK:90
d. reveals the eminent — SHAW:91
its mortification and my d. — SHAW:91
d. advertises the doctor — SHAW:91
ends in recovery or d. — SIGE:92
D., I suppose, may be a process — SIMON:93
about conquering diseases and d. — SKRA:93
D. that he had controlled — SMITH:93
D. must be distinguished from dying — SMITH:94
D. is not the greatest of ills — SOPH:94
to be jurors upon life and d. — SWIFT:98
in d. the same unknown will appear — TAGO:99
The reports of my d. — TWAIN:101
life well used brings happy d. — VINCI:102
sleep, so close to tranquil d. — VIRG:103
D. hath ten thousand several doors — WEBS:105
It is not the fear of d. — WEIN:105
survive everything . . . except d. — WILDE:106
D. from the bubonic plague — WILL:107

deaths

the intent of accelerating their d. — GILLO:39
All d. are hateful to miserable mortals — HOMER:49

debate

priorities and having a rational d. — ANON:5

decay

approaching and unavoidable d. — HEBE:44

decision

give the patient the benefit of your d. — HOLM:48
at least make a d. — PLATT:80

decrepit

not yet d. enough to turn them down — ELIOT:32
did not become d. in their activities — HUANG:50

deduction

then as much d. as you please — DARW:28

deductions

Re-examine your own d. — WHITF:106

deference

the collapse of d. — DICKS:29

deformed

D. persons commonly take revenge — BACON:8

delirious

The patient raves and roams d. — LUCR:62

delirium

When sleep puts an end to d. — HIPP:46

delusions

d. of the senses are the worst — LATH:58
childhood but a series of happy d. — SMITH:94

demand

what is thought to be the d. — ANON:5

demeanour

cool-headed and pleasant in his d. — SUSR:97

dentist

D., n. A prestidigitator	BIERC:13
depended on 'till a d. makes him one	TWAIN:101
I'd sooner go to my d. any day	WAUG:105

dermatologists

A rash of d.	ANON:3

dermatology

D. is the best specialty	ANON:3
can never be a thorough d.	DUHR:31

descended

the ape from which he is d.	WILB:106

desire

d. should so many years outlive	SHAK:90
It provoketh the d.	SHAK:90

despair

D. is better treated with hope	ASHER:7

destiny

fool lives as long as his d. allows him	ANON:3
The old acceptance of d. has gone	SAUN:87

developing countries

increasing importance in d.	JULI:55

device

seeming exactness of a mechanical d.	MACK:64

dexterity

where intellect and d. meet	SCHAU:87

diabetes

d. ('the siphon') or violent thirst	GALEN:38

diagnose

d. the present, foretell the future	HIPP:47
the disease that your friends d.	OSLER:74

diagnosed

Is sometimes d. with ease	ZETA:108

diagnoses

families will forgive you for wrong d.	ANON:4
For most d. all that is needed	ARAB:6
All d. are provisional formulae	COHEN:23

diagnosis

those most needed in d.	ADLER:1
lead to an unambiguous d.	ANON:4
mother makes often a better d.	BIER:13
above other men, understands d.	BIGE:13
used in arriving at the correct d.	BROOK:16
one who is shrewd in d.	CAIR:18
not only assist you in d.	CATH:19
D. by intuition is a rapid method	DA CO:23
The power of making a correct d.	DUHR:31
D. is not the end, but the beginning	FISC:35
In most cases the d. is easy	FITZ:35
Early d. of disease is the business	HALD:42
d. is where it happens	HILL:46
however clear the d. may appear	JONES:55
D. is a system	LEWIS:60
does not prove your d. was correct	MELT:68
no d. is complete or exact	PAGET:75
The d. of appendicitis requires	RUSSE:86
A d. is easy as long as you think of it	WEISS:105

diagnostic

So much of the d. process	MEANS:68
The d. problem of to-day	ZETA:108

diagnostically

the refuge of the d. destitute	OSLER:74

die

I am not afraid to d.	ALLEN:2
Man has an inalienable right to d.	ANON:4

It is as natural to d.   BACON:8
d. very nearly as privately   BENÉT:10
for tomorrow we d.   BIBLE:12
a place, not to live, but to d. in   BROW:16
to assure them they will not d.   BRUY:16
the children born in Great Britain d.   BUCH:17
costs a lot of money to d. comfortably   BUTL:18
In scarcely any house did only one d.   CLYN:23
do not always agree to d. together   COLT:24
more likely to d. on the first day   DAVIS:28
rather live, but I am not afraid to d.   DISR:30
D. well that live well   ENGL:33
unwilling to d. as tired-out children   FANU:34
we shall d. as usual   FONT:36
let me d. a natural death   GARTH:38
old men let them d.   GREGO:41
has caused the man to d.   HAMM:43
Grieve not that I d. young   HAST:43
man believes he shall ever d.   HAZL:43
d. suddenly   HIPP:46
fat are apt to d. earlier   HIPP:46
who will d.   HIPP:47
Remember you must d.   HORA:49
share the human condition and d.   ILLI:52
more than ever seems it rich to d.   KEATS:55
Rather suffer than d. is man's motto   LA FO:36
turn us to dust before we d.   MACAR:63
We begin to d. at birth   MANI:65
If you do not know how to d.   MONTA:70
One should d. proudly   NIET:73
Patients rarely d. of the disease   OSLER:75
D., my dear doctor   PALM:75
Whom the Gods love d. young   PLAU:80
live complaining, and d. disappointed   PROV:82
If you wish to d. soon   ROMAN:85
Spend all you have before you d.   SHAW:90
When men d. of disease   SHAW:91
To have to d. is a distinction   SMITH:93
it is worse to want to d.   SOPH:94
wisdom says: 'We must d.   UNAM:101
to d. beyond my means   WILDE:106

died

He d.; I dissected him   ANON:4
saving his money, he d. early   BARRY:9
man who d. from overwork   MAYO:67
I d. last night of my physician   PRIOR:82

dies

The patient never d.   ANON:3
He that d. before sixty   FIEL:34
d., in reality, by a violent death   FIEL:34
man always d.   FROMM:37

sticks to him till he d.   HOLM:48
wonders why his brother d.   HOLM:48
A man wounded in the abdomen d.   MACC:63
Whom the gods love d. young.   MENA:69
if he d. bury him.   SPAN:95
Every moment d. a man   TENN:99

diet

The best physicians are Dr. D.   ANON:4
neglects to d. himself   CHIN:21
regulation and administration of d.   COXE:26
The first rule to proper d.   FISC:35
neither exercise, nor d., nor physick   JOHNS:55
important part of a balanced d.   LEBO:59
careful and constant regulation of d.   MONTE:71

diets

D. were invented of the church   FISC:35

digest

To eat is human, to d. divine   COPE:25
more trouble to d. food   PROV:82

digestion

A good d. turneth all to health   HERB:45
for me is largely a matter of d.   LIN:60
d. is the great secret of life   SMITH:94
and strong stomachs for d.   VENN:102

digitalis

the fact that I use d.   WENC:105

dignity

think of the d. of your profession   MITC:70

dinner

After d. sit awhile   ENGL:33

diploma

passes between receiving his d.   DRAKE:30

directives

overwhelmed with inspections and d.   MORR:71

disability

the spectrum of d. problems   STOL:97

discover

To d. and to teach are distinct   NEWM:73

discoveries

vast importance of the d. of Pasteur   ALLB:2
instinct have produced many d.   BACON:8
ill prepared for making d.   BERN:11
the majority of d. in biology   BEVE:12
The greatest d. of surgery   FISC:35
increasing the number of d.   PAST:77
d. are met by captious criticism   POWE:81
d. are not usually not made   SIGE:92
Great d. which give a new direction   SMITH:94

discovery

Medicinal d.   AYRES:8
A d. is generally an unforeseen   BERN:11
No d. can be of general utility   BUCH:17
I have this day made a d.   DAVY:28
fifty years from the d. of a principle   FISC:35
research is the d. of the equations   MACH:63
The success of a d. depends upon   MITC:70
d. is rarely . . . a sudden achievement   MOYN:72
toward the d. of the unknown   PAST:77

discrimination

there is not enough d. in their use   GULL:41

disease

you choose your d.   ANON:3
It is not what d. the patient has   ANON:4
an immense hotbed of d.   ANON:5
Let out the blood, let out the d.   ANON:4
Cure the d. and kill the patient   BACON:8
The remedy is worse than the d.   BACON:8
The origin and the causes of d.   BAGL:8
There is no cure for this d.   BELLO:10

To the cure of this d.   BOCC:14
Acute d. must be seen at least once   BRIG:15
infallibly the symptom of d.   CARL:19
From the bitterness of d. man learns   CATA:19
D. is very old   CHARC:20
remedies are suggested for a d.   CHEK:21
When you treat a d.   CHEN:21
Before thirty, men seek d.   CHIN:21
The appearance of a d. is swift   CHIN:21
doctor treats the head of a d.   CHIN:22
When a d. relapses there is no cure   CHIN:22
man's d. is his personal property   CLARK:23
know the intractability of a d.   CLARK:23
The d. took at least half a million . . . lives   COLLI:24
explain our d., but cannot cure it   COLT:24
d. brought on by boredom   CONN:25
pyrexia as a part of the primary d.   CULL:26
d. may be distributed far beyond   DE MO:29
d. can pass from one individual   DUBOS:31
a pattern of d. peculiar to it   DUBOS:31
infection without d. is the rule   DUBOS:31
exchanging one d. for another   EDDY:32
D. is an experience   EDDY:32
the cause and prevent of d.   EDIS:32
prevention of d. is for the most part   EMER:33
deadly d. neither physician nor physic   ENGL:33
the d. is cured by nature   FORB:36
more to be feared than the d.   FRENC:37
The d. of an evil conscience   GLAD:40
I have learned much from d.   GOET:40
the daily observation of d.   GRAV:41
necessity for the removal of d.   HAES:42
A bodily d., may after all, be   HAWTH:43
ever had his d. themselves   HEROD:45
when immoderate, constitute d.   HIPP:46
in combating the d.   HIPP:47
Natural forces are the healers of d.   HIPP:47
d. not suited to surgical treatment   HOERR:48
a relapse of the old d.   HUANG:50
The physician must generalise the d.   HUFE:50
A long d. does not tell a lie   IRISH:52
suffering from the particular d.   JERO:54
When mean a dangerous d. did scape   JONS:55
Psychoanalysis is the d.   KRAUS:57
name of the drug to the name of a d.   LAUR:58
still uncertain of the nature of the d.   LATH:58
Perfect health . . . is perfect d.   LATH:58
leaves his d. to take care of itself   LATH:58
amount of irremediable d. in the world   LATH:58
some remedies worse than the d.   LATIN:58
a conception of health and d.   LIN:60
All interest in d. and death   MANN:65
D. has nothing refined about it   MANN:65
the observer must study d.   MART:66
fall by little and little into organic d.   MAUD:66
d. can scarcely keep pace   MAYOW:68
born with a deadly d. which is life   MOREA:71
unless organic d. can be excluded   MORR:71

To prevent d., to relieve suffering	OSLER:74
at times the d. is stronger	OVID:75
what sort of person has the d.	PARRY:76
When mediating over a d.	PAST:77
d. may be entirely impersonal	PEAB:77
same d. in an experimental animal	PEAB:77
Confront d. at its first stage	PERS:78
d. is the result of sin	PICKE:79
Medicine... has to examine d.	PLUT:80
Cured yesterday of my d.	PRIOR:82
A d. known is half cured	PROV:82
the d. is stronger than the patient	RHAZ:84
At the beginning of a d.	RHAZ:84
one particular aspect of a d.	SCHIC:88
D. is not of the body	SENE:89
A d. also is farther on the road	SENE:89
There is no d., bodily or mental	SHEL:91
D. creates poverty and poverty d.	SIGE:92
d. isolated its victims socially	SIGE:92
new weapons for the fight against d.	SIGE:92
D. is a dynamic process	SIGE:92
D. has social as well as physical	SIGE:92
a d. can be described and diagnosed	SKODA:93
what kind of a person has a d.	SMYTH:94
illness is man's reaction to d.	SOUT:94
A d., however much its course	SYDE:98
In the nineteenth century it was a d.	SZASZ:98
life's little ironies that surgical d.	THOMS:100
Decay and d. are often beautiful	THORE:100
D. often tells its secrets	TROT:101
element in d. is the key of medicine	TROU:101
muscles and tissues inflamed by d.	TWAIN:101
Wounds of the soul are a d.	VOLT:103
D. and sleep keep far apart	WELSH:105
write upon a d. than upon a remedy	WITH:107
ailment is worse than a d.	YIDD:108
Acute abdominal d.	ZETA:108

diseased

more than a d. organ	CUSH:27

diseases

d. as isolated disturbances	ALLB:2
coughs and sneezes spread d.	ANON:3
for detecting d. of the chest	AUEN:7
d. are revealed to the physician	BART:9
medicine is the art of understanding d.	BIGE:13
difference between particular d.	BROU:16
There are no such d.	BROU:16
D. crucify the soul	BURT:17
after thirty, d. seek men	CHIN:21
D. of the soul are more dangerous	CICE:23
do more for more d.	CLEN:23

d. which are so rare	DE GO:40
d. may also colour the moods	DUBOS:31
All d. run into one, old age	EMER:33
D. are but parts of a course	GULL:41
Similar d. are cured by similar things	HAHN:42
most appropriate for extreme d.	HIPP:46
chronic d. which do befall them	HIPP:46
As to d, make a habit of two things	HIPP:47
Many severe d.	HOFFM:48
has its special d.	HOFFM48
D. enter by the mouth.	JAPA:53
a prolific source of d.	JENN:54
Wind is the cause of a hundred d.	LÂO-T:58
Medicine heals doubt as well as d.	MARX:66
While there are several chronic d.	MAYO:67
For the most violent d.	MONTA:70
I do not want two d.	NAPO:72
worry over the great number of d.	PIEN:79
strange and new-fangled names to d.	PLATO:79
D. are the tax on pleasures	RAY:83
is the cause of all d.	SANTO:87
master incurable d.	SENE:89
you help make the d.	SHAK:90
die of the very d.	SHAW:90
doctor should come to know d.	SYDE:98

disinfectants

common sense are the best d.	OSLER:74

dissected

He died; I d. him	ANON:4

dissections

living d. any discovery	JOHNS:55

distinctions

all worldly d. are as nothing	LISTE:61

distinguish

can d. the possible from the impossible	HEROP:45

disuse

Use strengthens, d. debilitates	HIPP:47

divines

certainly be cleared up by the d. OULD:75

do

merely because we know how to d. FOX:36

doctor

If you are too smart to pay the d. AFRI:2
A d. who cannot take a good history ANON:3
D. says he would be a very sick man ANON:3
the successful d. was said to need ANON:3
Some d. full of phrase and fame ARNO:6
The blunders of a d. AR-RU:6
If my d. told me ASIM:7
d. is the servant and the interpreter BAGL:8
drinks more than his own d. BARA:8
The education of the d. BILLI:13
the d. will be made game of BRUY:16
The d. occupies a seat in the front BRAIN:15
a good d. is one who is shrewd CAIR:18
No man is a good d. CHIN:21
The unlucky d. treats the head CHIN:22
skillful d. treats those who are well CHIN:21
the human responsibility of the d. COMF:24
When a d. does go wrong CONAN:25
As a d. you would be well advised CRON:26
when a d. gets too lazy to work .... DA CO:23
Fresh air impoverishes the d. DANI:27
ye can always read a d.'s bill DUNNE:31
d. of the future will give no medicine EDIS:32
One d. makes work for another ENGL:33
A d. must work eighteen hours a day FISC:35
d. is often more to be feared FRENO:37
The silent d. shook his head GAY:38
A half d. near is better than a whole GERM:39
No d. is better than three. GERM:39
If a d. has treated a man HAMM:43
Ask the patient not the d. HINDU:46
Foolish the d. who despises HIPP:47
the duty of a d. to prolong life HORD:49
we demand in any d. HUGH:50
it is the d. who has killed him ITAL:53
d. was more concerned with healthy JAEG:53
patient tells you his d. has said JENN:54
the more restraint for the d. KORS:56
I often say a great d. kills more LEIB:59
able d. acts before sickness LIU:61
The able d. acts before sickness LIU:61
If you want to be a d. LORI:62
A good d. is equal to a good premier LU:62
considered the d. a gentleman MAUG:66

the d. must always be a student MAYO:67
change in the behaviour of the d. MEANS:68
d. has lost some of this ... omniscience MEANS:68
what the country d. is MITC:70
The religion of my d. MONTA:70
D. cures, if the sun sees it MONTA:70
how little reading a d. can practise OSLER:74
God and the D. we alike adore OWEN:75
You cannot be a perfect d. PAGET:75
D. and layman alike must learn PENF:78
not even a d. can kill you PERL:78
a d. is just to put your mind at rest PETRO:78
d. who desires the health PHILE:79
behoves the d. to become acquainted PINEL:79
A country d. needs more brains PITK:79
every Italian a d. POLI:81
as much as one d. hates another POLI:81
The d. demands his fees POLI:81
trained and highly motivated a d. POWIS:81
You tell your d., that ye're ill PRIOR:82
capable of deceiving the d. PROU:82
An apple a day keeps the d. away PROV:82
Beware of the young d. PROV:82
The presence of the d. PROV:82
the d. takes the fee PROV:82
less than the experience of a wise d. RHAZ:84
d. has to be within thirty inches RICHA:84
My d.'s issued his decree ROSS:85
steal a rouble from the d. RUSS:86
seldom needs the d. SCOT:88
the village d. SCOTT:88
or of a human in the hands of his d. SCRU:88
People pay the d. for his trouble SENE:89
death will seize the d. too SHAK:90
a sick d. SHAW:90
think no more of the condition of a d. SHAW:91
practising d. makes a contribution SHAW:91
a death advertises the d. SHAW:91
the d. gets the credit of curing them SHAW:91
Our d. would never really operate SHRI:92
give a d. less to do than one woman SPAN:95
a d. whom he trusts SPEN:95
d. does not give you a year STEV:96
with a young d. your health SWED:98
d. should come to know diseases SYDE:98
A. d. is a man who writes prescriptions TAYL:99
differs the surgeon from the d. UREN:101
nothing more laughable than a d. VOLT:103
Heaven defend me from a busy d. WELSH:105
It is the special vocation of the d. WHITT:106
The d. says there is no hope ZAVA:108

Doctor Slop

uncourtly figure of a D. STER:96

doctor-made

one nature-made, one d.   NAPOL:72

doctor–patient relationship

to fall short of the ideal d.   MEANS:68

doctors

d. are either good or bad	ALBR:2
D. should attend the sick	ANON:3
the d. who desert the dying	BARRE:9
The d. are too narrowly educated	BEVAN:11
who are the skilled lawyers and d.	BILLI:13
the d. know nothing	CELLI:20
D. are just the same as lawyers	CHEK:21
From d. and imagination flow	CHUR:22
The d. all say we all eat too much	COOK:25
I doubt if d. ever assault; they batter	DEVL:29
D. are always working	DIDE:29
Patients must be able to trust d.	GENE:38
D. must keep their knowledge	GENE:38
D cruelly and needlessly prolong	GILLI:39
D. are and should be natural leaders	GRUG:41
D. have a sense for things unseen	HECHT:44
secrecy is highly developed among d.	HECHT:44
I love the d., they are dears	HERB:45
D. think a lot of patients are cured	HEROL:45
exist for the convenience of d.	HILL:46
so little medicine as those of d.	HOLM:48
the d. are the most sensible	HOLM:48
D. are the best-natured people	HOLM:48
D. cannot cure their own complaints	HUAI:50
d. and patients	KIPL:56
The choice before d. is	LAUR:58
for d. imagine diseases	LUTH:62
The d. and nurses treated me	MAND:65
trained our young d. to consider	MEANS:68
best d. can make the worst mistakes	MILB:69
There are only two sorts of d.	OSLER:74
procession of four or five d.	OSLER:75
We d have always been a simple	OSLER:75
be struck between d. and society	PHILL:79
d. worry over the scarcity	PIEN:79
when d. disagree	POPE:81
The mistakes made by d.	PROU:82
if they are good d.	RUSK:86
D. are a social cement	SALI:87
the fact that d. themselves die	SHAW:90
No d. live on in the memory	SIGE:92
The best of d. will go to hell	TALM:99
the greatest deceivers? The d.?	VOLT:103
D. are mostly impostors	WILDE:106

hated by the best d.	WILDE:106
D. are generally dull dogs	WILS:107
The d. are a frightful race	WOLFE:107

doctrine

To have admitted the truth of a d.   JENN:54

dogmas

treat our own theories as d.   TOUL:100

dollars

d. spent on medical care   WILDA:106

dope

better treated with hope, not d.   ASHER:7

doses

d. the text books say are dangerous   WENC:105

double effect

pretending that the d. argument   DOYAL:30

doubt

many who died from d.	MAYO:67
When in d., drain	TAIT:99
to d. and to be ignorant	UNAM:101

doubter

The d. is a true man of science   BERN:11

doubts

to keep your d. to yourself	HOLM:48
Medicine heals d. as well as diseases	MARX:66

drain

When in doubt, d.   TAIT:99

drank

He neither d., smoked, nor rode   BARRY:9

dream

A d. which is not interpreted   TALM:99

dreams

D. are excursions into the limbo   AMIEL:2
D., Children of night   CHUR:22
D. in general originate   HEROD:45
more clearly in d. than the imagination   VINCI:102

dressed

I d. him and God healed him   PARÉ:76

drink

Let us eat and d.   BIBLE:12
D. because you are happy   CHES:21
generosity of men that d.   DAVIE:28
They that are thirsty d. silently   FRENC:37
the reason why I never d. it   JACK:53
then the d. takes the man   JAPA:53
We d. one another's health   JERO:54
The more you d., the more you crave   POPE:81
thirst vanishes as you d.   RABE:83
d. may be said to be an equivocator   SHAK:90
men eat and d. to live   SOCR:94
I can d. without danger   TOULO:100
D. makes men hungry   WILKI:107

drinking

to give up smoking, d. and loving   ANON:4
D. was much more general   BRUCE:16
D. strong wine cures hunger   HIPP:46
since my leaving d. of wine   PEPYS:78
Tis not the d. that is to be blamed   SELD:89

drinks

who d. as much as you do   THOMA:99

dropsy

So he whose belly swells with d.   OVID:75

drowned

a man who had been virtually d.   MAUR:67

drug

D. therapies are replacing a lot   BUSH:18
I will neither give a deadly d.   HIPP:47
A miracle d. is any d. that will do   HODG:48
D. therapy involves a great deal   LAUR:58
the incidence of needless d. use   SILV:93

drug companies

We trust the d. They wouldn't lie   RAMI:83

drugged

so d. that he cannot respond   BAIN:8

drugs

do not know the d. they use   BACON:8
nor the power of d. was of any effect   BOCC:14
the less confidence I have in d.   COXE:26
how do d. . . . heal   EDDY:32
in spite of d. or because of them   GADD:37
I do not say no d. are useful   GULL:41
no really 'safe' biologically active d.   KAMI:55
and for not assessing his d.   PENN:78
appropriately called 'wonder-d.'   STUM:97
one kills with his d.   UREN:101
A physician is one who pours d.   VOLT:103

drunk

especially when they are d.   CAPP:19
one should get d. at least once   FRENC:37

drunken

He uses statistics as a d. man   LANG:58

drunkenness

D., the ruin of reason   BASIL:9
D. spoils health   PENN:78
D. turns a man out of himself   PROV:82
D. is temporary suicide   RUSSE:86
D. is simply voluntary insanity   SENE:89

dull

I cannot think of anything more d.   BIER:13

duties

d. has been rigorously tested   SEEG:88
medicine recognises its tasks and its d.   WUND:108

duty

It is our d. . . . to resist old age   CICE:22
It is the d. of a doctor to prolong life   HORD:49
d. to seek medical aid   MAIM:64
Job was never on night d.   PAGET:75
It is our d. to remember at all times   SCHW:88
It was a son's d. to see his father   YOUNG:108

dying

d. with the help of too many   ALEX:2
Thou to whom the sick and d.   ANON:5
the doctors who desert the d.   BARRE:9
half the world's population is d.   CARRU:19
a most unconscionable time d.   CHARL:20
d., of course, but they look terrific   COSBY:25
Heal the sick and comfort the d.   DOUG:30
Poor honest sex, like d.   DURR:31
keep a d. patient's relatives busy   FRIPP:37
prolong the lives of the d.   GILLI:39
not his duty to prolong the act of d.   HORD:49
d. is more the survivors' affair   MANN:65
D. is a very dull, dreary affair   MAUG:67
who feel not themselves d.   MILT:69
and prolonging the act of d.   MINE:69
When a man lies d., he does not die   PÉGUY:78
observe many ways of d.   RHOA:84
Approaches to death and d.   SAUN:87
care of the d. and their families   SAUN:87
but d. well means d. gladly   SENE:89
Death must be distinguished from d.   SMITH:94
Rage, rage against the d. of the light   THOMA:99
Stop people d. of the illnesses   WHITE:106

dysentery

D. has been more fatal to armies   OSLER:74

dyspepsia

when they are troubled with d.   INGER:52

ear

and the other to my e.   LAËN:57
use too little hand and e. and eye   ZETA:108

ears

The e. should be kept perfectly clean   DE LA:57
to keep the e. from grating   VRIES:103
given man one tongue, but two e.   ZENO:108

eat

Let us e. and drink   BIBLE:12
Tell me what you e.   BRIL:15
One should e. to live   CICE:22
The doctors all say we e. too much   COOK:25
To e. is human, to digest divine   COPE:25
Short men e. more than tall ones   FRENC:37
I e. to live, to serve   GAND:38
e. moderately   HUTC:51
A person should not e.   MAIM:64
E. as much as you like   SECO:88
Base men live to e. and drink   SOCR:94

eaten

never repent of having e. too little   JEFF:54

eaters

Great e. and great sleepers   HENRY:45

eating

Excessive e. is like a deadly poison   MAIM:64
In e., a third of the stomach   TALM:99
a sign something is a. us   VRIES:103
e. dry food   WELSH:105

eats

He that e. till he is sick must fast   ENGL:33
even if he e. good foods   MAIM:64
choleric drinks, the melancholic e.   PROV:82
He that e. but one dish   SCOT:88

educated

The doctors are too narrowly e.   BEVAN:11
I take it that no man is e.   JAMES:53

education

most important part of his e.	BILLI:13
E. never ends, Watson	CONAN:24
e. should leave much to be desired	GREGG:41
The physician's continuing e.	HARR:43
The e. of most people ends	MARX:66
are two objects of medical e.	MAYO:67
The object of health e. is to change	MAYO:67
medical e. is not completed	WELCH:105

educational

take part regularly in e. activities	GENE:38

egg

Everything from an e.	HARV:43

elbow

Never rub your eye but with your e.	ENGL:33

elder

the life of our e. citizens	KENN:56

elderly

postponed in e. patients	COLE:24

elective

surgical therapy for e. conditions	COLE:24

embryo

are transmitted to the e.	BARA:9

emergency

It is the nature of e. surgery	JONES:55

emoluments

take position and e. as an accident	SMITH:94

empiricism

destined to get away from e.	BERN:11

employment

E. is nature's physician	GALEN:38

endoscopic

he can learn another e. technique	CLARK:23

enemy

who mishandles apparatus is my e.	ROEN:84

energies

handicaps release copious e.	PITK:79

English

E. physicians kill you	LAMB:57
language of medicine – broken E.	POPP:81

Englishmen

Many more E. die by the lancet	ARMS:6

enjoyment

I do not eat for the sake of e.	GAND:38

enteric sciences

Far too long the e., basic and clinical	PHILL:79

environment

interactions of man with his e.	BEAT:9
Heredity sets limits, e. decides	MACD:63

epidemic

snubbed if an e. overlooks them	HUBB:50

epidemics

history of e. is the history of wars   CHRI:22
E. have often been more influential   DUBOS:31

epidemiologist

An e. is a doctor broken down by age   ANON:3

epilepsy

e. may be called the reproach   HEBE:44

epitaph

I desire no other e.   OSLER:74

equal

In sleep we are all e   SPAN:95

error

they worship even e.   GOET:40
Amid many possibilities of e.   LATH:58
the public recantation of an e.   LISTE:61

errors

The medical e. of one century   CLARK:23
more harmful than reasoned e.   HUXL:52
E. in judgment must occur   OSLER:74

erysipelas

in every wound symptoms of e.   HAMI:42

erythrocytes

E. were primarily designed by God   COOM:25

ether

e. inhalation successfully practised   SIMP:93
chloroform and devoted to e.   SIMS:93
I commenced inhaling the e.   VENA:102

ethic

the service e. and clinical autonomy   HUNT:51

ethical

practice is steered by e. principles   LOPEZ:62

ethics

had lasting effect on e.   BRAIN:15
E. and Science need to shake hands   CABOT:18

eugenics

Men are not going to not embrace e.   CLEN:23

euthanasia

E. is a long, smooth-sounding word   BUCK:17
legalisation of active e.   DOYAL:30
e. is actually practised by . . . physicians   SIGE:92

events

the e. that happen around us   TROT:101

evil

Pain is in itself an e.   BENT:11
Death is the greatest e.   HAZL:43

evils

must expect new e.   BACON:8
Most of those e. we poor mortals   CHUR:22

evolution

Some call it E.
And others call it God   CARRU:19
our views one e.   HALD:42
E. is the most powerful   HUXL:52
error to imagine that e. signifies   HUXL:52
indifferent about what she is, viz., mere e.   JACO:53
E. is far more important than living   JÜNG:55
the end of their e.   WERT:105

evolved

have been and are being e.   DARW:28

examination

from want of a proper e.   HOWA:49
moment you have passed your final e.   MAUG:66

examinations

E. are formidable even to the best   COLT:24

examine

Always e. your cases thoroughly   WHITF:106

examiners

before our officials and e.   ROGER:84

excretory

the e. offices of the kidney   PETE:78

exercise

the Substitute for E. or Temperance   ADDI:1
E. is good for your health   ARAB:6
Bodily e. profiteth little   BIBLE:12
E. and temperance can preserve   CICE:22
e. acting as a pallbearer   DEPEW:29
E. is bunk   FORD:36
be devoted to bodily e.   JEFF:54
neither e., nor diet, nor physick   JOHNS:55
take their e. on an empty stomach   HIPP:47
The only e. I get   LARD:58
sedentary life and does not e.   MAIM:64
they have not time for bodily e.   STAN:95

existence

a precarious and limited e.   DOBOS:30

experience

e. is often a dreadful list   DA CO:23
E. comes from bad judgment   LILL:60

E. is the great teacher   MAYO:68
E. is the mother of science   PROV:82
E. is the mother of truth   SHIP:92

experiment

The men of e. are like the ant   BACON:8
scientific idea controlled by e.   BERN:11
E. is fundamentally only induced   BERN:11
not only what he seeks in an e.   BERN:11
everyone believes an e.   BEVE:12
do one e. in medicine to convince   DOCH:30
accuracy and precision in e.   EHRL:32
Why not make an e.   HUNTE:51
they should e. on their patients   LAUR:58
E. alone crowns the efforts   PAVL:77
by passing through the fire of e.   PAVL:77
a badly conceived e.   PLATT:80

experimental

same disease in an e. animal   PEAB:77
application of the e. method   WELCH:105

experimentation

complexity brings into e.   BERN:11
In e. it is always necessary to start   BERN:11

experimenter

What the e. is really trying to do   CANN:19
the e. questions and forces her   CUVI:27

experiments

teach himself by facts and e.   BOER:14
observes, e. and judges   FLEX:36

expert

An e. is one who known more   BUTL:18
An e. is a man who tells you   CAST:19
An e. is someone who is more   MEESE:68

expire

e. in a warm gush of sympathy   BEVAN:11

exploratory

E. operation   ANON:3

explore

the irresistible need to e.   BRON:15

eye

The e. is not satisfied with seeing   BIBLE:12
The light of the body is the e.   BIBLE:12
The e. altering alters all   BLAKE:14
A small hurt in the e. is a great one   ENGL:33
Never rub your e.   ENGL:33
devoted himself to the e. alone   MITC:70
the curious texture of the e.   NEED:73
The e. is bigger than the belly   PROV:82
The e. is a dark chamber   RUCK:85
E. is the window of the mind   SHAK:90
Why does the e. see   VINCI:102
use too little hand and ear and e.   ZETA:108

eyeballs

as if I was walking on my e.   SMITH:94

eyes

his e. were dim   BIBLE:12
The eyes are obliquely placed   DOWN:30
it prevents the e. from seeing   DUBOS:31
The e. must finish their work   SCHAT:87

eyesight

The precious treasure of his e. lost   SHAK:90

face

The f. is flat and broad   DOWN:30

fact

ultimate value of a new scientific f.   DOCH:30

facts

Today's f. are tomorrow's fallacies   ANON:5
whether f. can be established   CANN:19

a theory which he tries to fit to f.   DA CO:23
False f. are highly injurious   DARW:28
begin with a good body of f.   DARW:28
F. are not science   FISC:35
We must trust to nothing but f.   LAVO:59
substitute f. for appearances   RUSKI:86
F. are stubborn things   SMOL:94

faculties

the failing of one's f.   MAUG:67

fads

Most medical f. are like   FABR:34

failures

seeks the reason for certain of his f.   LERI:59

faith

The prayer of f. shall save the sick   BIBLE:12
the popular f. of the next   CLARK:23
an implicit or even a partial f.   HOLM:48
which is admitted through f.   RAMON:83
science and f. exclude one another   VIRC:103

fallacy

This is a popular f.   NIGH:73

fallopian

to cover cutting the F. tubes   HOLM:49
right F. tube was ruptured   TAIT:99

fame

and careless of f.   VIRG:103

families

Patients and their f. will forgive you   ANON:4
No f. take so little medicine   HOLM:48

family

his f. would wish to be treated   LOEB:61
each unhappy f. is unhappy   TOLS:100

famine

More die by food than f.   PROV:82

fart

the . . . most superbly stupendous f.   MAXW:67

fashion

we are not all formed in the same f.   RUFUS:86

fashions

like some women's f.   FABR:34

fast

He that eats till he is sick must f.   ENGL:33

fasting

f. is a medicine   CHRY:22

fat

Everybody loves a f. man   AMER:2
Nobody loves a f. man   AMER:2
Persons who are naturally very f.   HIPP:46
F people who want to reduce   HIPP:47
kindness is better than a f. pie   RUSSI:86

fatal

Doctor can foresee the f. outcome   BOER:14

fate

f. arrives the physician becomes   ARAB:6
Whom f. wishes to ruin   LATIN:58
The Angel of F.   ROSS:85

father

In illness the physician is a f.   BRAH:15
For they which share one f.'s blood   EURI:34

fault

what f. they commit   QUAR:83

faults

Physicians's f. are covered with earth   ENGL:33

fear

who f.s to suffer, suffers from f.   FRENC:37

fed

He f. fevers   GRAV:41

fee

no pain at all when he charges his f.   ANON:3
she . . . asks none of the f.   FISC:35
Despairing of his f. tomorrow   GAY:38
on fixing what your f. is to be   HIPP:47
they shall wish to learn it, without f.   HIPP:47
never take a higher f.   HOPE:49
God heals and the doctor takes the f.   PROV:82

feed

F. sparingly and defy the physician   ENGL:33

fees

The doctor demands his f.   POLI:81

feet

as is paid to their f.   ANON:4
Keep the head cool, the f. warm   BOER:14
The guts carry the f.   CERV:20
to come into the world with f. first   PLUT:80

felt

seldom think that it is f.   JOHNS:55

fertility

The management of f.   GREER:41

fever

Six weeks with a f. is an eternity   BALZ:8
puerperal f. raged violently   HAMI:42
that a f. succeed to a convulsion   HIPP:46
you frequently have to starve a f.   MACF:63
The f. is to the physicians   MILT:69
by far the most terrible, is f.   OSLER:75
nature induces f. and inflammation   STAHL:95

fevers

He fed f.   GRAV:41

fifty

After a man is f. you can fool him   HOWE:49

fighting

except when they get f. each other   HOLM:48

filthy

F. water cannot be washed   AFRI:2

financial

unconsciously by pressing f. need   LEHM:59

finds

He that seeks f.   SPAN:95

finger

it involves soiling the f.   MAYO:68

fingers

the instruments and the surgeon's f.   BLAND:14
eyes first and most; f. next   HUMP:51

fire

that the f. cures   HIPP:47

fish

dominion over the f. of the seas   BIBLE:12

fistula

health is often joined with a f. in ano   HEBE:44

fittest

Survival of the f.   SPEN:95

Fleming

Yet had F. not possessed   MAUR:67

flesh

the hard service of the f.   AURE:7
as f. of his own f.   ROUS:85

fleshy

proud office to tend the f. tabernacle   LISTE:61

food

Eat less fresh f.   CAND:19
F. is an important part   LEBO:59
distinction between f. and medicine   LIN:60
f. of a sucking child   PHAE:79
more trouble to digest f.   PROV:82
More die by f. than famine   PROV:82
no love sincerer than the love of f.   SHAW:91
channel for f.   VINCI:102
A f. is not necessarily essential   WHITE:106

foods

are due to bad f.   MAIM:64

fool

f. lives as long as his destiny allows	ANON:3
the greatest f. may ask more	COLT:24
I prefer to be called a f.	HOMA:49

forgotten

Physical pain is easily f.	RAMÓN:83

foxglove

The f.'s leaves with caution given	WITH:107

French

The F. let you die	LAMB:57

Frenchman

A F. will sooner part with his religion	SMOL:94
It was invented by a F.	WODE:107

Freud

F.'s discovery	BRAIN:15

friend

f. is the medicine of life	ANON:3
kindly indulgence of a considerate f.	BRADF:15

friendship

the f. they owe me	MONTA:70

friendships

an inability to form warm f.	ROBI:84

frog

Poison should be tried out on a f.	AFRI:2

function

the achievement of optimal f.	KOTT:57

functional

despise the little things of f. disorder	MAUD:66

functions

to disturb the f. in all the others	BICH:12

funeral

but guess how much his f. cost	ANON:4
the f. of his first patient	DRAKE:30
rejoice at a birth and grieve at a f.	TWAIN:101

funerals

f. discredit a physician	JONS:55

future

old age is that there is no f. in it	ANON:5

gadgets

g. can betray sound sense	SALT:87

Galen

Surgeon is a disciple of G.	BROOK:16
Did we not believe G. implicitly	OSLER:75
according to Hippocrates and G.	SANTO:87

gangrene

G. doth induce a certain death	HARV:43
pyaemia, hospital g. or erysipelas	LISTE:60
When g. is pronounced	PARÉ:76
g. and mortification are most likely	POTT:81
g. is pain and inconvenience	SMITH:94

garden

g. is the poor man's apothecary	GERM:39

gastroenterologist

The young g. of today	CLARK:23

general

The best surgeon, like the best g.   COOP:25
kills more people than a great g.   LEIB:59

General Medical Council

G. has called on his colleagues   BERN:11

general medicine

where I can learn something of g.   WIDAL:106

general practice

G. is at least as difficult   BASH:9

general practitioner

g. practicing in some rural area   HARR:43
no man needs it more than the g.   OSLER:75
A g. can no more become a specialist   PADD:75

generalisation

proceed to the g.   BERN:11

generations

the birthright of successive g.   GALT:38

genetics

The New G. and The Social Theory   LE FA:34
studied g. and natural selection   HALD:42

genitals

the case of the g. and the tongue   VINCI:102

genius

G. is one per cent inspiration   EDIS:32
G. seems to consist in the power   POLA:81
when g. is married to science   SPEN:95

gentleman

A tall thin, large bowed, old g.   DICKE:29
only four professions for a g.   MAUG:66

gentlemen

G., this is no humbug   WARR:104

geriatrics

study of g. begins with pediatrics   SEEG:89

Germany

In pre-Hitler G.   SIGE:92

glands

Today the g. may be free   DE MO:29

glasses

girls who wear g.   PARKE:76

globus hystericus

The g. in the throat   HEBE:44

gluttony

help to make the g.   SHAK:90
G. is an emotional escape   VRIES:103
The crime of our civilisation is g.   WILL:107

God

And others call it G.   CARRLI:19
primarily designed by G. as tools   COOM:25
The Act of G. designation   COREN:25
care not to make intellect our g.   EINS:32
G. gave his creatures light and air   HOLM:48
halfway between an ape and a g.   INGE:52
G. could not be everywhere   JEWI:54
People turn to G. in times of crisis   MANF:65

G. and the Doctor we alike adore   OWEN:75
I dressed him and G healed him   PARÉ:76
If G. operated on a hernia patient   RUTK:86
Imagine G. as tailor   SELZ:89
If you talk to G.   SZASZ:98
G.-like in our planned breeding   TOYN:100

gods

In a world controlled by g.   GRAH:41
Whom the g. love die young   PLAU:80

gold

would not give a little g.   ANON:4
Perfect health is above g.   ANON:5
G. that buys health   GEKK:38
made precious by the touch of g.   TROL:100

good

worst when he appeareth g.   PROV:82

gout

g., that incurred by the genteel   BELL:10
G., n. A physician's name   BIERC:13
There is no pain like the G.   BRET:15
The g. is so common a disease   CADO:18
Drink wine and have the g.   COGAN:23
It is with jealousy as with the g.   FIEL:34
the Gout will seize you   FRAN:36
G. is to the arteries   HUCH:50
With respect to the g.   ITAL:53
when I have the g.   SMITH:94
G., unlike any other disease, kills   SYDE:98
who are supposed to have died of g.   SYDE:98

government

It is poor g. that does not realize   MAYO:68
should not be a servant of any g.   PLATT:80

Grace

a double dose of G.   FISH:35

graduate

The first acts of a g. are   DRAKE:30

grandparents

an improper selection of g.   OSLER:75

grave

G., n. A place in which the dead   BIERC:13
Descend with ease into the g.   COTT:26
occurred on the way to the g.   CRISP:26
journey of man to the g.   SKRA:93
I had rather follow you to your g.   SHERI:91
a son's duty to see his father into the g.   YOUNG:108

graves

among the g. of their neighbours   EDWA:32

Great Britain

half of the children born in G. die   BUCH:17

Greek

prefers to describe in G.   ASHER:7

grief

G. is itself a medicine   COWP:26

grow

when you cease to g., you are old   HERR:45

growth

upon which all their g. depends   HARV:43

guild

merely a monopolistic g.   STARR:96

guinea pig

under the skin of a g.   LISTE:61

guts

The g. carry the feet   CERV:20

gynaecologists

G. are very smooth indeed   ASHER:7

gynaecology

determining point in the history of g.   SIGE:92

habit

Seldom of a plump and succulent h.   CULL:26

haematologist

The modern h.   ASHER:7

haemoglobin

and only secondarily as carriers of h.   COOM:25

hair

And you can't part the h.   BENN:10
A h. in the head   HERF:45
To heads whose h.   SALE:86
his h. that grows bald by nature   SHAK:90
loses his teeth, h. and ideas   VOLT:103
only one cure for grey h.   WODE:107

hand

the increment of the power of the h.   FISKE:35
his h. shall be cut off   HAMM:43
In a good h. every sword cuts well   MONTE:71
use too little h. and ear and eye   ZETA:108

handicaps

people are better off with grave h.   PITK:79

hands

They shall lay their h. on the sick   ANON:5
With thy healing h. replying   ANON:5
kept in the h. of a few   BUCH:17
Wash your h. often, your feet seldom   ENGL:33
movement of steady, experienced h.   GALEN:38
wash his h. before treating anyone   PFOL:78
without previously washing the h.   TALM:99

happiness

h. gives us the energy   AMIEL:2
H. lies, first of all in health   CURT:27
the foundation upon which all their h.   DISR:30
is essential to human h.   GALEN:38
The ground-work of all h. is health   HUNT:51
H. for me is largely a matter   LIN:60
H. is beneficial for the body   PROU:82

happy

He who is h. always gets well   PARA:76

Harley Street

inhabitants of H. and Wimpole Street   ANON:5

harm

at least not to h.   HIPP:47
h. comes to the strong   NIET:73
do the sick no h.   NIGH:73
First do no h. It is a good remedy   PROV:82

harmless

there is nothing that is h.   PARA:76

head

your h. sits on the other   ANON:5
Keep the h. cool, the feet warm   BOER:14
seize and turn the h.   CHUR:22
When the h. aches   ENGL:33
ought to have his h. examined   GOLDW:40
this differs from other pains of the h.   HEBE:44
h. is a thoroughly inefficient organ   MAUG:67

heads

they make our h. ache   ITAL:53

heal

Physician, h. thyself   BIBLE:12
Nature does not kill and does not h.   JACO:53

healed

I dressed him and God h. him   PARÉ:76

healer

The sharp compassion of the h.'s art   ELIOT:32

healers

Natural forces are the h. of disease   HIPP:47
The best of h. is good cheer   PIND:79

healing

from the bottom to ensure sound h.   ANON:5
With thy h. hands replying   ANON:5
For of the most High cometh h.   BIBLE:12
same relation to his power of h.   BUTL:18
buildings that are positively h.   CHARL:21
h. art enables one to make   CHIN:21
Hippocrates as first in the art of h.   GALEN:38
the h. art must be improved   HILL:46
H. is a matter of time   HIPP:47
The natural h. force within us   HIPP:47
important requirement of the art of h.   HUANG:50
The art of h. comes from nature   PARA:76
any h. discipline other than his own   PENN:78
medicine and the practice of h.   VIRG:103

heals

h., under the auspices of   EMER:33
God h. and the doctor takes the fee   PROV:82
Time h. what reason cannot   SENE:89
physician who h. for nothing   TALM:99

health

H. and cheerfulness naturally   ADDI:1
sick man who believes himself to be in h.   AMIEL:2
H. is the first of all liberties   AMIEL:2
He who has h. has hope   ARAB:5
contribute to h., wealth and wisdom.   ARIS:6
may be said to be in a state of h.   BENT:11
when h. is restored, he is a guardian   BRAH:15
Exercise is good for your h.   BRAH:15
H. indeed is a precious thing   BURT:17
man learns the sweetness of h.   CATA:19
soundness of h. is impossible   CICE:23
The origins of physical and mental h.   COCK:23

part with all their money for h.   COLT:24
Happiness lies, first of all, in h.   CURT:27
Gold that buys h.   DEKK:28
working to preserve our h.   DIDE:29
The h. of a people   DISR:30
H. is not a condition of matter   EDDY:32
H. is better than wealth   ENGL:33
H. is not valued till sickness comes   ENGL:33
deny the existence of h.   EMER:33
had been completely restored to h.   FRANK:36
Nothing is more fatal to H.   FRAN:36
master of his thirst is master of his h.   FRENC:37
careful of the h. of others   GALEN:38
A good digestion turneth all to h.   HERB:45
no avail if h. be lacking   HEROP:45
when h. is restored   HINDU:46
h. is his most valuable possession   HIPP:47
ground-work of all happiness is h.   HUNT:51
a major threat to h.   ILLI:52
H. without wealth is half a sickness   ITAL:53
H. is the first requisite after morality   JEFF:54
drink one another's h.   JERO:54
the h. and vitality of its population   KENN:56
Perfect h., like perfect beauty   LATH:58
a conception of h. and disease   LIN:60
secure h. for most of us   LUBB:62
but living in h.   MART:65
h. and happiness of its people   MAYO:68
Good h. is an essential to happiness   MAYO:67
kind of h. which can be preserved   MONTE:71
the quadrangle of h.   OSLER:74
sometimes snatches away h.   OVID:75
no two persons are exactly alike in h.   PAGET:75
Drunkenness spoils h.   PENN:78
not a doctor who desires the h.   PHILE:79
Attention to health   PLATO:79
best men when in the worst h.   PROV:82
H. is the poor man's riches   PROV:82
Sickness is felt, but h. not at all   PROV:82
Without h. life is not life   RABE:83
Sleep, riches, and h.   RICHT:84
To preserve one's h.   ROCH:84
the h. of its people   ROOS:85
H. is beauty   SHEN:91
task of medicine is to promote h.   SIGE:92
H. cannot be forced upon people   SIGE:92
h. is a symptom of unhealth   SKRA:93
H., like love, beauty   SKRA:93
The preservation of h. is a duty   SPEN:95
the h. of the nation   STAC:95
the infirmities of ill h.   STER:96
People ... taking care of their h.   STER:96
better to lose h. like a spendthrift   STEV:96
to restore the h. of the patient   SYDE:98
a decay of h., and hectic fever   TORR:100
the h. of the whole human race   TOYN:100
protection of the h. of the public   VIRC:103
the restoration of h. to other men   VOLT:103

Look to your h.   WALT:104
will be close to zero in improving h.   WILDA:106
H. is the primary duty of life   WILDE:106

health care

for more than 70% of h. services   CALI:18
H. professionals who always took   HUNT:51
greater access to h.   ILLI:52
the whole of h. will dissolve   LILF:60
the most crucial competency in h.   LILF:60
h. has changed from a private matter   LILF:60

health care system

Is the whole of the h.   CHARL:21

health program

whatever h. a country develops   SIGE:92

Health Service

a comprehensive H. for everyone   HAWTO:43

health-food stores

Did you ever see the customers in h.   COSBY:25

healthier

the h. Western society becomes   PORT:81

healthy

isolated disturbances in a h. body   ALLB:2
it is a h. habit   ARIS:6
the right to work as he is h.   BISM:14
He that goes to bed thirsty rises h.   ENGL:33
Every h. man is king   GAEL:37
he should look h.   HIPP:47
more concerned with h. people   JAEG:53
H. people need   ILLI:52
greatest danger for the h.   NIET:73
To desire to be h. is part of being h.   SENE:89
lives are different from h. people   SIGE:92
superfluous amongst the h.   TACI:98
h. to be sick sometimes   THORE:100
commonly a long time h.   VENN:102

heart

licks at the joints, but bites the h.   ANON:4
to be found in a melancholy man's h.   BURT:17
The h. is the most noble of all   CHRY:22
operates with his hand, not with his h.   DUMAS:31
The h. is the only organ   FISC:35
trade in a weak h. . . . for a better one   GILLI:39
the blood passes through the h.   HARV:43
The h. of animals is the foundation   HARV:43
The h. is the root of life   HUANG:50
A merry h. doeth good   HUBB:50
what rheumatism is to the h.   HUCH:50
Diseases of the h. and circulation   JULI:55
perceive the action of the h.   LAËN:57
not only the beating of the h.   LAËN:57
in every case of unsound h.   LATH:58
in illness is never to lose h.   LENIN:59
the study of diseases of the h.   MAJOR:65
practice of medicine is like h. muscle   SCHIC:88
The h. is in accord with the pulse   SU:97
veins and arteries proceed from the h.   VINCI:102

hell

work like h. and adverstise   BEYN:12
not threatened in h. itselfe   DONNE:30
The best of doctors will go to h.   TALM:99

help

some patients whom we cannot h.   BLOO:14

hemicrania

The h., or pain of one half of the head   HEBE:44

herbalist

The medical h. is at fault for clinging   PENN:78

hereditary

person suffering from a h. disease   GERM:39
diseases result from a h. disposition   HOFFM:48

heredity

H. sets limits, environment decides   MACD:63
H. is the last of the fates   WILDE:106

hernia

If God operated on a h. patient   RUTK:86

hiccup

a person afflicted with h.   HIPP:47

hidden

things are h., obscure and debatable   PAST:77

Hippocrates

H. more than 2000?   OSLER:75
according to H. and Galen   SANTO:87

histology

H. is an odd-tasting dish   HORT:49
to make h. experimental   RANV:83

history

it is necessary to know its h.   COMTE:24
The h. of medicine   GARR:38
The h. of medicine is a study   IBÁÑ:52
h. taker is he who can best interpret   WOOD:107

homeopathy

H. waged a war of radicalism   ANON:4
H. is insignificant as an act   EMER:33
H. . . . a mingled mass of perverse   HOLM:48

honour

essential to harmony and h.   ALLB:2
H. a physician   HEBR:44
regard for the h. of the profession   PRIT:82
noble scar, is a good liv'ry of h.   SHAK:90

hope

He who has health has h.   ARAB:5
He that lives upon h.   FRAN:36
Confidence and h. do me more good   GALEN:38
H. is the physician of each misery   IRISH:53

H. is necessary in every condition   JOHNS:55
Always give the patient h.   PARÉ:76
no other medicine. But only h.   SHAK:90

hopefulness

qualification for a physician is h.   LITT:61

hopes

man's insomnia . . . h. and aspirations   FITZG:35

horse

perhaps it be his h.   SCOTT:88

hospital

The h. is the only proper College   ABER:1
the poor devils in the h.   ABER:1
our M.D.'s and our h. appointments   BASH:9
I consider the h. to be a vestibule   BERN:11
cold altruism of a large h.   BEVAN:11
but an h., and a place, not to live   BROW:16
The purpose of a teaching h.   FAXON:34
After two days in h.   FIEL:35
his h. contained only twelve beds   MACP:64
depressing influence of general h.   MAYO:67
made the h. desirable for patients   MAYO:67
the first requirement in a H.   NIGH:73
as unlike my H. life   NIGH:73
fool who holds two h. appointments   RING:84
voluntary h. may not treat the poor   STARR:96
create havoc in the running of the h.   TWEE:101
A h. is an institution   WARR:104

hospitality

H. and medicine must be confined   INDI:52

hospitals

Big stools, small h.   BURKI:17
H. tend to weaken the family tie   GILL:39
H. are always touted as designed   HILL:46
trust h. may be overwhelmed   MORR:71

hours

doctor must work eighteen h. a day   FISC:35
have no working h.   KIPL:56

human

a semi-deliverance from the h. prison	AMIEL:2
front row of the stalls of the h. drama	BRAIN:15
The trouble with the h. body	FORD:36
psychoanalysis to h. progress	FROMM:37
H. life consists in mutual service	GILM:40
The h. race will be the cancer	HUXL:52
intimate knowledge of the h. body	JEFF:54
one brat into a decent h. being	KRUT:57
anthropoid apes and h. beings	LORE:62
The average h. has one breast	MCHA:63
my opinion of the h. race	MAUG:67
utterly beyond h. capability	MAXW:67
in the line of h. endeavour	MAYO:67
responsible actions in the range of h.	MILL:69
It is the h. touch after all	MORR:71
The essence of being h.	ORWE:74
light and help and h. kindness	SCHW:88
or of a h. in the hands of his doctor	SCRU:88
h. beings have come to the end	WERT:105

human body

The h. is the only machine	BIGGS:13
the secrets of the structure of the h.	FONT:36
The h. is a machine	OFFR:74
having the h. as a subject	PLATO:79

human condition

our fellow sufferers from the h.	BEAT:10

human form

The h. is a very delicate organization	CHEY:21

human investigation

No h. can be called true science	VINCI:102

human mind

far too recondite for the h. to unravel	BAGL:8
Our conception of h.	BRAIN:15

human nature

all our knowledge of h.	CHES:21

human race

the health of the whole h.	TOYN:100

human species

nature would lose the h.	VINCI:102

humane

the most h. of all professions	LISTE:61

humanity

point in the direction of pity and h.	JACO:53
the interests of h. ennoble	LAVO:59
Any lover of h. who looks back	LEAC:59
H. has but three great enemies	OSLER:75
the clinician is interest in h.	PEAB:77
joint exertion of skill and h.	VOLT:103

humbug

Gentlemen, this is no h.	WARR:104

humours

salt to remove salt h.	MILT:69

hungry

'tis Meat for the H.	CERV:20

Hunter

H. had never more than twenty	MACE:63

hurry

never appear to be in a h.	BILLR:13

hurt

A small h. in the eye is a great one	ENGL:33
He who complains is not h.	FRENC:37
so much misery and feel no h.	SELZ:89

hygiene

H. is the corruption of medicine · · · · · · · · · · · MENC:69

hygienist

from the point of view of the h. · · · · · · · · · · BILLI:13

hypertension

reeking with h. · · · · · · · · · · · · · · · · · CLEN:23

hypochondria

h. has always seemed to me to be · · · · · · · DIAM:29

hypochondriac

ennui the h. · · · · · · · · · · · · · · · · · · JEFF:54

hypochondriacs

H. squander large sums of time · · · · · · · COLLI:24
It is said to be the manner of h. · · · · · · · CULL:26
mathematics makes h. · · · · · · · · · · · · LUTH:62

hypotheses

of doctrines and h. · · · · · · · · · · · · · BEAUM:10
underpinning of h. · · · · · · · · · · · · · MEDA:68

hypothesis

scientific h. is merely a scientific idea · · · · BERN:11
no one believes an h. · · · · · · · · · · · · BEVE:12
to discard a pet h. every day before
breakfast · · · · · · · · · · · · · · · · · · LORE:62
The invention of an h. is a work · · · · · · PERC:78

hysteria

cannot be a symptom of h. · · · · · · · · · BRIS:15
Beware the diagnosis of h. · · · · · · · · · MORR:71
to enumerate all the symptoms of h. · · · · SYDE:98

hysteric

familiar symptoms with h. women · · · · · HEBE:44

hysterical

No laborious person was ever yet h. · · · · · JEFF:54

id

the care of the i. by the odd. · · · · · · · · · ANON:5

idea

If an i. presents itself · · · · · · · · · · · · BERN:11
the man to whom the i. first occurs · · · · DARW:28
give us a totally different i. · · · · · · · · · VALÉ:102

idealism

alcohol or morphine or i. · · · · · · · · · · JUNG:55

ideas

Whenever i. fail, men invent words · · · · · FISC:35
exclude the communication of i. · · · · · · INGLE:52
loses his teeth, hair and i. · · · · · · · · · VOLT:103

identity

with a perfect simplicity and i. · · · · · · · HUME:50

idiocy

The Mongolian type of i. occurs · · · · · · DOWN:30

idleness

I. begets ennui · · · · · · · · · · · · · · · · JEFF:54
I. is the parent of all psychology · · · · · · NIET:73

ignorance

in i., to refrain · · · · · · · · · · · · · · · BERN:11
Nothing is more terrible than to see i. · · · GOET:40
rather to remain in i. · · · · · · · · · · · · HOMA:49
to a plateau of i. · · · · · · · · · · · · · · PETE:78

ignorant

to doubt and to be i. · · · · · · · · · · · · UNAM:101

ill

let him get very i. first	AFRI:2
better be too smart to get i.	AFRI:2
The i. he cannot cure a name	ARNO:6
look after him when he is i.	BISM:14
i. as one of the greatest pleasures	BUTL:18
inferior doctor treats those who are i.	CH'IN:20
he usually discovers that he is i.	GOET:40
a man suffers from an i.	HIPP:47
One who is i. has not only the right	MAIM:64
pleasures in life is to be slightly i.	NICH:73
An i. man is worst	PROV:82
sage does not treat those who are i.	SU:97
They live i. who expect to live	SYRUS:98

ill-health

i. among labourers and their families	MCCR:63
real causes of i. were to be found	PLATT:80

illness

In the midst of your i.	AFRI:2
in every case of i.; well tried remedies	ASCL:6
fatal outcome of an incurable i.	BOER:14
In i. the physician is a father	BRAH:15
A long i. seems to be	BRUY:16
learn more about the i.	HERR:46
The map of mental i.	LE FA:34
The most important thing in i.	LENIN:59
irrespective of the nature of the i.	LONG:61
i. may become seriously aggravated	MEANS:68
stretch between i. and recovery	MOYN:72
Every i. has its natural course	PINEL:79
i. which it cannot counterfeit	PROU:82
I. is the doctor to whom we pay	PROU:82
part which makes the i. worth while	SHAW:90
I. . . . is not a good literary subject	SIGE:92
little i. is the beginning of the end.	SMITH:94
I. may precipitate a spiritual crisis	SOUT:94
have to find time for i.	STAN:95
to drive away the i.	SYLV:98
Old age is an i. in itself	TERE:99
I. isn't the only thing	VARRO:102
and there cause serious i.s	TURG:101
i. has not taken its place	WOOLF:107

illnesses

i. are already on the sperm	BARA:9
Of i. that no one's got	HERB:45
it is the principle cause of all i.	MAIM:64

not of their i.	MOLI:70
and give rise to grave i.	VARRO:102

ills

For major i., major remedies	CELS:20

illusions

the vicious circle of i.	ALLB:2

image

The i. of fulfilment	MUGG:72

imagination

Put off your i.	BERN:11
the products of a disordered i.	BROU:16
a new audacity of i.	DEWEY:29
more stimulating to the i.	HALD:42
work of no difficulty to a lively i.	PERC:78
never come to the end of our i.	WERT:105

imaginative

children are the most i.	MACAU:63

imbecility

to let them starve for their i.	HOLM:49

immoral

too i. for the pulpit.	GILM:40

immortal

do not strive for i. life	PIND:79

immortality

state of alarm about the i.	BOTS:15
desire for i. which causes the fear	WEIN:105

immunologist

designed by God as tools for the i. COOM:25

impossible

distinguish the possible from the i. HEROP:45

impotent

He also is i. DUNL:31

impressions

I. arriving at the brain make it CABA:18

inattention

so insignificant as to merit i. SYDE:98

incision

I made an i. about three inches MCDO:63

incomes

they have large i. GRAH:41

incurable

a man with his i. patient ARET:6
There are no such things as i. BARU:9
Life is an i. Disease COWL:26
it fails only in i. cases GALEN:38
master i. diseases SENE:89
to behave in cases of i. disease STIE:97
he has also declared him i. SUSR:97

India

the surgeons of I. MOTH:71

indigestion

Don't tell your friends about your i. s GUIT:41
I. is charged by God HUGO:50
He sows hurry and reaps i. STEV:96

indignity

The ultimate i. KUHN:57

individual

its chief responsibility is to the i. HOOT:49
Treatment is concerned with the i. LATH:58
on every i. in particular MOND:70
responsibility to their i. patient WALL:104

individuality

interact with the i. of the patient SCHW:88

individuals

Insanity in i. is something rare NIET:73
work in teams, but are blamed as i. POLL:81

indolence

We grow old more through i. CHRI:22

industrial relations

displaying a standard and style of i. HENDY:45

inequalities

aggravate i. in access to health care STARR:96

infancy

Marriage–a stage between i. and adultery ANON:4

infants

I. do not cry FERR:34

infection

that of any other known i. ANDR:3
i. without disease is the rule DUBOS:31

infections

Microbial i. are conveniently divided WRIG:108

infectious

I. Distempers   ARBU:6
I. diseases traverse the usual   MAND:65
just what relation i. agents bear   WELCH:105

inflammation

If nature induces fever and i.   STAHL:95

influenza

I. is something unique   ANDR:3

information

i. is a corollary of the patient's right   DODDS:30

infrastructure

if the i. is absent   POWIS:81

ingrafting

harmless by the invention of i.   MONTA:70

inhumanity

barbarous, illegal piece of i.   OULD:75

injury

part of the phenomena caused by i.   MALC:65

inoculation

a little i. of some microbe   LISTE:61

insane

pronounced i. by all smart doctors   FISC:35
An i. man is a sick man   FISC:35

insanity

must be credited to temporary i.   HUFE:50
a kind of temporary i.   MART:66
I. in individuals   NIET:73
Drunkenness is simply voluntary i.   SENE:89

insomnia

every man's i. is as different   FITZG:35
I. never comes to a man   HUBB:50

inspiration

Genius is one per cent i.   EDIS:32

instinct

Brutes by their natural i.   BACON:8

institutional

the i. autonomy of hospitals   STARR:96

institutionalized

deference and i. forms of dependence   STARR:96

instrument

increasing worship of the i.   SEEG:89

instrumentation

a new technique or i.   WATE:104

instruments

the i. and the surgeon's fingers   BLAND:14
make use of i. of precision   CATH:19
these new i. were absolutely free   THOMP:100

integrity

moral and intellectual i.   ANON:4
I. and rectitude in our profession   SCAR:87

intellect

take care not to make i. our god   EINS:32
there is too much pride of i.   ELIOT:32
not a thing of the i.   PLATT:80
where i. and dexterity meet   SCHAU:87

intellects

the senses and i. being uninjured PARKI:76

intellectual

It is i. and communication skills LILF:60
i. pre-eminence with nobility OSLER:74

intelligence

an ounce of i. ARAB:6

intercourse

should be restrained from i. FRANK:36
Every animal is sad after i. LATIN:58

interest

ceases to be a subject of i. HAZL:43

interne

The i. suffers HALS:42

internist

nobody can become a good i. LANF:57
the i. self sufficient MAYO:68

intestines

after the food is digested in his i. MAIM:64

intimacy

the i. of the consulting room SPEN:95

invalids

I. live longest GERM:39
one soon makes friends with i. IBSEN:52
healthy people than with i. JAEG:53

invasiveness

degree of i., the use of anaesthetic FOX:36

inventiveness

stimulate our i. POTT:81

investigating

I. such a lot
Of illnesses HERB:45

investigation

i. of the dead for the living EVANS:34
strictest attention to the methods of i. WUND:108

investigations

The . . . goal of i. is recognition of truth BILLR:13

investigator

The greatness of a scientific i. BAYL:9
not of the i., but of knowledge GORD:40
the i. should be free, independent NEWM:73

Italians

I. used to find their mate at a distance SMITH:93

itch

use sulphur for the i. ANON:4
difficult to stand an i. CHANG:20

itches

To scratch when it i. ANON:5

itching

A violent i. of the skin HEBE:44

jargon

Murder with j. GARTH:38

jaundice

eruption is familiar to the j.	HEBE:44
J. is the disease	OSLER:74

jejunum

The j. is more exempt	GULL:41

job

There is no better j. in the world	LORI:62

joints

Rheumatic fever licks at the j.	ANON:4

judge

his own j. jury and executioner	MARQ:65

judgment

experience treacherous, j. difficult	HIPP:46
Good j. comes from experience;	LILL:60
I desire j. and criticism	PAST:77
none of his j.	ROCH:84

kidney

prefer passing a small k. stone	ANON:4
the excretory offices of the k.	PETE:78

kidneys

the k. may go to the pathologist	ADDIS:1
the k. too are affected	GALEN:38
The k. are like the officials	HUANG:50

kids

K. They're not easy	MAHER:64

kill

Thou shall not kill	CLOU:23
many who dare not k. themselves	CONN:25

Young men k. their patients	GREGO:41
a single word of it may k. a man	HOLM:48
not even a doctor can k. you.	PERL:78

killed

Until a physician has k. one or two	INDI:52
it k. more than it cured	LAMB:57
If I am k., I can die but once	LINC:60

killing

is the same as k. him	HORA:49
as he does the k. he ought to know	ZAVA:108

kills

it k. at last	IRISH:52
but if he k., the earth hides it	MONTA:70
Gout, unlike any other disease, k.	SYDE:98

kind

we can always be k.	FRIPP:37

kindest

the k. man we have ever known	ELIOT:32

kindness

True k. presupposes the faculty	GIDE:39
light and help and human k.	SCHW:88
A word of k. is better	RUSSI:86
for his k. they still remain in his debt	SENE:89

king

the one-eyed man is k.	PROV:82

kinship

By many a bodily likeness k. show	EURI:34

knife

that the k. cures not	HIPP:47
I will not use the k.	HIPP:47
What does not come under the k.	MÜLL:72
nothing will help but the k.	PARÉ:76

know

When I was boy I wanted to k.	HUNTE:51
not necessarily k. them	SMITH:93

knowing

missed by not looking than by not k.	MCCRA:63

knowledge

real and useful k.	BEAUM:10
He has nerve and . . . k.	CONAN:25
not of the investigator, but of k.	GORD:40
Science is the father of k.	HIPP:47
the k. acquired by the ancients	HIPP:47
Specialised k. will do a man no harm	HOLM:49
Without this k. a man cannot	HUNTE:51
handing the cup of k. to the young	HUTC:51
the k. that proves it foolish and vain	IRISH:53
substitutes presumption for k.	JEFF:54
As no one can have perfect k.	MAUD:66
perfect k. of all parts of medicine	MAUD:66
K. makes the physician	PARA:76
It is not his possession of k.	POPP:81
Science is organised k.	SPEN:95
k. comes from noticing resemblances	TROT:101

laboratories

If you suppress l., physical science	PAST:77

laboratory

no short cut from chemical l. to clinic	ANON:5
spurious, precision of l. results	ANON:5
when you enter the l.	BERN:11
l. is the temple of science	BERN:11
All the world is a l.	FISC:35
l. of him who adds to our knowledge	GREEN:41
identified with scientific (l.) medicine	VIRC:103

labour

The l. we delight in physics pain	SHAK:90

ladies

complaints of indestructible old l.	WHITE:106

laity

conspiracies against the l.	SHAW:90

lame

If you dwell with a l. man	LATIN:58

lancet

more Englishmen die by the l.	ARMS:6

language

in the l. of the non-medical man	GOOD:40
international l. of medicine	POPP:81
The l. of the men of medicine	SAUN:87

laparoscopic

l. revolution remains the largest	HEALD:44
L. surgery	PETE:78

large bowel

have ignored the l.	PHILL:79

laryngologists

a gargle of l.	ANON:3

Latin

L. is the language	MEDI:68

laugh

A good l. and a long sleep	IRISH:52

law

considers itself above the l.	ADAMS:1
In science, l. is not a rule imposed	ALLB:2
a right recognised by l.	DODDS:30
absolutely clear that the l.	GILLO:39
Unlike the l. and the clergy	STARR:96

lawyer

my doctor or my l. cannot matter	MONTA:70
With a young l. you lose	SWED:98

lawyers

With the exception of l.	ADAMS:1
who are the skilled l. and doctors	BILLI:13
Doctors are just the same as l.	CHEK:21
l., like bread, when they are young	FULL:37
The l. are the cleverest men	HOLM:48
L. and physicians are a bad provision	MONTA:70

lay

arises from l. deference	STARR:96
irritated by l. knowledge	STEI:96

layman

cannot be appraised by a l.	HAMI:42

lean

Men of l. habit of body	VENN:102

learn

We shall have to l. to refrain	FOX:36
if they shall wish to l. it, without fee	HIPP:47
there is always more to l.	MAYO:68

learned

first, he should be l.	CHAU:21
the most l. men I know	POPE:81

learning

pursuit of l. has been	ANON:5
L. without thinking is useless	CONF:25
That l., thine ambassador	DONNE:30

leeches

L. should be kept a day	AVIC:7

leg

Any fool can cut off a l.	ROSS:85

legal

In strict l. terminology I doubt	DEVL:29

legislate

You cannot l. a new layer	BILLI:13

legislation

only opposition to effective medical l.	MILLA:69

legs

the l. have muscles for walking	OFFR:74
a sturdy pair of l.	WANG:104

lengthening

thinks too much about l. it	SENE:89

leper

The l. in whom the plague is	BIBLE:12

lepers

with l. alone	ANON:5

lie

A long disease does not tell a l.	IRISH:52
it makes them l.	WILKI:107

lies

Here l. one who for medicines would	ANON:4
l., damned l. and statistics	DISR:30

life

and so his l. he lost	ANON:4
from things lifeless to animal l.	ARIS:6
said to be the time of a man's l.	BARA:9
L. is the sum of the functions	BICH:12
I divided my l. into three parts	BLAND:14
the decencies, whether of l. or of death	BORR:14
displayed during l.	BRIG:15
birth, l. and death	BRUY:16
placed between l. and death	BRUY:16
There's nothing certain in man's l.	BULW:17
There are two things in l.	BULW:17
L. is one long process of getting tired	BUTL:18
novice at each age of his l.	CHAM:20
to prolong l. worry less	CHU:22
to re-establish a purpose in l.	CONN:25
L. is an incurable Disease	COWL:26
mechanism by which l. comes from l.	CRICK:26
L. was a funny thing	CRISP:26
spends his l. as an operating surgeon	DA CO:23
L. was originally	DARW:28
likely to die on the first day of your l.	DAVIS:28
the only rational position to take on l.	DIAM:29
To reject them is to reject l. itself	ELLIS:33
show respect for human l.	GENE:38
l. could have never taught me	GOET:40
ere l. hath lost its brightness	HAST:43
to set a just value on l.	HAZL:43
The love of l., or fear of death	HEBE:44
Where L. and Death . . . meet	HENL:45
L. is made up of sobs	HENRY:45
Walking makes for a long l.	HINDU:46
L. is short, the art long	HIPP:46
To save a man's l.	HORA:49
duty of a doctor to prolong l.	HORD:49
The art of l.	JEFF:54
the real experiences of l.	KEY:56
the l. of man	LATH:58
limit living to prolong l.	LONG:61
merely to extend l. in old age	LONG:61
another expression of interest in l.	MANN:65
L. is not living, but living in health	MART:65
The transition between l. and death	MATAS:66
There were just facts. It was l.	MAUG:67
to prolong l. for the sole purpose	MEANS:68
actions in the range of human l.	MILL:69
born with a deadly disease which is l.	MOREA:71
L. is a great surprise	NABO:72
One of the minor pleasures in l.	NICH:73
we may deprive a man of l.	NIET:73
Breathing is the greatest pleasure in l.	PAPI:75
it deals with the very processes of l.	PARA:76
He dies from his whole l.	PÉGUY:78
wine is l.	PETRO:78
assumption that human l. is sacred	PHILL:79
do not strive for immortal l.	PIND:79
greatest hindrance to l.	PLATO:79
divide l. from death	POE:80
Without health, l. spells but languor	RABE:83
L. is not a spectacle or feast	SANTA:87
The purpose of human l.	SCHW:88
single out a dull day in their way of l.	SEEG:88
for him the last bubbles of his l.	SELZ:89
No man can have a peaceful l.	SENE:89
L. levels all men	SHAW:91
digestion is the great secret of l.	SMITH:94
the ultimate concerns of l.	SOUT:94
Success in l. depends on the three I's	STOC:97
And because I love this l.	TAGO:99
long passed the peak of l.	TEGN:99
aim not at the destruction of l.	TREV:100
l. well used brings happy death	VINCI:102
L. well spent is long	VINCI:102
the utmost respect for human l.	WORLD:108

lifestyle

demand a more balanced l.	SANF:87

light

to transmit the rays of l.	NEED:73

limbs

the cruel cold cuts off the l.	SILI:93

limp

you will learn to l.	LATIN:58

liquor

I like I – its taste and its effects	JACK:53

Lister

L. saw the vast importance	ALLB:2
more worthy of remembrance than L.	MOYN:72

literary

Illness . . . is not a good l. subject	SIGE:92

literature

medical l. is stuffed to bursting	BEAN:9
in l., the many. In science, the few	BULW:17
l. my mistress	CHEK:21
The physician ought to know l.	ISID:53
formal scientific l. is hardly ever read	MADD:64

live

you will l. to ninety-nine	ANON:3
you don't actually l. longer	ANON:4
I had only six minutes to l.	ASIM:7
Man shall not l. by bread alone	BIBLE:12
hath but a short time to l.	BOOK:14
a place, not to l., but to die in	BROW:16
they help you l. longer	CAND:19
to think he cannot l. one more year	CICE:22
One should eat to l.	CICE:22
rather l, but I am not afraid to die	DISR:30
Die well that l. well	ENGL:33
Invalids l. longest	GERM:39
your temporal affairs – you may l.	GOUR:41
to have someone to l. for	IBSEN:52
l. in an unlivable situation	LAIN:57
to l. in constant dread of it	LINC:60
no longer possible to l. proudly	NIET:73
All would l. long	PROV:82
desire to l. increases as life itself shortens	RAMON:83
to l. rather than avoid death	ROUSS:85
Do not try to l. forever	SHAW:91
They l. ill who expect to live always	SYRUS:98
Science says: 'We must l.'	UNAM:101

lived

| people l. to be over a hundred years | HUANG:50 |

liver

| A man's l. is his carburettor | ANON:3 |
| a cirrhosed l. | BILLI:13 |

lives

fool l. as long as his destiny allows	ANON:3
Surgeons get long l.	ANON:4
half of our l. is ruined by our parents	DARR:28
Who l. medically l. miserably	LATIN:58
more l. to answer for	NAPO:72
He l. long that l. till all are weary	PROV:82
l. are different from those of healthy people	SIGE:92

living

difficult chapters in the great art of l.	AMIEL:2
the more l. it becomes	BUTL:18
L. is a sickness	CHAM:20
in her care for l. beings	ERAS:33
investigation of the dead for the l.	EVANS:34
whole of the l. world around us	GALT:38
care for science so far as they get a l.	GOET:40
far more important than l.	JÜNG:55
Plain l. and high thinking	LUBB:62
with some chance of making a l.	MAUG:66
it is indecent to go on l.	NIET:73
the l. image of perpetual movement	OFFR:74
L. well and beautifully	SOCR:94
A l. thing is distinguished	SPEN:95
the ultimate units of the l. cell	WEAV:105

lobotomy

| a full frontal l. | NICH:73 |

loin

| An artificial anus in the l. | CURL:26 |

loneliness

| The arctic l. of age | MITC:70 |

longevity

There is no short-cut to l.	CRICH:26
a most unfortunate tendency to l.	DA CO:23
In spite of increasing l.	JASP:53

louse

| the l. will defeat socialism | LENIN:59 |

love

L. and pregnancy and riding	ARAB:5
You may give them your l.	GIBR:39
L. is an acute psychosis	PICK:79
the best l. that of children	PROV:82
Work and l. – these are the basics	REIK:83
L. as a relation between men	RUSSE:86
painful, healing and full of l.	SELZ:89
no l. sincerer than the l. of food	SHAW:91

loved

When you have l. as she   MAUG:66

lover

To lose a l. or even a husband   WHEE:106

lucrative

That salutary and l. profession   GIBB:39

lunatics

All are l.   BIERC:13

lungs

in the discharge from the l. alone   ARET:6
dangerous to the l.   JAMES:53
through the medium of the l.   LATH:58

machine

Learn that your are a m.   STILL:97

mad

We all are born m.   BECK:10
There is pleasure, sure,
In being m.   DRYD:31
fate wishes to ruin she first makes m.   LATIN:58
they first drive m.   PROV:82
to destroy she first makes m.   SYRUS:98
Men will always be m.   VOLT:103
I am going m. again   WOOLF:107

madman

A m. has no free will   LEGAL:59
m. thinks the rest of the world crazy   SYRUS:98

madmen

which none but m. know   DRYD:31
world is so full of simpletons and m.   GOET:40

madness

sorts of m. are innumerable   AVIC:7
a dash of m.   EMER:33
Anger is short-lived m.   HORA:49
The greatest proof of m.   NAPO:72
Though this be m.   SHAK:90
Science is m. if good sense does not   SPAN:95
suicide always comes from m.   VOLT:103

magic

indistinguishable from m.   COMF:24
an almost medieval belief in m.   DIAM:29

mail

by m. patients he has never seen   ADAMS:1

maladies

thoughts bring on physical m.   LUTH:62
there are m.   ROCH:84

malady

All pain is one m. with many names   ANTI:5
not to aggravate the sick person's m.   BOER:14
distinction between one m.   BROU:16
to remedy a severe m.   CELS:20
m. is more easily cured   JOHNS:55
regime is in itself a tedious m.   ROCH:84
the close resemblance of the m.   SEMM:89

malariologists

the eradication of m.   DUBOS:31

malignancy

issuing from a m. of the abdomen   SCHIL:88

malnutrition

form of m. in the western world   DEIT:28

man

management

managers

manhood

mankind

manly

manslaughter

marriage

This we call m.	DARL:27
M.s are not normally made	VIRC:103
teeth and m. spoil a woman's beauty	AFRI:2

marry

No man should m.	BALZ:8

masturbation

M.: the primary sexual activity	SZASZ:98

maternity

M. is a matter of fact	WELLS:105

mathematical

without passing through m. tests	VINCI:102

matter

Mind over m.	ANON:4

maturity

deliberately defer m.	GREGG:41
to the experience of m.	POLA:81

meaning

some m. in the ritual of surgery	SELZ:89

measles

The physical signs of m.	AVIC:7
Love is like the m.	JERO:54

meat

man's m. is another man's	LUCR:62

mechanical

seeming exactness of a m. device	MACK:64

mechanism

m. by which life comes from life	CRICK:26

medical care

the cost of m.	KENN:56
one billion-dollars spent on m.	WILDA:106

medical career

a necessary hurdle in a m.	ASHER:7

medical centre

made of it the m. of Europe	MACP:64

medical education

The future of American m.	GARR:38
two objects of m.	MAYO:67

medical establishment

The m. has become a major threat	ILLI:52

medical ethics

M. are a bargain that has to be struck	PHILL:79

medical expertise

m. to sluggish ignorance	HILL:46

medical history

cancer extend to the dawn of m.	SHIM:91

medical instruction

M. does not exist	VIRC:103

medical insurance

only genuine m. for this country	BOK:14

medical knowledge

the attainment of m.	ABER:1
The road to m.	GULL:41
to add to the store of m.	MCGE:63

medical man

seldom a m. has true religious views   ELIOT:32

medical management

The principles of m. are   ATCH:7

medical men

M. do not know the drugs they use   BACON:8

medical people

m. will have more lives to answer for   NAPO:72

medical practice

at any point in m.   HILL:46
requisites for proficient m.   MAIM:64
The human lessons which m. teaches   PLATT:80
The essential unit of m.   SPEN:95

medical practitioners

in disease is indispensable to m.   WUND:108

medical profession

heals, under the auspices of the m.   EMER:33
Meanwhile the m.   GILLO:39
cause the m. of today to fear   HERR:46
character of the regular m.   MORR:71
the excrescences of the m.   SAUN:87
members of the m. might agree   SEEG:88
a well-organised and united m.   STAC:95
The m. has had (a) persuasive claim   STARR:96
rationality and power as has the m.   STARR:96
The m. is unconsciously irritated   STEI:96
The m. is a noble and pleasant one   SYMI:98

medical progress

The true test of national m. is   MITC:70

medical revolution

A m. has extended the life   KENN:56

medical school

absolutely essential to a m.   WARR:104
education is not completed at the M.   WELCH:105

medical science

between m. and the physician's art   BILLR:13
dawn of m. to the present moment   COOP:25
M. must cease to regard its function   HOOT:49
the achievements of m.   LEAC:59
M. aims at the truth   MAYO:68
Progress in m. depends   SEEG:89
M. is as yet very imperfectly   SHAW:90

medical scientists

M. are nice people   BIER:13

medical student

await the coming of the m.   BIERC:13
m. is likely to be one son   GILM:40
criterion should prevail for the m.   SEEG:88

medical subjects

a difference of opinion upon m.   RUSH:86

medical universe

The patient is the centre of the m.   MURP:72

medical work

I look over twenty five years of m.   CABOT:18

medicalization

The m. of early diagnosis   ILLI:52

medically

Who lives m. lives miserably   LATIN:58

médicine

L'amour de la m. fait le savant   FRENC:37

medicine

M. would be the ideal profession ADAMS:1
he may see the benefit of your m. AFRI:2
faithful friend is the m. of life ANON:3
the qualities of a good teacher of m. ANON:4
M., like every useful science, should ANON:4
every m. is an innovation BACON:8
fulcra of m. are reason BAGL:8
In the practice of m. more mistakes BELL:10
M. is destined to get away BERN:11
discoveries in biology and m. BEVE:12
M. is like a woman who changes BIER:13
m. is the art of understanding diseases BIGE:13
M. is the only profession BRYCE:17
m., on account of its eminent utility BUCKL:17
m. has almost no constant rule CELS:20
Philosophy, like m., has plenty CHAM:20
m. is like the celebrated tower of Pisa CHARL:21
M. is my lawful wife CHEK:21
He that takes m. and neglects to diet CHIN:21
M. cures the man CHIN:21
Fasting is a m. CHRY:22
Grief is itself a m. COWP:26
practice of m. depends on CUSH:27
M. cannot be practised DAAR:27
M. discusses diseases DE GO:40
changing in the state of m. DICKS:29
As long as m. is an art DIETL:29
one experiment in m. to convince DOCH:30
In m. even more than in other fields DUBOS:31
Patience is the best m. FLOR:36
The history of m. GARR:38
where his m. fails GARTH:38
M. absorbs the physician's whole GOET:40
one m. can cure various kinds GOGA:40
a distinct art to talk m. GOOD:40
M. is my hobby GRACE:41
M. is as old as the human race HAES:42
The art of m. is intricate HAMI:42
the art of m. still falls HECHT:44
M. with them is distributed HEROD:45
I like to think of m. in our day HERT:46
m. has skidded off the path HILL:46
the means at the disposal of m. HIPP:47
m., professedly found HOLM:48
No families take so little m. HOLM:48
but m. goes on forever HORD:49
dangerous – in m. to be too clever HUTC:51
indirectly with the pursuits of m. IBÁÑ:52
Domestic m. is preferable INDI:52
Hospitality and m. must be confined INDI:52
Bed is a m. ITAL:53
Better go without m. JAPA:53
Good m. always has a bitter taste JAPA:53
The only sure foundations of m. are JEFF:54
m. to be as inoffensive JEFF:54
appeared in the annals of m. JENN:54

M. has been caught up KEEN:56
the practice of m. LATH:58
Common sense is in m. the master LATH:58
M. is a strange mixture LATH:58
constitutes the fall of modern m. LE FA:34
M. is not a lucrative profession LETT:60
as m. loses its professional hegemony LILF:60
any distinction between food and m. LIN:60
healed and changed by m. LUCR:62
M. makes sick patients LUTH:62
Boys, don't study m. MCMU:64
M. is a science in the making MAGE:64
M. heals doubts as well as diseases MARX:66
m. has united the aims and aspirations MARX:66
perfect knowledge of all parts of m. MAUD:66
The aim of m. is to prevent disease MAYO:68
While m. is a science MAYO:67
m. deals with the tomorrows MAYO:68
The glory of m. MAYO:68
M. is a profession for social service MAYO:67
M. is not a perfect science MILB:69
The true rate of advance in m. is MITC:70
m. is practised not on mankind MOND:70
M. indeed never cures a disease MOND:70
well prepared for the study of M. MONT:71
M. is a collection NAPO:72
M. is the only world wide profession OSLER:74
A desire to take m. OSLER:74
educate the masses not to take m. OSLER:74
M. sometimes snatches away health OVID:75
M. is not only a science PARA:76
m. to follow the will of nature PARA:76
This basis of m. is sympathy PAYNE:77
M. is not yet liberated PICKE:79
M. is an art PLATO:79
M., to produce health PLUT:80
international language of m. POPP:81
the more m. it craves PORT:81
M. for the dead is too late QUIN:83
such is the basis of future m. RANV:83
out of m. the fullest enjoyment RIES:84
The axiom of m. ROKI:85
M. is a noble profession ROLL:85
false declamations made against m. ROUSS:85
bad for the soul of m. RYLE:86
give to their patients the least m. SAUN:87
The language of the men of m. SAUN:87
practice of m. is like heart muscle SCHIC:88
those pillars from which m. started SCHÖ:88
frequent changes of m. SENE:89
It is m. not scenery SENE:89
miserable have no other m. SHAK:90
the most noble branch of m. SIEF:92
the world's first and foremost m. SLOV:93
Sleep is the only m. SOPH:94
Modern m. is one of those STARR:96
But m. is also, . . . , a world of power STARR:96
M. can never abdicate STRA:97

The art of m.	SYDE:98
Nothing in m. is so insignificant	SYDE:98
died of the m. rather than the disease	SYDE:98
The status and progress of m.	THORO:100
element in disease is the key of m.	TROU:101
M. consists of a science	TROU:101
Should m. ever fulfill its great ends	VIRC:103
to learn the powers of m.	VIRG:103
m. must have something to hand on	WALS:104
mystery about the practice of m.	WARN:104
M. is not a field in which sheep	WHITE:106
m. recognises its tasks and its duties	WUND:108

medicines

The Lord hath created m.	BIBLE:12
therapies are replacing a lot of m.	BUSH:18
when m. cannot save	COTT:26
The poisons are our principal m.	EMER:33
worthlessness of the most m.	FRAN:36
M. are not meat to live by	GERM:39
much on the efficacy of m.	GOLDS:40
Poisons and m.	LATH:58
to avoid sicknes, than to wishe for m.	MORE:71
wine is the most profitable of m	PLUT:80
Wine is the foremost of all m.	TALM:99
m. in too large doses are poisonous	WITH:107

meditation

M. is not a means to an end	KRIS:57

melancholic

things of a m. hue	MILT:69

melancholy

it is to be found in a m. man's heart	BURT:17

memories

Surgeons get long lives and short m.	ANON:4
the burden of one's m.	MAUG:67

memory

Everyone complains of his m.	ROCH:84

men

great m. are recognised	BERN:11
the m. of Sodom were wicked	BIBLE:12
glory of young m. is their strength	BIBLE:12
What m. call gallantry	BYRON:18
Nine out of every ten m. have piles	CHIN:21
M. have expended infinite ingenuity	ELLIS:33
M. resemble their contemporaries	EMER:33
Short m. eat more than tall ones	FRENC:37
Whenever ideas fail' m. invent words	FISC:35
Old m.'s heads are just as bare	HOFFE:48
m. of eminence lie like the devil	HUNTE:51
M. have broad and large chests	LUTH:62
M. seldom make passes	PARKE:76
coveted by all m.	PROV:82
Life levels all m.	SHAW:91
to ourselves young m. and women	STEIN:96
For m. to take their exits	WEBS:105

menstrual

the history of a missed m. period	MORR:71

mental

When a man lacks m. balance	FISC:35
our approach to m. affliction	KENN:56
The map of m. illness	LE FA:34
the blunting of my m. edge	MILT:69
in a perpetual m. restlessness	TEMP:99

mesmerism

gentlemen, beats M. hollow	LISTO:61

metaphysical

Health . . . is a m. concept	SKRA:93

method

to take a m. and try it	ROOS:85

microbe

The M. is so very small	BELLO:10
a m. is composed of only one	CHRI:22
a little inoculation of some m.	LISTE:61

microbes

and acquired a fear of m.	ANON:4
There are more m. per person	BENN:10

microbial

M. infections are conveniently divided	WRIG:108

microorganisms

m. have always been ready to take	CHRI:22

middle age

M. has been said to be the time	BARA:9
M. is youth without its levity	DEFOE:28
Senescence begins	
And m. ends	NASH:72

middle years

In a man's m.	WHITE:106

middle-aged

When a m. man says in a moment	DAVIS:28

midwife

then must the m. do all her diligence	ROSL:85

midwifery

the vast bulk of m.	CLAYT:23
Meddlesome m. is bad	PROV:82

midwives

When there are two m.	PERS:78

military

m. doctor is an unwillingly tolerated	ZINS:108

millionaire

a m. with a positive Wassermann	ANON:4

mind

the obstetrician of the m.	ANON:5
M. over matter	ANON:4
the m. at about forty-nine	ARIS:6
the good ordering of the m.	AURE:7
The more a thing knows its own m.	BUTL:18
It is the m. which is really alive	CHARC:20
first treat the m.	CHEN:21
body may be healed but not the m.	CHIN:21
In a disordered m.	CICE:23
to prolong the youth of the m.	COLLI:24
Body and m., like man and wife	COLT:24
The m. can be a piercing search-light	DUBOS:31
experience of mortal m.	EDDY:32
not a condition of matter, but of M.	EDDY:32
Bodies devoid of m. are as statues	EURI:34
laboratory to the inquiring m.	FISC:35
The conscious m. may be compared	FREUD:37
Sickly body, sickly m.	GERM:39
What we call a m. is nothing	HUME:50
the m. will not be strong	JEFF:54
uninformed m. with a healthy body	JEFF:54
most abhorrent is body without m.	JEFF:54
The natural course of the human m.	JEFF:54
with an unquiet m.	JOHNS:55
if his m. grows turgid in old age	JOHNS:55
sound m. in a sound body	JUVE:55
a wandering m.	LUCR:62
m. is begotten along with the body	LUCR:62
The m. like a sick body	LUCR:62
Master Surgeon must be a man of m.	MATAS:66
m. has great influence over the body	MOLI:70
Our m. grows constipated	MONTA:70
functions of the m. are dependent	MOTT:72
I am no better in m. than in body	OVID:75
chance only favours the prepared m.	PAST:77
the powers of the human m.	PAVL:77
no method of controlling the m.	PENF:78
dismounts the m., and unmans men	PENN:78
just to put your m. at rest	PETRO:78
M. is ever the ruler of the universe	PLATO:79
to be found largely in the m.	PLATT:80
In sickness the m. reflects upon itself	PLINY:80
preserve the m. in all its vigour	PLINY:80
develops the powers of the m.	PROU:82
transforming power the m. can exert	PUTN:83
m. as an organ of conscious thought	PUTN:83
which enters the m. through reason	RAMON:83
to have a very confused state of m.	RHAZ:84
and the traditional civilized m.	ROBI:84
unless your m. is in a splint	SCUL:88
Eye is the window of the m.	SHAK:90
body is a product of the sound m.	SHAW:91
If it is for m. that we are searching	SHERR:91
The care of the human m.	SIEF:92
Pain of m. is worse than pain of body	SYRUS:98

minds

attention is paid to our children's m.   ANON:4
People whose m. are not disciplined   BEVE:12
Little m. are interested   HUBB:50
Sick m. must be healed as well   MILLE:69
Old age puts more wrinkles in our m.   MONTA:70
people will not weed their own m.   WALP:104

ministers

the m. are the most learned   HOLM:48

miracle

A m. drug is any drug that will do   HODG:48

miracles

the tiny m. wrought day in day out   CHARL:21

mirror

an image in a m.   MARX:66

mirth

other evils of life, by m.   STER:96

miserable

never because you are m.   CHES:21
secret of being m. is to have leisure   SHAW:91

miserably

Who lives medically lives m.   LATIN:58

misery

in some degree the sum of human m.   LISTE:61
But pain is perfect m.   MILT:69
so much m. and feel no hurt   SELZ:89

missed

m. by not looking than by not knowing   MCCRA:63

mistake

fact of his having never made a m.   BAYL:9

mistakes

more m. are made   BELL:10
one who makes fewest m.   COOP:25
a dreadful list of ghastly m.   DA CO:23
More m. are made from want   HOWA:49
no m. or neglect occurs   HUANG:50
best doctors can make the worst m.   MILB:69
The m. made by doctors   PROU:82
The physician can bury his m.   WRIG:108

moderation

Abstinence . . . should always be practised
in m.   ANON:3

modern medicine

the most agonising dilemmas in m.   PHILL:79

molecular biology

m. – which is beginning to uncover   WEAV:105

money

with the soul of a m. changer   BROW:16
costs a lot of m. to die comfortably   BUTL:18
a mere art for the acquisition of m.   GISB:40
Get your m. when the patient is in pain   PROV:82
their competition for business and m.   RUSH:86
If he didn't need the m.   SHRI:92

moneymaker

is not a mere m.   PLATO:79

Mongolian

The M. type of idiocy occurs   DOWN:30

moral

m. luminaries are those who forego	RUSSE:86
individual's degraded m. character	SELV:89

morality

Health is the first requisite after m.	JEFF:54
the corruption of medicine by m.	MENC:69
there is such a thing as physical m.	SPEN:95

morgue

one that passes too close to the m.	ANON:5

morning

in the m. feeling just plain terrible	KERR:56

mortal

shuffled off this m. coil	SHAK:90

mortality

Reduce the m. rate	CATH:20
there is so high a m. in childbed	SEMM:89

mosquitoes

of malariologists than of m.	DUBOS:31
stomachs of a thousand m.	ROSS:85

mother

A smart m. makes	BIER:13
However strong a m. may be	CHIN:21
to squeal on your m.	CONN:25
The m. – child relationship	FROMM:37
therefore he made m.s	JEWI:54
destroy the m. to save the child	OULD:75
m.'s milk is more convenient	ROSL:85
from his m.'s womb	
Untimely ripp'd	SHAK:90
his m's age	SPOCK:95
near my m.	WHIS:106
the doctor slapped my m.	YOUN:108

mouth

Diseases enter by the m.	JAPA:53
into our bodies through m.	VARRO:102

multidisciplinary

harmonious islands of m. practice	LILF:60

murder

Suicide is the worst form of m.	COLLI:24
guilty of m. by omitting to fulfil	HAVE:43

murders

The m. fed Shipman's fascinating	SMITH:93

muscle

by m., speed, or physical dexterity	CICE:22
Voluntary, or skeletal, m. is by far	MAYER:67
The function of m. is to pull	VINCI:102

music

surgery is like m.	GRAH:41
Keep up you patient's spirits by m.	MOND:70

mystery

As long as our brain is a m.	RAMÓN:83
m. about the practice of medicine	WARN:104

mystic

The m. sees the ineffable	MAUG:67

Nagasaki

even in the ruins of N.	BRON:15

name

Though we n. the things we know	SMITH:93

names

new-fangled n. to diseases	PLATO:79

narcotic

The amount of n. you use — FISC:35
n.s, alcohol and Christianity — NIET:73

National Health Service

The N. is rotting before our eyes — ANON:5
signalize the inauguration of the N. — CHUR:22
in the intricate network of the N. — GRUG:41
N. seemed to spend inordinate time — HENDY:45
only a belief in the N. — LAWS:59

natural

allocate causes of disease to n. laws — ARIS:6
the term of N. Selection — DARW:28
let me die a n. death — GARTH:38
diseases are but parts of a course or
n. history — GULL:41
studied genetics and n. selection — HALD:42
The n. healing force within us — HIPP:47

nature

N. does nothing without a purpose — ARIS:6
N. proceeds little by little from things — ARIST:6
persons commonly take revenge on n. — BACON:8
if he follows not in n.'s footsteps — BAGL:8
n. can do a great deal better than you — BELLE:10
the powers of n. — CELL:20
The observer listens to N. — CUVI:27
N. heals' under the auspices of — EMER:33
N. is the great artist — ERAS:33
the disease is cured by n. — FORB:36
Nothing in n. stands alone — HUNTE:51
N. does not kill and does not heal — JACO:53
originally placed by n. — JENN:54
presented to us by N. — LAVO:59
In n. those who cry out with pain — MARX:66
sweetest gratifications of n. — MONTA:70
N. will tell you what to do — MONTA:70
to redress the defects of n. — PARÉ:76
N., time and patience — PROV:82
what method N. might take — SYDE:98
N. has given man one tongue — ZENO:108

nature-made

one n., one doctor-made — NAPOL:72

nectar

Even n. is poison if taken to excess — HINDU:46

need

what is seen to be the n. — ANON:5

needle

work without his hypodermic n. — FISC:35

needs

The n. of children — KENN:56

neglect

curiosity and experiment, or by n. — BLAC:14

neglectful

Poor medical workmanship is n. — HUANG:50

negligence

the n. they have received — HINT:46

neighbours

for fear of what the n. will say — CONN:25

nerves

must be credited to the n. — CLARK:23
When you suffer an attack of n. — HOBAN:47

nervous

approaching n. breakdown — RUSSE:86

nervous system

enclose the central n. in a bony case — CUSH:27
your n. won't — KORZ:57

neurologists

the n. just talk and do nothing — WIDAL:106

neuroses

to comprehend, under the title of n.   CULL:26

neurosis

the task of forming a personal n.   FREUD:37
N. has an absolute genius   PROU:82
Without them there is n.   REIK:83

neurotic

Psychiatrists classify a person as n.   SZASZ:98
A n. is the man who builds a castle   WEBB:105

neurotics

about n.   CONN:25
great in the world comes from n.   PROU:82

news

If your n. must be bad   BASH:9

newspapers

n. modify new   ADAMS:1

night

at the beginning of the n.   MAIM:64
Job was never on n. duty   PAGET:75
get you up in the middle of the n.   YOUNG:108

night-call

only thing wrong with every other n.   SANF:87

nitrous

freed from nitric phosoxyd (n. gas)   DAVY:28

nose

The wringing of the n.   BIBLE:12
he will immediately scratch his n.   MIRF:69

nostrums

large sums of time in search of n.   COLLI:24

novels

nurses have been getting into n.   MITC:70

nurse

better to be sick than to be a n.   EURI:34
took a turn for the n.   FIEL:35
trained n. has given nursing   MAYO:67
The n. should never neglect   NIGH:73
n. has become one of the great   OSLER:74
patience of Job, said a Hospital n.   PAGET:75
who so fit a n. as woman!   STILL:97
person alone is fit to n.   SUSR:97

nurses

a giggle of n.   ANON:3
under constant watch of n.   JANET:53
The doctors and n. treated me   MAND:65
N, therefore, are in a unique position   MANF:65
n. have been getting into novels   MITC:70
N. and doctors who accompany   RHOA:84

nursing

N., sometimes a trade   GULL:41
n. the chief agent in the cure   STILL:97

nutrition

only an ecological approach to n.   BEAT:9

nutritional

the accumulation of n. deficits   RHOA:84

obesity

O. is a mental state   CONN:25
malnutrition in the western world is o.   DEIT:28

obscure

things are hidden, o. and debatable   PAST:77

observation

O. is the clue to guide the physician   BAGL:8
made from lack of accurate o.   BELL:10

fundamentally only induced o.   BERN:11
Solitary, meditative o. is the first   BILLR:13
to be taught o. by a physician   GILLI:39
equipped with the gift of keen o.   MAIM:64
an unremitting gift of o.   MAUR:67
In the field of o.   PAST:77

observations

they also make very poor o.   BERN:11
Clinical o., classifications, and theories   SHIM:91

observe

above all one must o.   BERN:11
the Art is to be able to o.   HIPP:47
O. methodically and vigorously   MARF:65

observer

The o. listens to Nature   CUVI:27
only competent o. is yourself   HOWA:49
the o. must study disease   MART:66

obstetrician

o. is there to look   MORG:71

obstruction

set or rise on a small bowel o.   ANON:4

occupation

what o. does he follow   RAMA:83
The cure for it is o.   SHAW:91

occupations

also among all other o.   STAC:95
There are worse o. in the world   STER:96

offspring

waiting to execute degenerate o.   HOLM:49

old

To know how to grow o.   AMIEL:2
take care of him when he is o.   BISM:14
Become o. early if you wish to stay o.   CATO:20
grow o. more through indolence   CHRI:22
so o. as to think he cannot live   CICE:22
I grow o....I grow o.   ELIOT:32

would be young when they are o.   ENGL:33
O. persons are sometimes   FANU:34
best when they are o.   FULL:37
No skill or art is needed to grow o.   GOET:40
when you cease to grow, you are o.   HERR:45
O. people, on the whole, have fewer   HIPP:46
the misery of an o. man   HUGO:50
grow o. beautifully   MAUG:66
Growing o. is a bad habit   MAUR:67
sluggish as it grows o.   MONTA:70
Growing o. is   POWE:81
live long but none would be o.   PROV:82
It is idle to dispute with o. men   RAMÓN:83
Few people know how to be o.   ROCH:84
Before I became o. I tried to live   SENE:89
so few who can grow o.   STEE:96
A man is as o. as his arteries   SYDE:98

old age

The principal objection to o.   ANON:5
premature o., momentary death   BASIL:9
strength even in o.   CICE:22
o. is usually not only not poorer   CICE:22
to resist o.   CICE:22
manhood a struggle; o. a regret   DISR:30
All diseases run into one, o.   EMER:33
If youth but know,
And o. only   ESTI:34
the discomforts of o.   HEBE:44
Adultery brings on early o.   HEBR:44
if his mind grows turgid in o.   JOHNS:55
The sins of youth are paid for in o.   LATIN:58
merely to extend life in o.   LONG:61
What makes o. hard to bear   MAUG:67
O. puts more wrinkles in our minds   MONTA:70
O., though despised, is coveted by all   PROV:82
O. is a disease   SENE:89
One evil in o. is   SMITH:94
That sign of o.   SMITH:94
greatest problem about o. is the fear   TAYL:99
O. is an illness in itself   TERE:99
your o. will not lack sustenance   VINCI:102
a doctor who does not die of o.   VOLT:103

old people

the burden of supporting o.   METC:69

older

one is to grow o., the other not   ANON:3
as men grow o.   CICE:22
no longer ask its o. people to live   KENN:56
As I grow o., I have less and less   LONG:61
part of the hygiene of o. people   SMITH:93
The o. a doctor is   WILDE:106

operate

We are entitled to o. — BILLR:13
A surgeon is a doctor who can o. — KOCH:56

operated

If God o. on a hernia patient — RUTK:86

operating

witnessed in the o. room — AYER:7
o. should be the achievement — HOWA:49

operation

A minor o. — ANON:3
Exploratory o. — ANON:3
good o. done poorly is still a poor o. — ANON:3
in which the o. was performed — AYER:7
dangerous items in a surgical o. — BLAND:14
surgical o. begins with an incision — CALN:18
The feasibility of an o. — COHEN:23
It is easy to agree to do a beauty o. — GILLI:39
The o. is a silent confession — HUNT:51
The o. itself is but one incident — MOYN:72
o. is an experiment in bacteriology — MOYN:72
the slightest pain from the o. — VENA:102
Immediate o. for its cure — ZETA:108

operations

o. can now be performed painlessly — DIEF:29
The last part of surgery, namely o. — HUNTE:51
It is less important to invent new o. — LANGE:58
the performance of o. — PEAR:78

operative

abolished the need for o. speed — LISTE:61

operators

skilful o. are not good surgeons — MAYO:68

ophthalmologist

an eyeful of o.s — ANON:3

ophthalmology

may be of the utmost importance in o. — HELM:45

opinions

Their o., like their cranial sutures — RAMÓN:83

opposites

O. are cures for o. — HIPP:47

opposition

o. to effective medical legislation — MILLA:69

optimism

The place where o. most flourishes — ELLIS:32

organ

change in just one of an o.'s tissues — BICH:12
Always aid the o. that suffers most — CELS:20
the only o. that takes no rest — FISC:35
the mystery of o. transference — GILLI:39
All o. systems may be involved — MAND:65

organic

fall by little and little into o. disease — MAUD:66
unless o. disease can be excluded — MORR:71

organism

concerned with the entire human o. — GOET:40
the energies of the o. to drive away — SYLV:98

organisms

there will still be o. in the sweat — ANNA:3
unproving the cycles of their own o. — ELLIS:33

organization

Our hospital o. has grown up	BEVAN:11
The human form is a very delicate o.	CHEY:21
So far as o. exists in every system	STRA:97

organs

she had her o. removed one by one	ABBO:1
the cry from suffering o.	CHARC:20

orgasm

excitement and was climaxed by o.	KAPL:55
The o. has replaced the Cross	MUGG:72

origin

indelible stamp of his lowly o.	DARW:28

orphans

Late children, early o.	PROV:82

orthopaedic

A cast of o. rheumatologists	ANON:3

orthopaedics

O. is a medical and surgical science	TUREK:101

osteopathy

Quit your pills and learn from O.	STILL:97

overfed

are over clothed and o.	CADO:18

overfeeding

it is due to o.	CHIN:21

overwork

a man who died from o.	MAYO:67

paediatrician

the p. is there to look after the baby	MORG:71

paediatricians

Children are not little adults but p. are	WILL:107

paediatrics

study of geriatrics begins with p.	SEEG:89

paid

will be made game of and well p.	BRUY:16

pain

it did not involve giving p.	ADAMS:1
A surgeon should give as little p.	ANON:3
To their wearied cry of p.	ANON:5
All p. is one malady	ANTI:5
chronic abdominal p. in a child	APLE:5
greatest evil is physical p.	AUGU:7
if he remains in severe p.	BAIN:8
so much to be learned about p.	BARRE:9
sovereign masters, p. and pleasure	BENT:10
P. is in itself an evil	BENT:11
There is no p. like the Gout	BRET:15
It is easy to stand a p.	CHANG:20
Where a man feels p. he lays his hand	DUTCH:32
may feel too much p.	ELIOT:32
P. and death are part of life	ELLIS:33
its limit in the removal of all p.	EPIC:33
where the p. is	HINDU:46
thousands in sorrow and p.	IRISH:53
the art of avoiding p.	JEFF:54
Those who do not feel p. seldom think	JOHNS:55
cease upon the midnight with no p.	KEATS:55
No remedies cause so much p.	LATIN:58
In nature those who cry out with p.	MARX:66
But p. is perfect misery	MILT:69
by poultices, not by words, that p. is	PETRA:78
p. is by words both eased	PETRA:78
p. we obey	PROU:82
begins with pleasure and ends with p.	PROV:82
your money when the patient is in p.	PROV:82
uneasy at every little p.	PROV:82
Physical p. is easily forgotten	RAMÓN:83
P. is a more terrible lord of mankind	SCHW:88
p. has this most excellent quality	SENE:89
The labour we delight in physics p.	SHAK:90
P. of mind is worse than p. of body	SYRUS:98
therapy specifically directed at p.	WALL:104

painful

his death had not been p.	MAUR:67

painlessly

operations can now be performed p.   DIEF:29

pains

what shift and p.s   BROW:16
A weary thing is sickness and its p.   EURI:34
name for many aches and p.   HEBE:44
what sort of p.s he has   RAMA:83

pallbearer

I get my exercise acting as a p.   DEPEW:29

palliate

We p. what we cannot cure   JOHN:54

pancreatitis

surgical discussion of acute p.   GEOK:38

paper

to presenting a p.   ANON:4
is a logical order for a scientific p.   HILL:46

paralysis

p. is nervousness   SMITH:94

parasite

Every man carries a p. somewhere   JAPA:53

parent

An observant p.'s evidence   ANON:3
p. had unlimited claims on the child   SUMN:97

parenthood

P. is the only profession   ANON:4
p., which is also a kind of servitude   HARD:43

parents

P.s are the last people on earth   BUTL:18
half of our lives is ruined by our p.   DARR:28
p. do not count their child their own   PASH:76
only illegitimate p.   YANK:108

partnership

go into p. with nature   FISC:35

parturition

p. is a physiological process   CHIP:22

passion

same symptoms as p.   ANON:3
the third thing necessary is p.   PAVL:77

passions

natural man has only two primal p.   OSLER:75

past

against living in the p.   LERN:59

patent

beck and call of the p. medicines   ADAMS:1

paternity

p. is a matter of speculation   WELLS:105

pathological

knowledge is through the p. museum   GULL:41
p. anatomy must be the foundation   ROKI:85

pathologist

A p. is someone who knows   ANON:3
a pessimistic p.   WILS:107

pathologists

pathology

patience

patient

patients

private matter between doctors and p.   LILF:60
the relationship between p.   LISTE:60
what we tell our p.   LOPEZ:62
to bring spiritual aid to their p.   MANF:65
little time left to look after p.   MORR:71
in our relation with our p.   MORR:71
P. should have rest, food, fresh air   OSLER:74
P. rarely die of the disease   OSLER:75
The best practitioners give to their p.   SAUN:87
P. must be adjusted socially as well   SIGE:92
P. themselves cannot escape   SILV:93
the greatest fools? The p.   VOLT:103

paupers

the government of p.   NIGH:73

pecuniary

To give a surgeon a p. interest   SHAW:91

penis

the functional role of the p.   MAST:66
he also has he biggest p.   MORR:71

people

Objectionable p. are numerous   DA CO:23
in ancient times the p. lived   HUANG:50
Some p. are so sensitive   HUBB:50
much more taking with the p.   HUME:50
used only for the good of the p.   HUNA:51
P. should be very free with sex   JOHN:54
P. ask you for criticism   MAUG:66
Few p. know how to be old   ROCH:84
The common p. say   SALI:87
I love mankind – it's p. I can't stand   SCHU:88
p. will not weed their own minds   WALP:104
In former times p. treated themselves   WESL:106

perception

nothing but developed p.   SANTA:87

perceptions

safer to appeal to men's p.   LATH:58

percussion

consists in p. of the human thorax   AUEN:7

perfect

P. health is above gold   APOC:5

perfection

a constant tendency to increased p.   HUXL:52
one does not seek p.   ORWE:74

performance

science is power of p.   VIRC:103

period

a missed menstrual p.   MORR:71

peritoneum

I scratched through the p. on the left   COOP:25

person

what kind of a p. has a disease   SMYTH:94
what sort of disease the p. has   PARRY:76

personal

man's disease is his p. property   CLARK:23

personality

subsequent development of the p.   BRAIN:15
greater or lesser upheaval of p.   SCHIL:88

persons

must be interested in things, not in p.   CURIE:26

perspiration

precise amount of that insensible p.   SANTO:87

persuasion

to use either p. or compulsion   ARIS:6

phagocytes

Stimulate the p.   SHAW:91

pharmacologist

a biologist, a p., and an electrician   MACP:64

phenomena

if the cause of the p. be unknown   PAST:77
the very essence of p.   PAST:76

philosopher

delusion is called a p.   BIERC:13

philosophers

The poets and p. before me   FREUD:37

philosophy

they are the parents of p.   BROWN:16
P., like medicine, has plenty of drugs   CHAM:20
Aristotle and all p. may say   MOLI:70

physic

P., for the most part, is nothing   ADDI:1
For p. made, from poison be exempt   DONNE:30
hope do me more good than p.   GALEN:38
The practice of p.   LATH:58
Temperance is the best p.   PROV:82

physician

Any p. who advertises a positive cure   ADAMS:1
The p. should look upon the patient   ALEX:2
A p. is someone who knows   ANON:3
No man is a good p.   ARAB:5
p. becomes a fool   ARAB:6
the p. alone can mourn   ARET:6
The p. himself, if sick, actually calls   ARIS:6

It is no part of a p.'s business to use   ARIS:6
A man is a poor p.   ASCL:6
clue to guide the p. in his thinking   BAGL:8
diseases are revealed to the p.   BART:9
P.' heal thyself   BIBLE:12
Honour a p.   BIBLE:12
They that be whole need not a p.   BIBLE:12
He is a great p.   BIGE:13
medical science and the p.'s art.   BILLR:13
preparatory school for the p.   BILLR:13
The p. can do all he has to do   BILLR:13
the party had placed in his p.   BLAC:14
It is extremely difficult for a p.   BOOR:14
good p. is a disciple of Paracelsus   BROOK:16
A p.'s physiology has much the same   BUTL:18
The p. is the central decision maker   CALI:18
It is a good thing for a p. to have   CANN:19
divests the p. of his proper prestige   CATH:19
wastes the skill of the p.   CHIN:21
p. who fails to combine pathological   CORV:25
to change often their p.   CULL:26
A p. is obligated to consider more   CUSH:27
A p. should not be judged   DIETL:29
Time is a p. that heals every grief   DIPH:30
Time is the great p.   DISR:30
The p. must look beyond the picture   DOCK:30
disease neither p. nor physic can ease   ENGL:33
Feed sparingly and defy the p.   ENGL:33
The p. today seems athirst for blood   FERN:34
so do the p. and surgeon   FLEX:36
The p. is not the servant of science   FOX:36
He's the best p.   FRAN:36
a p. who is naturally wise   FRAN:36
A surgeon should be young, a p. old   FRENC:37
A young p. fattens the churchyard   FRENC:37
p. is bound to take up the position   FREUD:37
That p. will hardly be thought   GALEN:38
to be taught observation by a p.   GILLI:39
look upon his p. as his friend   GISB:40
skilful p. distinguishes the symptoms   GOLDS:40
The p.'s continuing education   HARR:43
Honour a p. before thou has need   HEBR:44
a city whose governor is a p.   HEBR:44
every p. is for one disease   HEROD:45
The best p. is he who can distinguish   HEROP:45
In illness the p. is a father   HINDU:46
A p. who is a lover of wisdom   HIPP:47
The p. is the servant of the art   HIPP:47
p. must have a worthy appearance   HIPP:47
may be a good p.   HOLM:48
having found a good p.   HOLM:48
The best a p. can give   HOLM:48
The p. must generalise the disease   HUFE:50
Medicine's preferable to that of a p.   INDI:52
Until a p. has killed one or two   INDI:52
Hope is the p. of each misery   IRISH:53
Death is the poor man's best p.   IRISH:52
The p. ought to know literature   ISID:53

the p. is but a lout   ITAL:53
call in an unskilful p.   JAPA:53
The adventurous p. goes on   JEFF:54
Many funerals discredit a p.   JONS:55
qualification for a p. is hopefulness   LITT:61
nor does a p. work cures   LOGIA:61
better after the p.'s visit   LONG:61
duty of the p. to bring contentment   LONG:61
there is no time to make a p. of him   MACP:64
p. means a lifetime of incessant study   MARX:66
The examining p. often hesitates   MAYO:68
eliminate the need for a p.   MAYO:68
A good p. appreciates the difference   MINE:69
A p. and a priest ought not   NAPO:72
a good man can be a great p.   NOTH:73
The first figure of a p.   OSLER:74
a place beside the p.   OSLER:74
A p. who treats himself   OSLER:74
One of the first duties of the p.   OSLER:74
'Tis not always in a p's power   OVID:75
A sick person who lies to his p.   PAUD:77
from nature not from the p.   PARA:76
The p. is only the servant of nature   PARA:76
There are two kinds of p.   PARA:76
knowledge makes the p.   PARA:76
a p. seldom obtains bread   PARKI:76
p. can sometimes parry the scythe   PIOZ:79
for the true p. is also a ruler   PLATO:79
A p. should not be a servant   PLATT:80
died last night of my p.   PRIOR:82
he does not need a p. at all   RHAZ:84
to die soon, make your p. your heir   ROMAN:85
palpation to which the p. is trained   RUSSE:86
The p. that bringeth love   SAVO:87
The p.'s best remedy   SCHIC:88
p. that should be the patient   SHAK:90
surgeon should be something of a p.   SHEP:91
a regular-bred p.   SHERI:91
the p. as scientist, educator   SIGE:92
supercilious self-conceit of a p.   SMOL:94
p. must not try to counteract nature's   STAHL:95
follows the instructions of the p.   SUSR:97
an implicit faith in his own p.   SUSR:97
The p. is superfluous   TACI:98
A p. who heals for nothing   TALM:99
house ... will be opened to the p.   TALM:99
where the strength of the p. lies   TOLS:100
A p. should take his fee   TROL:100
A p. is one who pours drugs   VOLT:103
The p. can bury his mistakes   WRIG:108

physicians

dying with the help of too many p.   ALEX:2
like other doctrines advanced by p.   ANON:4

Many p. would prefer   ANON:4
P. and politicians resemble one   ANON:4
P. are like undescended testicles   ANON:4
by p. no longer forced to practise it   ANON:4
Conscientious and careful p.   ARIS:6
We are p. It is a proud title   BEAT:10
P. of the Utmost Fame   BELLO:10
P. should be consulted when needed   BUCH:17
Keep away from p.   BURG:17
P., when the cause of disease   CICE:23
his p. cannot cure   COLLI:24
there will be no scientific p.   DIETL:29
P. and public health officials   DUBOS:31
P.' faults are covered with earth   ENGL:33
p. are generally sceptics   FEUC:34
p., like beer, are best   FULL:37
proportion of cases treated by p.   FORB:36
Most p. are like athletes who aspire   GALEN:38
beyond the practice of all the p.   GLAD:40
called the reproach of p.   HEBE:44
They have no p.   HEROD:45
P. who meet in consultation   HIPP:47
little liked by p.   HORT:49
P. live by rich patients   INDI:52
There are only 'safe' p.   KAMI:55
P. think they do a lot   KANT:55
English p. kill you   LAMB:57
p. have abandoned operative   LANF:57
P. see many 'diseases'   MARX:66
The p. are here' too   MAYO:68
The fever is to the p.   MILT:69
older p. refused to recognise socially   MITC:70
Lawyers and p. are a bad provision   MONTA:70
The most dangerous p.   NIET:73
assigned in some degree to p.   PARR:76
Only p. and advocates can kill   PHILE:79
P. are in general the most amiable   POPE:81
P. are costly visitors   PROV:82
three great p.   PROV:82
P. of all men are the most happy   QUAR:83
odium of the hostility of p. to each   RUSH:86
p. are the class of people who kill   SALI:87
euthanasia is actually practised by p.   SIGE:92
p. must thus also play a social role   SIGE:92
If consumption is too powerful for p.   SMITH:94
P. cure little or nothing   SPOD:95
deprive p. of much of the influence   STARR:96
instruct p. how to behave   STIE:97
women should be p.   STILL:97
The sick man is the garden of the p.   SWAH:98
P. ought not to give their judgment   SWIFT:98
Take care not to fancy that you are p.   TROU:101
p. are the natural attorneys   VIRC:103
Even in the hands of the greatest p.   VIRC:103
P. are like kings   WEBS:105
p. then concocted complicated theories   WESL:106

physics

He who p. himself poisons a fool   PROV:82

physiology

In pathology, as in p.   BERN:11
pathological p. with his anatomy   CORV:25
real investigations on p.   DARW:28
Anatomy is for p. what geography is   FERN:34
lectures on the P. of the Sense-organs   HELM:45

pick

It will never get well if you p. it   AMER:2

piles

p. to give an Anxious Expression   ANON:3
prematurely grey hair and itching p.   CANN:19
Nine out of every ten men have p.   CHIN:21
are peculiarly subject to the p.   HEBE:44
riding bare-back causes nasty p.   MART:65

pills

It is an age of p.   MUGG:72
Quit your p. and learn   STILL:97

place

not of the body but of the p.   SENE:89

placenta

from it a p. was protruding   TAIT:99

plague

The leper in whom the p. is   BIBLE:12
from p., pestilence and famine   BOOK:14
Death from the bubonic p.   WILL:107

planet

the cancer of the p.   HUXL:52

plastic surgeon

The great ignominy to the p.   GILLI:39
The p. works with living flesh   WEBS:105

pleasure

two sovereign masters, pain and p.   BENT:10
temptation of denying himself a p.   BIERC:13
The p. is momentary   CHES:21
The magnitude of p. reaches its limit   EPIC:33

pleasures

Diseases are the tax on p.   RAY:83
those who forego ordinary p.   RUSSE:86

pneumonia

Never forget that it is not a p.   GULL:41
p. is an easy second, to tuberculosis   OSLER:74
p. as the immediate prelude to death   RHOA:84

poetry

p., for those who know   ROUX:85

poison

P. should be tried out on a frog   AFRI:2
For physic made, from p. be exempt   DONNE:30
Even nectar is p. if taken to excess   HINDU:46
The treatment with p. medicines   HUANG:50
directions for using p.   KRAUS:57
man's meat is another man's rank p.   LUCR:62

poisonous

All things are p.   PARA:76

poisons

The p. are our principal medicines   EMER:33
P. and medicines   LATH:58
He who physics himself p. a fool   PROV:82
P. in small doses are the best   WITH:107

political

p. will to make the tough choices — ANON:5
be divested of all p. opinions — NAPO:72
becomes a symptom of p. sickness — SKRA:93
enter into the larger p. and social life — VIRC:103

politician

too lazy to work he becomes a p. — DA CO:23

politicians

Physicians and p. resemble one — ANON:4
medical profession of today to fear the p. — HERR:46
Put not your faith in p. — HORD:49

politics

in p. they are one and the same — MARX:66

pomposity

invented out of p. rather than utility — HEIS:45

poor

Death is the p. man's best physician — IRISH:52
the p. and destitute — MOTH:71
The p. are cured by work — POLI:81
natural attorneys of the p. — VIRC:103

poorest

p. man would not part with health — COLT:24

population

service for an ever more demanding p. — ANON:5
Children are one third of our p. — ANON:3
the entire p. of the world — BENN:10

position

the p. ridiculous — CHES:21

posterity

People will not look forward to p. — BURKE:17

post-mortem

In the p. room — BRAIN:15
in the p. room is the truth — HORD:49

poultices

by p., not by words that pain is ended — PETRA:78

poverty

P. is a virtue greatly exaggerated — ANON:4
dying as a result of diseases of p. — CARRU:19
The miseries of p., sickness — JOHNS:55
Disease creates p. and p. disease — SIGE:92
The real public health problem . . . is p. — WILKI:107

power

also, unmistakably, a world of p. — STARR:96
science is p. of performance — VIRC:103

practical

but by the p. capacity of the mass — MITC:70

practice

p. of medicine depends on — CUSH:27
medical p. of the time — EMER:33
to set an example of p. — FAXON:34
Here's good advice for p. — FISC:35
the beginning of p. — FISC:35
to its adoption in p. — FISC:35
True science is the key to wise p. — HARL:43
be at the heart of good p. — HUGH:50
the p. of medicine — LATH:58
p. is steered by ethical principles — LOPEZ:62
from its p. and its exercise — SYDE:98
enamoured of p. without science — VINCI:102

practise

wishes to p. medicine — ROGER:84

practitioner

p. must preserve and exercise — BRAD:15

practitioners

The best p. give to their patients   SAUN:87

pray

always p. for your patients   HOPE:49

prayer

The p. of faith shall save the sick   BIBLE:12

pregnancy

she wishes to avoid p.   ANON:4
Love and p. and riding on a camel   ARAB:5
Certainly p. is a form of servitude   HARD:43
Women during the state of p.   HEBE:44
p. the progress of the consumption   HEBE:44
avoid p. by a resort to mathematics   MENC:69

pregnant

afraid when she is p.   CHIN:21

prehistoric

India's p. clay   KIPL:56

prejudices

patients' interests if not their p.   CRON:26

premier

A good doctor is equal to a good p.   LU:62

prescription

ye niver can read his p.   DUNNE:31

prescriptions

It is easy to get a thousand p.   CHIN:21
A doctor is a man who writes p.   TAYL:99

present

the past at the expense of the p.   SMITH:94

preservatives

Eat more things containing p.   CAND:19

preserve

To p. a man alive   TAYL:99

press

the p. of the United States   ADAMS:1

prestige

divests the physician of his proper p.   CATH:19

preventative

discourages p. health care   ILLI:52

prevention

in the cause and p. of disease   EDIS:32
p. of disease is for the most part   EMER:33
The p. of disease today   MAYO:67
P. of disease must be the goal   SIGE:92

preventive

it is a branch of p. medicine   CRICH:26
only one ultimate and effectual p.   CUSH:27

pride

for Shame, for your P. has a Fall   ANON:5

priest

A physician and a p. ought not   NAPO:72

primitive peoples

even p. realized that loss of blood   WINT:107

principles

with p. we learn the cause of disease   HUNT:51

private

so taken up with their p. s

P. patients . . . can go elsewhere	ABER:1
exclusively a disease of p. patients	ABRA:1
The essence of p. medical practice	LISTE:60

private practice

so taken up with their p. s	ANON:5
P. and marriage	BROCA:15

probabilities

consists largely in balancing p.	OSLER:74

problem

It never solves a p.	SHAW:91

problems

To solve p.	MINOT:69
Children . . . have their own specific p.	SCHIC:88

procedures

allow time for careful p.	LISTE:61

procreation

When one contemplates p.	DAVIS:28
given to living beings for p.	FIRM:35
rendered incapable of p.	GERM:39
The act of p. and the members	VINCI:102

proctologists

a pile of p.	ANON:3

productive

set up by persons no longer p.	STARR:96

profession

Medicine would be the ideal p.	ADAMS:1
so widely as the medical p.	ADAMS:1
Parenthood is the only p.	ANON:4
A young man entering upon the p.	BEAUM:10
in the first I learned my p.	BLAND:14
The one eternal jibe at our p.	BROW:16

p. that labours incessantly to destroy	BRYCE:17
can know his own p. perfectly	COLLE:24
Nothing is known in our p. by guess	COOP:25
the medical p. and the public	DICKS:29
we as a p. have a duty	GENE:38
That salutary and lucrative p.	GIBB:39
the disgrace of their p.	GISB:40
cricket is my p.	GRACE:41
sometimes a p.	GULL:41
even more than of the medical p.	HALD:42
For the honour of the P.	HARV:43
in the course of my p.	HIPP:47
research is now regarded as a p.	JEVO:54
medicine is not a lucrative p.	LETT:60
medical p. is the only one	MAUG:66
Medicine is a p. for social service	MAYO:67
comes from the p. itself	MILLA:69
Do not think of the dignity of your p.	MITC:70
In the records of no other p.	OSLER:74
the only worldwide p.	OSLER:74
In no p. does culture count	OSLER:74
seldom obtains bread by his p.	PARKI:76
hear it often said of the medical p.	POWE:81
regard for the honour of the p.	PRIT:82
the excrescences of the medical p.	SAUN:87
Integrity and rectitude in our p.	SCAR:87
power as has the medical p.	STARR:96
medical p. were merely	STARR:96
to go on practising their base p.	WOLFE:107

professional

assigned his long p. rides	DICKE:29
delivery of p. illusions and torts	ILLI:52
The magnetic needle of p. rectitude	JACO:53
as medicine loses its p. hegemony	LILF:60
p. patriotism amongst medical men	PRIT:82
There is only one rule of p. conduct	SMITH:94
a long p. life in medicine	WALS:104

professions

the most humane of all p.	LISTE:61
only four p. for a gentleman	MAUG:66
Of the three learned p.	PARR:76
All p. are conspiracies	SHAW:90

professor

A p. is one who talks	AUDEN:7

professors

P. in every branch of the sciences	COLLI:24

profit

Hold fast to reputation rather than p.   HIPP:47
those who work for their own p.   PARA:76
P.-making enterprises are not   STARR:96

profits

as true parasites, they share the p.   SKRA:93

progenitors

even more than their p.   EMER:33

prognoses

rarely forgive you for wrong p.   ANON:4

prognosis

that may always be given a good p.   PICK:79

progress

sign of the rapid p. of our time   BILLR:13
Despite all our toil and p.   HECHT:44
The status and p. of medicine   THORO:100
unparalleled p. in physiology   WELCH:105

promiscuity

through a period of playfulness or p.   DARL:27

promptly

tell it soberly and p.   BASH:9

prophet

A p. is not acceptable   LOGIA:61

proprietary

the market for most p. remedies   ADAMS:1

prosector

adroit, diligent and patient p.   CORV:25

protest

weakens the force of real p   GREGG:41

prove

If I set out to p. something   SPAL:95

psychiatric

obviously needs p. attention   CHUR:22

psychiatrist

A p. is someone who knows   ANON:3
p. is the obstetrician of the mind   ANON:5
each conversation with a p.   ARTA:6
P.: A man who asks you a lot   BARD:9
Anybody who goes to see a p.   GOLDW:40
Don't refer a patient to a p.   PALM:75
p. is the man who collects the rent   WEBB:105

psychiatrists

P. are often amusing company   CAPP:19
P. classify a person as neurotic   SZASZ:98

psychiatry

p. is the care of the id by the odd   ANON:5
being explored by p.   PLATT:80

psychoanalysis

P. is confession without absolution   CHES:21
P. is spending forty dollars an hour   CONN:25
most significant contribution of p.   FROMM:37
P. is the disease it purports to cure   KRAUS:57

psychological

settled p. habits   ARIS:6

psychology

pity that p. should have destroyed   CHES:21
Popular p. is a mass of cant   DEWEY:29
P. has a long past, but only a short history EBBI:32

The separation of p. | JUNG:55
P. is as unnecessary as directions | KRAUS:57
Idleness is the parent of all p. | NIET:73
There is no p. | SZASZ:98
The object of p. | VALÉ:102

psycho-pathologist

the p. the unspeakable | MAUG:67

psychotherapist

clergyman and the p. to join forces | JUNG:55

psychotic

committed to a public hospital as 'p'. | JANET:53
p. if he makes others suffer | SZASZ:98
A p. is the man who lives in it | WEBB:105

public

we are merely the servants of the p. | BASH:9
p. is not always sagacious | BILLI:13
the medical profession and the p. | DICKS:29
the business of the general p. | HALD:42
In the minds of the p. | WARN:104

public health

Physicians and p. officials | DUBOS:31
import to a State than its p. | ROOS:85
The real p. problem . . . is poverty | WILKI:107

public opinion

work not in the light of p. | ALLB:2
the aristocracy of an enlightened p. | GARR:38

public trust

must continue to earn that p. | GILLO:39

publication

p. of a long list of authors' names | ANON:5
man who submits his paper for p. | BEVE:12

publicity

p. given to what goes wrong | CHARL:21

published

a p. article is a tedious duty | ASHER:7

puerperal

p. fever raged violently | HAMI:42

pulmonary

powerful channel of p. absorption | SIMP:93

pulse

The heart is in accord with the p. | SU:97
The rapid p. it can abate | WITH:107

pupil

A p. who is pure, obedient | SUSR:97

purgative

Englishman believes that a p. can | GOGA:40

purge

Bleed him and p. him | SPAN:95

purse

his p. lies open to thee | BURT:17

quack

patients he has never seen is a q. | ADAMS:1
It is better to have recourse to a q. | COLT:24

quackery

Q. gives birth to nothing | CARL:19

quacks

number was increased by q. | BOCC:14
Q. are the greatest liars | FRAN:36

physic is jostled by q. on the one side   LATH:58
The number of q. in a locality   MORR:71

quality of life

The highest q. attainable   KOTT:57
energies of man to improving the q.   LASA:58

quarrels

controversies without personal q.   VIRC:103

question

interpret the answer to a leading q.   WOOD:107

questioning

about who you are q.   EINS:32

questions

to make two q. grow   VEBL:102

quiet

Dr. Q. and Dr. Merryman   ANON:4

rabbit

any white r. on earth   COBB:23

radicalism

Homeopathy waged a war of r.   ANON:4

rarely

but they should be needed very r.   BUCH:17

rationality

position is this new world of r.   STARR:96

read

R. little, see much, do much   DUPU:31

reading

how little r. a doctor can practise   OSLER:74

reads

too much trust in what he r.   BOOR:14

reality

never quite in touch with r.   CONN:25

reason

R., Observation' and Experience   INGER:52
limits which divide the province of r.   PRES:81
which enters the mind through r.   RAMÓN:83
Time heals what r. cannot   SENE:89
of those extraordinary works of r.   STARR:96

reasoners

the r. resemble spider   BACON:8

reasoning

a process of r.   MACK:64

reasons

think about the r. for what you are   EINS:32

recover

help of a surgeon he might yet r.   SHAK:90

recovered

but when you have r.   AFRI:2

recovery

surgery to get minor r.   ASHER:7
ends in r. or death   SIGE:92

rectal

To sing of r. carcinoma   HALD:42

rectum

developing within the anus in the r.   JOHN:54
for colostomy over resection of the r.   VOLK:103

regimen

administration of diet and r.   COXE:26

rehabilitate

and to r. the people   SIGE:92

relapses

When a disease r. there is no cure   CHIN:22

relatives

keep a dying patient's r. busy   FRIPP:37
from their homes and their r.   GILL:39

religion

ought to be a r.   GULL:41
people think they have r.   INGER:52
r. deals with why   REZN:84
Frenchman will sooner part with his r.   SMOL:94
to give their judgment of r.   SWIFT:98

religions

founded our r. and composed   PROU:82

religious

a medical man has true r. views   ELIOT:32

remedies

market for most proprietary r.   ADAMS:1
two or three r. ready for use   ASCL:6
he that will not apply new r.   BACON:8
For major ills, major r.   CELS:20
a disease by its long list of r.   CLARK:23
too fond of new r.   COOP:25
Extreme r. are most appropriate   HIPP:46

No r. cause so much pain   LATIN:58
Most men die of their r.   MOLI:70
the most violent r.   MONTA:70
worry over the scarcity of effective r.   PIEN:79
some r. worse than the disease   PROV:82
such r. as will not lessen the patient's   RHAZ:84
accepted r. serve only to aggravate   ROCH:84
no one tries extreme r.   SENE:89
Our r. oft in ourselves do lie   SHAK:90

remedy

It is better to employ a doubtful r.   ANON:4
The r. is worse than the disease   BACON:8
a sovereign r. to all disease   BURT:17
unless by a r. likewise severe   CELS:20
r. for everything except death   CERV:20
hard to get one single r.   CHIN:21
All who drink of this r.   GALEN:38
Suicide is not a r.   GARF:38
be sure of the success of your r.   LATH:58
If superstition were curable, the r.   MARX:66
Better a tried r.   PARÉ:76
never think of finding a r.   PAST:77
a good r. sometimes to do nothing   PROV:82
There is a r. for everything   PROV:82
write upon a disease than upon a r.   WITH:107

repent

We never r. of having eaten too little   JEFF:54

repentance

it leaves no opportunity for r.   COLLI:24

reputation

Hold fast to r. rather than profit   HIPP:47

research

The faculties developed by doing r.   ADLER:1
from advances made in surgical r.   BELL:10
first step in the poetry of r.   BILLR:13
R., though toilsome, is easy   BRADL:15
do r. for the fun of doing it   BROWN:16
Scientific r. is not itself a science   GEOR:38
The object of r. is the advancement   GORD:40
r. is now regarded as a profession   JEVO:54

cripple, and hamper r.   KIPL:56
exercise for a r. scientist   LORE:62
The aim of r. is the discovery   MACH:63
Such is the supreme goal of our r.   RANV:83
r. committee can do one useful thing   TOPL:100
The outcome of any serious r.   VEBL:102

researcher

it brings joy to the r.   LESS:60

responsibility

the human r. of the doctor   COMF:24
has no r. for implementing   MEESE:68

restraint

less r. for the patient, the more r.   KORS:56

results

spurious, precision of laboratory r.   ANON:5

retina

first to see a living human r.   HELM:45

retinitis

an old case of albuminuric r.   GUNN:42

retire

Calmly r., like the evening light   COTT:26

retiring

Don't think of r. from the world   JOHNS:55

retreat

a quieter or more untroubled r.   AURE:7

rheumatic fever

R. licks at the joints, but bites at the heart   ANON:4

rheumatism

r. is the tax most frequently paid   BELL:10
the r. of a rich patient   BIERC:13
r. is a common name for many aches   HEBE:44
what r. is to the heart   HUCH:50

rheumatologists

a cast of orthopedic r.   ANON:3

rich

the r. by the doctor   POLI:81
the r. man's bliss   PROV:82

riches

a sound body before r.   APOC:5

richest

r. would gladly part with all   COLT:24

ridiculous

to be certain is to be r.   CHIN:22

riding

r. bare-back causes nasty piles   MART:65

right

Man has an inalienable r. to die   ANON:4
to be always in the r.   LATH:58

rising

R. before daylight   ARIS:6

risks

The patient takes the r.   MARC:65

roentgenology

anaesthesia, asepsis, and r.   FISC:35

Röntgen

comprehend R.'s pallid shades   CAFF:18

rotting

To lose a r. member is a gain   BAXT:9

routines

above the r. of the daily ward round   MCGE:63

rust

It is better to wear out than to r. out   CUMB:26

sadness

Sickness is better than s.   PROV:82

sage

s. does not treat those who are ill   SU:97

saints

it is the s. who have cured him   ITAL:53

sane

Show me a s. man.   JUNG:55
An asylum for the s. would be empty   SHAW:91

sanity

S. is very rare   EMER:33

savages

S. explain, science investigates   GULL:41

scar

wounds ever closed without a s.   BYRON:18
A wound heals but the s. remains   ENGL:33
his inability to remove a s.   GILLI:39
He who scratches a s. is wounded   RUSSI:86
A s. nobly got, or a noble s.   SHAK:90

scars

s. grow with us   LEC:59
experience leaves mental s.   MAYO:68

scene

the most sublime s. ever witnessed   AYER:7

scepticism

The solemn s. of science   HOLM:48
from credulity to s.   JEFF:54

sceptics

physicians are generally s.   FEUC:34

schizophrenia

if God talks to you, you have s.   SZASZ:98
S. is a special strategy   LAING:57

school

makes the physician, not the name or the s.   PARA:76

sciatica

cold s.
Cripple our senators   SHAK:90

science

In s., law is not a rule imposed   ALLB:2
Medicine, like every useful s.   ANON:4

sciences

scientific

scientist

part craftsman, part practical s.	ADDIS:1
exercise for a research s.	LORE:62
The s. is not content to stop	MAYO:67
the s. is like a traveler	PAST:77
physician as s.	SIGE:92
I am no real s.	SPAL:95

scientists

the ablest s. go back to medicine	ARIS:6
society of s. is more important	BRON:15
S. should be on tap, but not on top	CHUR:22
The Republic has no need for s.	COFF:23

scleroderma

s. is one of the most terrible of all	OSLER:75

Scotland

There is no harder worker in all S.	SCOTT:88

scratch

To s. when it itches	ANON:5

scratches

He who s. a scar is wounded twice	RUSSI:86

scratching

S. is one of the sweetest	MONTA:70
S. is bad because it begins	PROV:82

scribble

keep pace with the itch to s. about it	MAYOW:68

seasick

nearly all his comrades are s.	TWAIN:101

sea-sickness

The only cure for s.	ENG:33

secrecy

but in the s. of the bed chamber	ALLB:2
s. is highly developed among doctors	HECHT:44

secret

holding such things to be holy s.	HIPP:47

see

so that he could not s.	BIBLE:12
we s. only what we are ready to s.	CHARC:20
Read little, s. much, do much	DUPU:31

seeing

The eye is not satisfied with s.	BIBLE:12

seeks

He that s. finds	SPAN:95

self-contemplation

s. is infallibly the symptom of disease	CARL:19

self-deception

no guesswork or s.	EHRL:32

self-destruction

S. is the effect of cowardice	DEFOE:28

senescence

S. begins:	
and middle age ends	NASH:72

senility

true s. announces itself by trembling	RAMÓN:83

senses

most delightful of all our s.	ADDI:1
The keenest of all our s.	CICE:22
The knowledge of the s. is the best	LATH:58
the s. and intellects being uninjured	PARKI:76
things given to it by the other s.	VINCI:102

sensibility

excess of s. to the presence	CARL:19

sensitive

as s. to outside influences	HOLM:48

sepsis

S. is an insult to a surgeon	ANON:4

septicaemias

divided into s. and intoxications	WRIG:108

services

give your s. for nothing	HIPP:47

seventy

To be s. years	HOLM:48

severe

if s. it cannot be prolonged	SENE:89

sex

a doctor broken down by age and s.	ANON:3
Poor honest s., like dying	DURR:31
each s., has its special diseases	HOFFM:48
People should be very free with s.	JOHN:54
there has to be some penalty for s.	MAHER:64
S. is not an antidote for loneliness	ROBI:84
s. plays a more important part	SIGE:92

sexes

the union of the two s.	FIRM:35

sexual

the human s. response	KAPL:55
He who immerses himself in s. intercourse	MAIM:64

sexuality

S. is the lyricism of the masses	BAUD:9

shadows

S. are but dark holes	CAFF:18

Shipman

The murders fed S.'s	SMITH:93

shock

S. is more a part of the phenomena	MALC:65

short

S. men eat more than tall ones	FRENC:37

shortage

There is no bed s.	ANON:5

short-winded

long-winded about the s.	BIRD:14

sick

they heal the s.	AFRI:2
makes the s. well and the well s.	AMER:2
no curing a s. man	AMIEL:2
s. man if he were still alive today	ANON:3
My friend was s.	ANON:4
They shall lay their hands on the s.	ANON:5
The s. are still in ... Workhouses	ANON:5
Thou to whom the s. and dying	ANON:5
who has never been s.	ARAB:5
When you are called to a s. man	BELLE:10
not slow to visit the s.	BIBLE:12
they that are s.	BIBLE:12
The prayer of faith shall save the s.	BIBLE:12

Those who are well get s. BRUY:16
has never been s. himself CHIN:21
Heal the s. and comfort the dying DOUG:30
The multitude of the s. EMER:33
It is dainty to be s. EMER:33
An insane man is a s. man FISC:35
Let your entrance into the s. room FISC:35
Be not s. too late, nor well too soon FRAN:36
helping nature to get a s. man well GEDD:38
the burden of the s. GILL:39
The indigent s. of this city HOPK:49
to attend the s. and dissect the dead HUNTE:51
S. minds must be healed MILLE:69
The s. are the greatest danger NIET:73
The s. man is a parasite to society NIET:73
do the s. no harm NIGH:73
care and government of the s. poor NIGH:73
to heal the s. OSLER:74
doctors into the s. man's room OSLER:75
A s. person who lies to his physician PAUD:77
a s. man neglecting himself ROMA:85
desire to cure the s. RUSK:86
bringeth love and charity to the s. SAVO:87
a s. man must go searching SENE:89
a s. doctor SHAW:90
occasion the s. to be deserted SNOW:94
in the kingdom of the s. SONT:94
Time cures the s. man SPAN:95
s. man is the garden of the physicians SWAH:98
to be s. sometimes THORE:100

sickness

To avoid s. eat less CHU:22
S. comes riding on a hare CREO:26
There is something in s. DICKE:29
S. comes on horseback and departs DUTCH:32
Health is not valued till s. comes. ENGL:33
In the hour of sorrow or s., a wife is EURI:34
A weary thing is s. and its pains EURI:34
S. poses only one problem EURI:34
witness the progress and effects of s. GRAV:41
Bathe every day and s. will avoid you INDI:52
Health without wealth is half a s. ITAL:53
just get them over a s. JARV:53
companions in the chamber of s. JOHNS:55
Preventable s., disability KENN:56
dignity in s. as well as in health KENN:56
How s. enlarges the dimensions LAMB:57
lose more of their men by s. LIND:60
able doctor acts before s. comes LIU:61
a wise mans part, rather to avoid s. MORE:71
In s. the mind reflects upon itself PLINY:80
S. is better than sadness PROV:82
S. is felt, but health not at all PROV:82
In regard to s., I shall not repeat ROUSS:85

sight

Our s. is the most perfect ADDI:1
is the sense of s. CICE:22
bear gently the deprivation of s. MILT:69

signs

s. are in a foreign language BROWN:16

sin

disease is the result of s. PICKE:79

sing

I do not think that they will s. to me ELIOT:32

sins

God may forgive you your s. KORZ:57
s. of omission veneal TRON:100

sister

s. puts all her patients back to bed ASHER:7

skeletal muscles

largest complex of s. MAYER:67

skill

inversely proportional to your s. FISC:35

skills

we need to maintain diversity of s. HUGH:50

skin

knowledge of the healing of s. wounds CALN:18
scabby s. from which matter oozed FRAS:36
A violent itching of the s. HEBE:44
S. is like wax paper LINK:60
slowly contracting s. of steel OSLER:75

His shelves are lined with rolls of s.   SELZ:89
Woollen clothing keeps the s. healthy   VENE:102

sleep

The s. of the just   ANON:5
one who talks in someone else's s.   AUDEN:7
S. covers a Man all over   CERV:20
sickness from which s. provides relief   CHAM:20
Oh s.! it is a gentle thing   COLER:24
Six hours s. for a man   ENGL:33
When s. puts an end to delirium   HIPP:46
S. and watchfulness   HIPP:46
anaesthetics . . . s., fainting, death   HOLM:48
S. and Death, are twin brothers   HOMER:49
troubles only those who can s.   HUBB:50
A good laugh and a long s.   IRISH:52
A person should not s. on his face   MAIM:64
put you to s., wake you up   MUGG:72
S., rest of things, O pleasing Deity   OVID:75
S. is the nourishment and food   PHAE:79
S., riches, and health   RICHT:84
To s. – perchance to dream   SHAK:90
In s. we are all equal   SPAN:95
S. is the only medicine   SOPH:94
a well-spent day brings happy s.   VINCI:102
That sweet, deep s.   VIRG:103
Disease and s. keep far apart   WELSH:105

sleepers

Great eaters and great s.   HENRY:45

sleeping

All this fuss about s. together   WAUG:105
s. on hairy mattresses   WELSH:105

sleeps

He that s. feels no toothache   SHAK:90

sleepy

He may be hungry, weary, s.   SHAW:91

slimming

if you insist on s.   SECO:88

smallpox

nearly the same as those of s.   AVIC:7
only that the loathsome s. has existed   JEFF:54
take the s. here by way of diversion   MONTA:70
Until he gets over the s.   PASH:76

smoke

Don't screw around, and don't s.   CURRI:27
but a good cigar is a s.   KIPL:56

smoker

What difference is there between a s.   BALDE:8

smoking

resolve to give up s.   ANON:4
absolutely sacred rite s. cigars   CHUR:22
cease s. is the easiest thing   TWAIN:101

sneezes

And beat him when he s.   CARRO:19

sneezing

S. coming on   HIPP:47

soap

S. and water and common sense   OSLER:74

social

s., ethical and political circumstances   BILLR:13
reference to s. and cultural values   DAAR:27
The New Genetics and The S. Theory   LE FA:34
Doctors are a s. cement   SALI:87
devise a plan of s. intercourse   WATE:104

social life

enter into the larger political and s.   VIRC:103

social medicine

him who adds to our knowledge of s.   GREEN:41

social problems

s. should largely be solved   VIRC:103

social science

medicine as basically a s.   SIGE:92

social service

Medicine is a profession for s.   MAYO:67

socialism

the louse will defeat s.   LENIN:59

socially

Patients must be adjusted s. as well   SIGE:92

society

the breath of life to human s.   HOLM:48
s. can prevent those who are . . . unfit   HOLM:49
to the individual rather than s.   HOOT:49
be struck between doctors and s.   PHILL:79
the healthier Western s. becomes   PORT:81
dangerous to s. an unskilled surgeon   SIGE:92
to the abstract claims of s.   SPER:95
single cell to the s. of nations   STRA:97

sociology

technology . . . has outrun its s.   SIGE:92

soldier

not a s. who desires the peace   PHILE:79

solitude

S. is a torment   DONNE:30

solution

I believe your s. is right   HUNTE:51

son

It was a s.'s duty to see his father   YOUNG:108

sore

pitiful surgeon makes a dangerous s.   MARS:65

sore throats

My s., you know, are always worse   AUST:7

sorrow

comfort to thousands in s. and pain   IRISH:53

soul

the death of the s.   ANON:4
Diseases of the s. are more   CICE:23
when the s. is oppressed   LUTH:62
the physicians separate the s.   PLATO:79
Wounds of the s. are a disease   VOLT:103

souls

their bodies but not their s.   GIBR:39

sound

a s. mind in a s. body   JUVE:55

spare

for which there are no s. parts   BIGGS:13

speak

hear twice as much as we s.   ZENO:108

special practice

as any s. can be   BASH:9

specialisation

S. is proof of how far medicine   HILL:46
That is the genius of s.   HILL:46

specialise

One must s. these days   SAKI:86

specialised

S. knowledge will do a man no harm   HOLM:49

specialism

extremely conservative and hates s.   MACK:64

specialisms

too rapid subdivisions into s.   RYLE:86

specialist

Choose your s.   ANON:3
practitioner can no more become a s.   PADD:75
No man can be a pure s.   SHAW:91

specialists

Consultant s. are . . . more remote   FISH:35

specialties

has fragmented the s.   OSLER:75

species

another prerogative of the human s.   LICH:60

speeches

S. are like babies easy to conceive   ARIST:6

speed

S. in operating should be   HOWA:49

sperm

illnesses are already on the s.   BARA:9

spinal

musculature involved in s. movement   MAYER:67

spine

The s. is a series of bones   ANON:5

spirit

The s. needs healing as well   CHARL:21
to release anxiety from his s.   HAZM:44
fleshy tabernacle of the immortal s.   LISTE:61
they have never s. enough to enjoy   STER:96

spiritual

some ailment in the s. part   HAWTH:43
Nurses . . . bring s. aid   MANF:65
Illness may precipitate a s. crisis   SOUT:94
a belief in the s. nature of man   WALLA:104

spleen

digest the venom of your s.   SHAK:90

sprain

worse to s. an ankle than to break it   WATS:105

squint

How is it that animals do not s.   LICH:60

staff

by an expert, kind and dedicated s.   CHARL:21

stammering

A s. man is never a worthless one   CARL:19

standards

Too much emphasis on s.   STARR:96

starve

the most pitiable death of all is to s.   HOMER:49

state

what a loss to the s.   CATH:20
power as a S. depend   DISR:30
his physical and moral s.   GOET:40

state's

the S. paramount concern   ROOS:85

statistical

A s. analysis, properly conducted   MORO:71
S. evidence shows   RANU:83

statistics

Medical s. are like a bikini   ANON:4
S. are like women   BILLR:13
lies, damned lies and s.   DISR:30
He uses s. as a drunken man   LANG:58
the handling of evidence and s.   SHAW:91
vast quantities of figures and s.   SMITH:94
There are two kinds of s.   STOUT:97
S. may be defined   WALLI:104

status

The s. and progress of medicine   THORO:100

sterility

techniques and its emphasis on s.   FOX:36

stethoscope

In order for the s. to function   RICHA:84

stimulate

S. the phagocytes   SHAW:91

stomach

the hole in a man's s.   ANDE:2
use a little wine for thy s.'s sake   BIBLE:12
a patriot on an empty s.   BRANN:15
the coats of his s.   BULW:17
enforcing morality on the s.   HUGO:50
The s. is the distinguishing part   HUNTE:51
eat until his s. is replete   MAIM:64
a third of the s. should be filled   TALM:99
have his s. behave itself   TWAIN:101

stone

prefer passing a small kidney s.   ANON:4
not even on the sufferers from s.   HIPP:47

stone-attack

To alleviate a s.   LOWE:62

stool

you look but on a s.   SHAK:90

stools

small s., big hospitals   BURKI:17

stoutness

I see no objection to s.   GILB:39

strangers

should make him kinder to s.   SELZ:89

strangle

I knew I could not s. him   ARTA:6

strength

glory of young men is their s.   BIBLE:12
Three things give hardy s.   WELSH:105

stroke

heart disease, s., respiratory diseases   ANON:3

stubborn

Facts are s. things   SMOL:94

student

the s. should set out to witness   GRAV:41
essential part of a s's instruction   HOLM:48
s. must be converted   MACP:64
the doctor must always be a s.   MAYO:67
The involved s. may thus come   SEEG:88

students

had never more than twenty s.   MACE:63
I taught medical s. in the wards   OSLER:74
be s. all your lives   RIES:84
cannot teach s. clinical medicine   STRA:97

studies

a physician hot from his s.   SMOL:94

study

to the observation and s. of all   ANON:4
a lifetime of incessant s.   MARX:66

success

The s. of a discovery depends upon   MITC:70
S. in life depends on the three I's   STOC:97

suckle

giving of s. to the child   ROSL:85

suffer

who fears to s., s.s from fear   FRENC:37
If we must s., let us s. nobly   HUGO:50
Rather s. than die is man's motto   LA FO:36
You s., this is enough for me   PAST:77

sufferer

sympathy that every human s. feels   TOLS:100

suffering

to judge his own condition while s.   ARIS:6
goal is to alleviate s.   BARN:9
too often s. fellow creature   BROWN:16
the s. and joy of others   GIDE:39
I am s. from the particular disease   JERO:54
accompanied by a little pain and s.   KIPL:56
To prevent disease, to relieve s.   OSLER:74
about the alleviation of s.   SKRA:93
the point of view of the s. patient   THORO:100
learn to relieve the s.   VIRG:103
grow familiar to s.   WHITT:106

sufferings

Amid the s. of life on earth   PLINY:80

suffers

Always aid the organ that s. most   CELS:20

sugar

the victim of his blood s.   OAKL:74

suicide

the s. braves death   ARIS:6
between a smoker and a s.   BALDE:8
If you must commit s.   BORR:14
S. is the worst form of murder   COLLI:24
a steady and consistent rise in s.   DUBL:31
S. is not a remedy   GARF:38
dallied with the thought of s.   JAMES:53
man responds by s.   LUDW:62
A s. is a person who has considered   MARQ:65
Thought of s. is a great consolation   NIET:73
ever lacks a good reason for s.   PAVE:77
s. is God's best gift to man   PLINY:80
Drunkenness is temporary s.   RUSSE:86
s. always comes from madness   VOLT:103

suicides

the greater is also the number of s.   RANU:83

sulphur

use s. for the itch   ANON:4

summary

close with a strong s.   MAYO:68

superstition

of slush and s.   DEWEY:29
If s. were curable, the remedy for   MARX:66
poison of enthusiasm and s.   SMITH:93

surgeon

A s. is someone who does everything   ANON:3
A s. should give as little pain   ANON:3
Sepsis is an insult to a s.   ANON:4
a subject for the s.'s knife   AYER:7
good s. is a disciple of Galen   BROOK:16
Now a s. should be youthful   CELS:20
same way as a s. on the body   CHAU:21
conditions necessary for the s.   CHAU:21
The best s., like the best general   COOP:25
s. somewhere who had no hands   CUSH:27
A fashionable s.   DA CO:23
spends his life as an operating s.   DA CO:23
A good s. operates with his hand   DUMAS:31
The wounded s. plies the steel   ELIOT:32
That s. whose fine tact   ELIOT:32
none was made by a s.   FISC:35
so do the physician and s.   FLEX:36
A s. should be young, a physician old   FRENC:37
There is no better training for a s.   GILLI:39
A s. should have three   HALLE:42
the incompetent s.   HALS:42
The s. is a man of action   HOERR:48
confession of the s.'s inadequacy   HUNTE:51
a man cannot be a s.   HUNTE:51
The office of s. has been considered   JEFF:54
A s. is a doctor who can operate   KOCH:56
a s. should have a temperate   LANF:57
nobody can become a good s.   LANF:57
difference between the physician and the s.   LANF:57
a s.'s judgment may not be influenced   LEHM:59
Every s. carries about him   LERI:59
A pitiful s. makes a dangerous sore   MARS:65
Master S. must be a man of mind   MATAS:66
The s. is often intolerant   MAYO:68
If the s. cuts a vessel   MORG:71
training of the s.   MOYN:72
qualifications of a good s.   PARA:76
deserve to be treated as a good S.   PEAR:78
best s. is he that has been well hacked   PROV:82
it takes a s. to save one   ROSS:85
and the s. may be capable   RUSSE:86
The s. knows all the parts of the brain   SELZ:89
With the help of a s.   SHAK:90
the safe side for the s.   SHAW:91

To give a s. a pecuniary interest   SHAW:91
s. should be something of a physician   SHEP:91
dangerous to society an unskilled s.   SIGE:92
differs the s. from the doctor   UREN:101
useful equipment for a successful s.   WILS:107
And each good s. eagerly desires   ZETA:108

surgeons

S. get long lives and short memories   ANON:4
You S. of London, who puzzle   ANON:5
The glory of s. is like that of actors   BALZ:8
the instruments and the s. fingers   BLAND:14
'Tis the S. praise, and height of Art   HERR:46
Other s. only tie them   HOLM:48
The s. have arrived   MAYO:68
skilful operators are not good s.   MAYO:68
people have believed s. to be thieves   MOND:70
one little touch of a s.'s lancet   MONTA:70
the s. of India   MOTH:71
assassination, I shall start with the s.   THOMA:99
S. and anatomists   TWAIN:101
S. have little knowledge   TWEE:101

surgery

worth the discomforts of major s.   ASHER:7
to prostitute the beautiful art and
science of s.   BILLR:13
It is with coarctation s. as with love   BROM:15
S. does the ideal thing   CLEN:23
The greatest discoveries of s   FISC:35
Three elements of s. define it as different   FOX:36
S. is the unceasing movement   GALEN:38
s. is like music   GRAH:41
desires to practise s.   HIPP:47
S. is an art, and the best way   HUMP:51
In s., eyes first and most; fingers next   HUMP:51
the insufficiency of s.   HUNTE:51
It is the nature of emergency s.   JONES:55
to find ways and means to avoid s.   LANGE:58
S. cures diseases that cannot be cured   MOND:70
As art s. is incomparable   MOYN:72
There are five duties in s.   PARÉ:76
S. has undergone many   POTT:81
In the s. of the future   RAVD:83
S. is the endeavour where intellect   SCHAU:87
some meaning in the ritual of s.   SELZ:89
For the difficult s. of today   WANG:104

surgical

from advances made in s. research   BELL:10
dangerous items in a s. operation   BLAND:14

s. therapy for elective conditions   COLE:24
s discussion of acute pancreatitis   GEOK:38
Before undergoing a s. operation   GOUR:41
the refinement of s. instrumentation   HEALD:44
In every s. intervention   HEIS:45
may require s. or medical treatment   HOPK:49
life's little ironies that s. disease   THOMS:100

S. are the body's mother tongue   BROWN:16
S., then are in reality nothing   CHARC:20
S. which cannot be readily marshalled   CLARK:23
know all the s.   HIPP:47
enumerate all the s. of hysteria   SYDE:98
the causes and to mitigate the s.   SYLV:98
s. of disease are marked by purpose   TREV:100

survival

S. of the fittest   SPEN:95

survivors

dying is more the s.' affair   MANN:65

sweat

It is not manly to fear to s.   SENE:89

Swift

The appearance of a disease is s.   CHIN:21

swooning

frequent and severe attacks of s.   HIPP:46

sympathy

This basis of medicine is s.   PAYNE:77

symposia

S., like hard liquor, should be taken   WALS:104

symptom

A s. that cannot be simulated   BRIS:15
it is a bad s.   HIPP:46
A misleading s. is misleading only   OGIL:74
intention of subduing the s.   SYDE:98

symptoms

s. where her organs used to be   ABBO:1
have to listen to woeful and sordid s.   ASHER:7

syphilis

The epidemic of s. which spread   DUBOS:31

system

attacked by the nervous s.   HOBAN:47

tabetic

t. has the power of holding water   DUNL:31

tailor

Imagine God as a t.   SELZ:89

tall

Short men eat more than t. ones   FRENC:37

taste

Good medicine always has a bitter t.   JAPA:53
especially pleasant to the t. buds   MASOR:66

taught

in the second I t. it   BLAND:14

teach

To discover and to t. are distinct   NEWM:73
Many of those who can t., can do   SEEG:89

teacher

the qualities of a good t. of medicine   ANON:4
to take up the position of t.   FREUD:37
In order to be a t. of medicine   MAYO:67

teaches

lessons which medical practice t.   PLATT:80

teaching

the true centre of medical t.   HOLM:48
In t. the medical student   JACK:53
a man engaged in t. medicine   MAYO:67

teams

in t., but are blamed as individuals   POLL:81

technical

specialised knowledge, t. procedures   STARR:96

technique

good for the t. but bad for the soul   RYLE:86
When applying a new t.   WATE:104

technology

avarice and passion for t.   GILLI:39
t. . . . has outrun its sociology   SIGE:92

teenager

father died of cancer when I was a t.   ACE:1

teeth

Loss of t. and marriage   AFRI:2
Removing the t. will cure something   ANON:4
Writers, like t., are divided   BAGE:8
the enamel of his t.   BULW:17
knocked out the t. of a man   HAMM:43
until he has no t. to eat it   PARKI:76
Sans t., sans eye, sans taste   SHAK:90
everyone happy whose t. are sound   SHAW:91
physician of the t.   SIGE:92
animals get their t. without pain   TWAIN:101
loses his t., hair and ideas   VOLT:103
to lose one's t. is a catastrophe   WHEE:106

teething

they escaped t.   TWAIN:101

teetotallers

T. lack the sympathy and generosity   DAVIE:28

teleology

T. is a lady   BRÜC:16

temperance

the Substitute of Exercise or T.   ADDI:1
T. is the best physic   PROV:82

temperate

t. in wine, in eating, girls, and sloth   FRAN:36

temperature

t. can neither be feigned nor falsified   WUND:108

testicle

human has one breast and one t.   MCHA:63

testicles

rather like undescended t.   ANON:4

text-books

our best t. become antiquated   BILLR:13

theories

have excessive faith in their t.   BERN:11
prefer their own t. to truth   COLLI:24
t. of our predecessors as myths   TOULM:100

theory

Any t. is better than no t.   ALBR:2
unforeseen relation not included in t.   BERN:11
logical deductions of a reigning t.   BERN:11
which will support some t.   CANN:19
A man who has a t.   DA CO:23
based upon a sound knowledge of t.   VINCI:102

therapeutics

and t. at once cease to hold   DUHR:31

thieves

believed surgeons to be t.   MOND:70

thin

The one way to get t.   CONN:25
T. women live long   WELSH:105

think

better to t. and sometimes to t. wrong   MAYO:68
A diagnosis is easy as long as you t.   WEISS:105

thinking

Learning without t. is useless   CONF:25
Plain living and high t.   LUBB:62
t. and feeling are identical   WEIN:105

thirst

master of his t. is master of his health   FRENC:37

thirstier

the more he drinks, the t. he grows   OVID:75

thirsty

He that goes to bed t. rises healthy   ENGL:33
They that are t. drink silently   FRENC:37

thoracic

producing sound in the t. cavity   LAËN:57

thoroughness

intelligence, and a pound of t.   ARAB:6

thought

sometimes best to slip over t.s   SÉVI:90
The brain secretes t.   VOGT:103

thread

its disappearance slow, like a t.   CHIN:21

throats

my sore t. are always worse   AUSTE:7

time

sign of the rapid progress of our t.   BILLR:13
T. is a physician that heals   DIPH:30
T. is the great physician   DISR:30
loss of adaptability as t. passes   EVANS:34
allow yourself enough t.   HIPP:47
Healing is a matter of t.   HIPP:47
best remedy is Tincture of T.   SCHIC:88
T. heals what reason cannot   SENE:89
T. cures the sick man   SPAN:95
T. carries all things   VIRG:103

tired

Life is one long process of getting t.   BUTL:18

tobacco

T., divine, rare, superexcellent   BURT:17
T. surely was designed   FRENE:37
there's nothing like t.   MOLI:70

today

T.'s facts are tomorrow's fallacies   ANON:5

tomb

From the womb to the t.   ENGL:33

tongue

t. is ever turning to the aching tooth   FULL:37
Teach they t.   MAIM:64

The t. is ever turning to the aching   PROV:82
the case of the genitals and the t.   VINCI:102
Nature has given man one t.   ZENO:108

tongues

those who practise with their t.   OSLER:74

tool

As he picks up his beautiful new t.   SALT:87

tooth

An aching t. is better out than in   BAXT:9
Every t. in a man's head   CERV:20
He looks like a t.-drawer   ENGL:33
tongue is ever turning to the aching t.   FULL:37
tongue is ever turning to the aching t.   PROV:82

toothache

He that sleeps feels no t.   SHAK:90
endure the t. patiently   SHAK:90
man with t. thinks everyone happy   SHAW:91

torts

professional illusions and t.   ILLI:52

towns

The fact is that in creating t.   ANON:5

tradition

in the best t. of medical excellence   MCGE:63

tragedy

neither of t. nor of comedy   MAUG:67

tragic

most t. thing in the world   SHAW:90

trained

well t. and highly motivated a doctor   POWIS:81

trainees

Today's t. have different values   SANF:87

training

minds are not disciplined by t.   BEVE:12
improve and extend my t.   MAIM:64
No t. of the surgeon   MOYN:72

tranquiliser

The t. of greatest value   MASOR:66

tranquilizers

T. at times do much more   BERG:11

treat

you should not let them t. you   BIER:13
first t. the mind   CHEN:21

treated

same ward where they cannot be t.   ANON:5

treating

It is not a case we are t.   BROWN:16

treatment

giving and receiving bad t.   ANON:3
t. should be stopped   BARN:9
the success of his t.   DIETL:29
may require surgical or medical t.   HOPK:49
The t. with poison medicines   HUANG:50
For too long the shabby t.   KENN:56
T. is concerned with the individual   LATH:58
the case which requires t.   MORR:71
to forego prolonged and costly t.   PENFI:78
optimism as to t.   PROU:82
to compare two regimens of t.   SCHIC:88
The aim of t. must be to maintain   SYLV:98

tremulous

Involuntary t. motion   PARKI:76

tropics

When medicine is practised in the t.   BROOK:16

trouble

People pay the doctor for his t.   SENE:89

trust

because it breaks the t.   BLAC:14
t. hospitals may be overwhelmed   MORR:71

truth

the t. may be in conflict   BILLR:13
He that desires to learn t.   BOER:14
be sure you know the 't.'   CHIN:21
the t. is common stock   COLLI:24
must be daring and search after T.   GALEN:38
T. is the breath of life   HOLM:48
in the post-mortem room is the t.   HORD:49
The scientific t. may be put   HUTC:51
To have admitted the t. of a doctrine   JENN:54
It is a t.   LATH:58
t. we may get by scientific study   LEAKE:59
Not the possession of t.   LESS:60
Next to the promulgation of the t.   LISTE:61
T. is a constant variable   MAYO:68
Medical science aims at the t.   MAYO:68
to the gradual disclosure of t.   MOYN:72
and in your search for t.   PAVL:77
recklessly critical quest for t.   POPP:81
Experience is the mother of t.   SHIP:92

truths

t may be more harmful   HUXL:52

try

above all, t. something   ROOS:85

tuberculosis

One rarely records pulmonary t.   MARF:65
pneumonia is an easy second, to t.   OSLER:74

from septic abortion than from t.   SIGE:92
responsible for the treatment of t.   WALK:104

tumour

a t. developing within the anus   JOHN:54
could not believe the t. was removed   VENA:102

tumours

T. destroy man   ROUS:85

twin

Sleep and Death, who are t. brothers   HOMER:49

typhoid

In t. treat the beginning   CHIN:21

ugly

I was so u. when I was born   YOUN:108

ulcer

a peptic u. may be the hole   ANDE:2

uncertain

To be u. is to be uncomfortable   CHIN:22

uncertainties

a delicate dissection of u.   MORO:71

uncertainty

wise decisions in the face of u.   WALLI:104

unconscious

discovery of u. motivation   BRAIN:15
have discovered the u.   FREUD:37
u. patient can immediately retaliate   HALS:42

understanding

ten cents worth of human u.   FISC:35
will have recourse to his U.   HAY:43

unemployed

hear people talk about u. women   NIGH:73

unhealth

pursuit of health is a symptom of u.   SKRA:93

unhealthy

they will leave the u. to die   PLATO:79

unintelligibility

seethe in restless u.   BEAN:9

United States

most obviously visible in the U.   HALD:42
The population of the U.   MCCR:63

urine

while he lives the u. is ours   ADDIS:1
by taking a small quantity of u.   BRIG:15
consequent retention of u.   LOWE:62
a man suffers from honey u.   SUSR:97

urologists

a flood of u.   ANON:3

use

U. strengthens, disuse debilitates   HIPP:47

uterine

never result from accidents in u. life   DOWN:30

uterus

after-burden be left sticking to the u.   HARV:43
swellings are the pregnant u.   MORR:71

vaccine

converting it into a v.   RAMÓN:83
the 1954 trials of the Salk v.   STARR:96

vegetable

between an animal and a v.   HUNTE:51
adoption of v. diet and pure water   SHEL:91

vegetables

Persons living very entirely on v.   CULL:26

vegetarianism

V. is harmless enough   HUTC:51

veins

it enters the v. and the pores   HARV:43
Varicose v. are the result   OSLER:75
V. which by the thickening   VINCI:102
v. and arteries proceed from the heart   VINCI:102

venereal

infected with v. disease should be   FRANK:36
consider v. diseases to be shameful   SELV:89

Venus

V. found herself a goddess   GRAH:41

victim

also the v. of his blood sugar   OAKL:74

victims

disease isolated its v.   SIGE:92

vision

imaginative v., though delightful   BRADL:15

visitors

V., footfalls are like medicine   AFRI:2
V. are no proper companions   JOHNS:55

vital

what they conceal is v.   ANON:4

vivisection

V. is justifiable   DARW:28

vocation

It is the special v. of the doctor   WHITT:106

voice

no index of character so sure as the v.   DISR:30

voices

I am always hearing v.   WOOLF:107

walk

after supper w. a mile   ENGL:33

walking

W. makes for a long life   HINDU:46
as if I was w. on my eyeballs   SMITH:94

war

must go to w.   HIPP:47
while they do the fighting in w.   EURI:34

ward

often in the same w.   ANON:5

ward round

rise above the routines of the daily w.   MCGE:63

wash

W. your hands often   ENGL:33

washes

doesn't matter how long one w.   ANNA:3

washing

without previously w. the hands   TALM:99

Wassermann

a millionaire with a positive W.   ANON:4

water

Filthy w. cannot be washed   AFRI:2
w. flowed like champagne   EVAR:34
cleanliness lies in w. supply   NIGH:73
Blood is thicker than w.   PROV:82
Pure w. the world's first   SLOV:93
causes the w. to smell bad   ZINS:108

wax

due to w. and is not curable   WILDE:106

wealth

Health is better than w.   ENGL:33
Wisdom and art, strength and w.   HEROP:45
Health without w. is half a sickness   ITAL:53
all classes are striving after w.   MCCR:63

wear

It is better to w. out than to rust out   CUMB:26

weariness

often leads to periods of w.   SEEG:88

weary

delightful hiding place for w. men   HEROD:45

well

It will never get w. if you pick it	AMER:2
leave the w. alone	ANON:3
Cut w., get w., stay w.	DEAV:28
Be sick not too late, nor w. too soon	FRAN:36
men who do not feel quite w.	GALB:37
It is a lot harder to keep people w	JARV:53
He who is happy always gets w.	PARA:76
Every man who feels w.	ROMA:85
those who are w.	SU:97

wheezes

All that w. is not asthma	JACK:53

whisk(e)y

hot w. at bedtime	FLEM:35
kill a live man put w. in him	GUTH:42
What butter and w. will not cure	IRISH:53
the w. which kills	JEFF:54

white

a black gets a w. woman with child	VINCI:102

wife

to escape from his w.	ANDE:2
expensive questions your w. asks	BARD:9
a w. is a man's greatest blessing	EURIP:34

will

against his w.	HORA:49
A madman has no free w.	LEGAL:59

wind

man with w. and self-righteousness	HUTC:51
W. is the cause of a hundred diseases	LÃO-T:58
are suffering from w.	YOUNG:108

wine

use a little w. for thy stomach's sake	BIBLE:12
Drink w. and have the gout	COGAN:23

Drinking strong w. cures hunger	HIPP:46
Happy with a bottle of Falernian(w.)	HORA:49
temperate in w., in eating	FRAN:36
Honey and w. are bad for children	MAIM:64
Good w. lights the candelabra	MERE:69
W. is the most healthful	PAST:76
since my leaving drinking of w.	PEPYS:78
w. is life	PETRO:78
w. is the most profitable	PLUT:80
That too much w. is killing me	ROSSE:85
Drink a glass of w. after your soup	RUSSI:86
Drink not much w.	SALE:86
W. is the foremost of all medicines	TALM:99

wisdom

w. is the equal to a god	HIPP:47
from putting knowledge before w.	HUTC:51
by experience we learn w.	SHIP:92
learned by rote, but W. not	STER:96
age has w. for its food	VINCI:102

wise

he that is w. will not abhor them	BIBLE:12
physician who is naturally w.	FRAN:36
Death never takes the w. man	LA FO:36

wisest

more than the w. man can answer	COLT:24

witchcraft

from common curemongering w.	SHAW:90

wits

even our w., away	VIRG:103

woman

marriage spoil a w.'s beauty	AFRI:2
longer time than a w. is a w.	BALZ:8
dissected at least one w.	BALZ:8
One is not born a w	BEAU:10
A w. when she is in travail	BIBLE:12
Unto the w. he said	BIBLE:12
Medicine is like a w. who changes	BIER:13
Man, that is born of W.	BOOK:14

The man 's desire is for the w.   COLER:24
a w. as old as she looks   COLLI:24
advice I would give to any young w.   CURR:27
seven for a w., and eight for a fool   ENGL:33
sail and a big-bellied w.   FRAN:36
w. without man is body   GERM:39
his hands the hands of a w.   HALLE:42
for the best years of a w.'s life   HARD:43
Knowledge of a w. whose back aches   KAHUN:55
A w. is only a w   KIPL:56
every w. has the same aura   PAST:76
no w. ever produced a child   PLUT:80
more important part in the life of w.   SIGE:92
give a doctor less to do than one w.   SPAN:95
than feeling a w.'s pulse   STER:96
With the w., thinking and feeling   WEIN:105

womb

From the w. to the tomb   ENGL:33
it is the falling of the w.   KAHUN:55
from his mother's w.,
Untimely ripp'd   SHAK:90

women

Statistics are like w.   BILLR:13
but doesn't know any w.   DENNI:29
W. during the state of pregnancy   HEBE:44
are very common in w.   HEBE:44
more understanding than w.   LUTH:62
talk about unemployed w.   NIGH:73
numbers of w. perish after childbirth   SEMM:89
to ourselves young men and w.   STEIN:96
w. should be physicians   STILL:97
Thin w. live long   WELSH:105

words

Whenever ideas fail, men invent w.   FISC:35

work

w. like hell and advertise   BEYN:12
not obliged to w. until one is better   BUTL:18
One doctor makes w. for another   ENGL:33
Much of the world's w.   GALB:37
ennoble the most disgusting w.   LAVO:59
to heal the sick—this is our w.   OSLER:74
w. in teams, but are blamed   POLL:81
appreciate that w., w., and more w.   SEEG:88
applies himself steadily to his w.   SUSR:97

workers

w. lose all sense of proportion   OSLER:75

workhouses

sick are still in General Mixed W.   ANON:5

working

have no w. hours   KIPL:56

world

his presence calls the w. into question   BEAU:10
whole of the living w. around us   GALT:38
This is the boundary of the w.   GREEK:41
Don't think of retiring from the w.   JOHNS:55
irremediable disease in the w.   LATH:58
We come into the w. with the mark   LESA:60

worry

to prolong life w. less   CHU:22
W., doubt, fear and despair   MACAR:63

worship

increasing w. of the instrument   SEEG:89

wound

The w. is granulating well   ANON:5
A w. heals but the scar remains   ENGL:33
The irritation of the w. by antiseptic   LISTE:61
The w. that bleedseth inward   LYLY:63
w. should be bound   PFOL:78

wounded

to bayonet the w.   ANON:3
A man w. in the abdomen dies   MACC:63
A man deep-w. may feel too much   ELIOT:32
He who scratches a scar is w. twice   RUSSI:86

wounds

Million have died of medicable w.   ARMS:6
deep w. ever closed without a scar   BYRON:18

W. heal and become scars   LEC:59
twenty w. with a sword   MONTA:70
W. of the soul are a disease   VOLT:103

writers

W., like teeth, are divided   BAGE:8

wrong

publicity given to what goes w.   CHARL:21

X-ray

Unless you are a fool, X. them all   CATH:19
Treat the patient, not the X.   HUNTE:51

X-rays

I shall call them 'x'.   ROEN:84

Yankee

This Y. dodge, gentlemen   LISTO:61

years

shall be to one hundred and twenty y.   BIBLE:12
The y. between fifty and seventy   ELIOT:32
lived to be over a hundred y.   HUANG:50
revolution of the last hundred y.   KEEN:56
so many y. outlive performance   SHAK:90

young

the old y. and the y. old   AMER:2
Let the y. know they will never find   BAGL:8
would be y. when they are old   ENGL:33
To be seventy years y.   HOLM:48
the cup of knowledge to the y.   HUTC:51
Whom the gods love dies y.   MENA:69
Y. men ought to come   MONTE:71
Beware of the y. doctor   PROV:82
The denunciation of the y.   SMITH:94
Always seek out a bright y. doctor   WILDE:106

younger

wished to be y.   SWIFT:98

yourself

only competent observer is y.   HOWA:49

youth

to prolong the y. of the mind   COLLI:24
Y. is a blunder; manhood a struggle   DISR:30
If y. but know,
And old age only   ESTI:34
The sins of y. are paid for in old age.   LATIN:58
applying the originality of y.   POLA:81
or that y. would sleep out the rest   SHAK:90
Y. is a wonderful thing   SHAW:91